Nutriomics

Food Analysis & Properties

Series Editor
Leo M.L. Nollet
University College Ghent, Belgium

This CRC series **Food Analysis and Properties** is designed to provide a state-of-art coverage on topics to the understanding of physical, chemical and functional properties of foods: including (1) recent analysis techniques of a choice of food components; (2) developments and evolutions in analysis techniques related to food; (3) recent trends in analysis techniques of specific food components and/or a group of related food components.

Fingerprinting Techniques in Food Authenticity and Traceability
Edited by K.S. Siddiqi and Leo M.L. Nollet

Hyperspectral Imaging Analysis and Applications for Food Quality
Edited by Nrusingha Charan Basantia, Leo M.L. Nollet, and Mohammed Kamruzzaman

Ambient Mass Spectroscopy Techniques in Food and the Environment
Edited by Leo M.L. Nollet and Basil K. Munjanja

Food Aroma Evolution: During Food Processing, Cooking and Aging
Edited by Matteo Bordiga and Leo M.L. Nollet

Mass Spectrometry Imaging in Food Analysis
Edited by Leo M.L. Nollet

Proteomics for Food Authentication
Edited by Leo M.L. Nollet and Otles, Semih

Analysis of Nanoplastics and Microplastics in Food
Edited by Leo M.L. Nollet and Khwaja Salahuddin Siddiqi

Chiral Organic Pollutants: Monitoring and Characterization in Food and the Environment
Edited by Edmond Sanganyado, Basil Munjanja, and Leo M.L. Nollet

Sequencing Technologies in Microbial Food Safety and Quality
Edited by Devarajan Thangadurai, Leo M.L. Nollet, Saher Islam, and Jeyabalan Sangeetha

Nanoemulsions in Food Technology: Development, Characterization, and Applications
Edited by Javed Ahmad and Leo M.L. Nollet

Mass Spectrometry in Food Analysis
Edited by Leo M.L. Nollet and Robert Winkler

Bioactive Peptides from Food: Sources, Analysis, and Functions
Edited by Leo M.L. Nollet and Semih Ötleş

Nutriomics: Well-being through Nutrition
Edited by Devarajan Thangadurai, Saher Islam, Leo M.L. Nollet, and Juliana Bunmi Adetunji

For more information, please visit the Series Page: www.crcpress.com/Food-Analysis – Properties/book-series/CRCFOODANPRO

Nutriomics

Well-being through Nutrition

Edited by
Devarajan Thangadurai
Saher Islam
Leo M.L. Nollet
Juliana Bunmi Adetunji

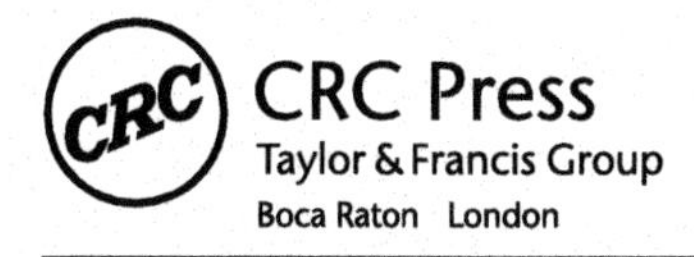

CRC Press is an imprint of the
Taylor & Francis Group, an **informa** business

First edition published 2022
by CRC Press
6000 Broken Sound Parkway NW, Suite 300, Boca Raton, FL 33487–2742

and by CRC Press
4 Park Square, Milton Park, Abingdon, Oxon, OX14 4RN

CRC Press is an imprint of Taylor & Francis Group, LLC

Library of Congress Cataloging-in-Publication Data
Names: Thangadurai, D. (Devarajan), 1976- editor. | Islam, Saher, editor. |
Nollet, Leo M. L., 1948- editor. | Adetunji, Juliana, editor.
Title: Nutriomics : well-being through nutrition / edited by Devarajan Thangadurai, Saher Islam, Leo Nollet and Juliana Adetunji.
Description: First edition. | Boca Raton : CRC Press, 2022. | Series: Food analysis and properties | Includes bibliographical references and index. | Summary: "This book enhances scientific evidence based on omics technologies and effectiveness of nutrition guidelines to promote well-being. It provides advanced understanding towards nutrients and genotype effects on disease and health status. Helps to design the precise nutritional recommendations for prevention or treatment of nutrition-related syndromes. Discusses impact of genetics on food ingestion, metabolism, and food-drug interactions. Describes potential of transcriptomic, genomic, proteomic, metabolomic, and epigenomic tools within nutrition research. Explores state-of-the-art tools to identify safety and quality of nutrition and development of personalized nutrition to improve health status"-- Provided by publisher.
Identifiers: LCCN 2021055509 (print) | LCCN 2021055510 (ebook) |
ISBN 9780367694814 (hardback) | ISBN 9780367695415 (paperback) |
ISBN 9781003142195 (ebook)
Subjects: LCSH: Nutrition--Research. | Food--Analysis.
Classification: LCC TX537 .N785 2022 (print) | LCC TX537 (ebook) | DDC
363.8--dc23/eng/20211230
LC record available at https://lccn.loc.gov/2021055509
LC ebook record available at https://lccn.loc.gov/2021055510

ISBN: 978-0-367-69481-4 (hbk)
ISBN: 978-0-367-69541-5 (pbk)
ISBN: 978-1-003-14219-5 (ebk)

DOI: 10.1201/9781003142195

Typeset in Times LT Std
by Apex CoVantage, LLC

It is a great pleasure to work with my co-editors Devarajan Thangadurai, Saher Islam, and Juliana Bunmi Adetunji.

They did a great job. It is always nice to work with colleagues you can rely on.

This creates possibilities for the future.

Leo M.L. Nollet

Contents

Series Preface

There will always be a need to analyze food compounds and their properties. Current trends in analyzing methods include automation, increasing the speed of analyses, and miniaturization. Over the years, the unit of detection has evolved from micrograms to pictograms.

A classical pathway of analysis is sampling, sample preparation, cleanup, derivatization, separation, and detection. At every step, researchers are working and developing new methodologies. A large number of papers are published every year on all facets of analysis. So there is a need for books that gather information on one kind of analysis technique or on the analysis methods for a specific group of food components.

The scope of the CRC Series on Food Analysis & Properties aims to present a range of books edited by distinguished scientists and researchers who have significant experience in scientific pursuits and critical analysis. This series is designed to provide state-of-the-art coverage on topics such as the following:

1. Recent analysis techniques on a range of food components.
2. Developments and evolution in analysis techniques related to food.
3. Recent trends in analysis techniques for specific food components and/or a group of related food components.
4. The understanding of the physical, chemical, and functional properties of foods.

The book *Nutriomics* is volume number 19 of this series.

I am happy to be a series editor of such books for the following reasons:

- I am able to pass on my experience in editing high-quality books related to food.
- I get to know colleagues from all over the world more personally.
- I continue to learn about interesting developments in food analysis.

Much work is involved in the preparation of a book. I have been assisted and supported by a number of people, all of whom I would like to thank. I would especially like to thank the team at CRC Press/Taylor & Francis, with a special word of thanks to Randy Brehm and Steve Zollo, senior editors.

Many, many thanks to all the editors and authors of this volume and future volumes. I very much appreciate all their effort, time, and willingness to do a great job.

I dedicate this series to the following people:

- My wife, for her patience with me (and all the time I spend on my computer).
- All patients suffering from prostate cancer; knowing what this means, I am hoping they will have some relief.

Dr. Leo M.L. Nollet (Retired)
University College Ghent
Ghent, Belgium

Preface

Consumers around the globe are increasingly concerned about the safety and quality of the nutritional elements and are passionate about knowing how diets influence their health. The field of nutrition and its applications are mainly the subjects of nutritional biomarkers discovery, nutrition-related disease analysis, and dietary intervention research in the past several decades. Nutrition is greatly intricate due to the underlying diverse external and internal factors that model it. Therefore, revealing this complexity demands more network and holistic-based strategies. Understanding nutritional science has become more significant from both clinical and translational perspectives. Moreover, these challenges demand robust and sensitive molecular research initiatives to expose the pathways and interactions of a variety of nutrients. Depending on genotypes, nutrients modify their metabolic pathways through regulating gene expressions and protein translation that ultimately lead to distinct health status. The existing omics era, along with high-throughput sequencing data generation, embraces this complexity greatly.

With the introduction of diverse omics approaches into nutrition research, a new discipline has emerged as nutriomics. Transcriptomics, proteomics, metabolomics, and genomics are major platforms for omics analysis in nutritional science. Other omics tools, including epigenomics, miRomics, and metabonomics are also subject of great concern. The constant use of omics approaches is due to recent advancements in nutritional science and bioinformatic technologies. These novel and advanced approaches offer vast potential to explore the complex associations of dietary elements. Omics technologies tremendously facilitate the novel biomarkers discovery associated with particular dietary factors. These methodologies are also increasingly applied as powerful tools to recognize the biochemical changes related to human nutrition. Human nutriomics mainly involves the findings of nutritional intervention mechanisms and dietary health measurements at both population and molecular levels to formulate and personalize nutrition recommendations for disease prevention. Human genetics has a strong impact on nutrient absorption, distribution, metabolism, excretion, and even drug-nutrient interactions. Currently, a most influential topic in food science provides a lot of evidence that has revealed that not only do nutrients influence human genetics, but genetics also greatly modulates the metabolism of nutrients. Several research works have increasingly exploited the distinct omics technologies toward a more in-depth understanding of such processes.

This book *Nutriomics* presents a comprehensive overview and novel insights of omics tools for nutrition-based studies. First, two chapters discuss the basic principles, applications, and analysis pertaining to traditional and high-throughput nutriomic tools. Chapters 3 to 5 have a special focus on current practices of nutriepigenomics, nutriproteomics, and nutrimetabolomics for nutritional safety and disease prevention. These chapters also discuss the future prospects and limitations of omics technologies in relation to nutrition science. Chapters 6 and 7 provide new perspectives to understand the role of nutritional care practices to deal with diabetics and other clinical implications. Chapter 8 extensively reviews the integrative omics approaches to customize the dietary recommendations. Chapters 9 and 10 elaborately discuss the uses of nutriomic approaches to analyze natural food products for human healthcare. The last two chapters deal with the metabolomic markers for food authenticity, quality, and composition.

Nutriomics is intended to advance the understanding of researchers, industrialists, nutritionists, and graduate and postgraduate students about the molecular influences of routine diets on common nutrition-related diseases. Delivering detailed knowledge on nutritional science and nutriomic technologies, this book serves as a valuable and vital source to explore state-of-the-art tools to identify safety and quality of nutrition and development of personalized nutrition to improve health status.

Devarajan Thangadurai
Saher Islam
Leo M.L. Nollet
Juliana Bunmi Adetunji

Editors

Devarajan Thangadurai is Associate Professor at Karnatak University, in Dharwad, India, and did his postdoctoral research at the University of Madeira, Portugal; University of Delhi, India; and ICAR National Research Centre for Banana, India. He is the recipient of the Best Young Scientist Award with a Gold Medal from Acharya Nagarjuna University, India, and the VGST-SMYSR Young Scientist Award from the Government of Karnataka, India. He has a keen interest and expertise in the fields of biodiversity and biotechnology, genetics and genomics of food crops, and beneficial microbes for crop productivity and food safety. He has authored/edited more than 30 books, including *Genetic Resources and Biotechnology* (three vols.), *Genes, Genomes and Genomics* (two vols.), *Genomics and Proteomics*, *Biotechnology of Microorganisms*, *Mycorrhizal Biotechnology*, *Nanotechnology for Food, Agriculture and Environment*, *Functional Bionanomaterials*, and *Bioprospecting Algae for Nanosized Materials* with international publishers in the United States, Canada, Switzerland, and India. He has authored/coauthored 250 publications inclusive of journal articles, book chapters, books, and invited presentations. He has extensively traveled to many universities and institutes in Africa, Asia, Europe, and the Middle East for academic works, scientific meetings, and international collaborations. He is also a peer reviewer for several reputed journals, including *Comprehensive Reviews in Food Science and Food Safety*, *Food Science and Technology International*, *Journal of Agricultural and Food Chemistry*, *Journal of Food Science*, *Journal of the Science of Food and Agriculture*, and *International Journal of Plant Production.*

Saher Islam is Visiting Lecturer at the Department of Biotechnology of Lahore College for Women University, Pakistan. She received her PhD in molecular biology and biotechnology from the University of Veterinary and Animal Sciences, Lahore, Pakistan. She was an IRSIP Scholar at Cornell University, New York, and Visiting Scholar at West Virginia State University, West Virginia. She has keen research interests in genetics, molecular biology, biotechnology, and bioinformatics and has ample hands-on experience in molecular marker analysis, whole genome sequencing, and RNA sequencing. She has visited the United States, the UK, Singapore, Germany, Italy, and Russia for academic and scientific trainings, courses, and meetings. She is the recipient of the 2016 Boehringer Ingelheim Fonds Travel Grant from European Molecular Biology Laboratory, Germany. She is an author/coauthor of 70 publications, including journal articles, book chapters, books, and conference presentations.

Leo M.L. Nollet earned an MS (1973) and a PhD (1978) in biology from the Katholieke Universiteit Leuven, Belgium. He is an editor and associate editor of numerous books. He edited for M. Dekker, New York – now CRC Press of Taylor & Francis – the first, second, and third editions of *Food Analysis by HPLC* and *Handbook of Food Analysis*. The last edition is a two-volume book. Dr. Nollet also edited the *Handbook of Water Analysis* (first, second, and third editions) and *Chromatographic Analysis of the Environment* (third and fourth editions;

CRC Press). With F. Toldrá, he coedited two books published in 2006, 2007, and 2017: *Advanced Technologies for Meat Processing* (CRC Press) and *Advances in Food Diagnostics* (Blackwell Publishing – now Wiley). With M. Poschl, he coedited the book *Radionuclide Concentrations in Foods and the Environment*, also published in 2006 (CRC Press). Dr. Nollet has also coedited with Y.H. Hui and other colleagues on several books: *Handbook of Food Product Manufacturing* (Wiley, 2007), *Handbook of Food Science, Technology, and Engineering* (CRC Press, 2005), *Food Biochemistry and Food Processing* (first and second editions; Blackwell Publishing – now Wiley – 2006 and 2012), and the *Handbook of Fruits and Vegetable Flavors* (Wiley, 2010). In addition, he edited the *Handbook of Meat, Poultry, and Seafood Quality* (first and second editions; Blackwell Publishing – now Wiley – 2007 and 2012). From 2008 to 2011, he published five volumes on animal-product-related books with F. Toldrá: *Handbook of Muscle Foods Analysis*, *Handbook of Processed Meats and Poultry Analysis*, *Handbook of Seafood and Seafood Products Analysis*, *Handbook of Dairy Foods Analysis*, and *Handbook of Analysis of Edible Animal By-Products*. Also, in 2011, with F. Toldrá, he coedited two volumes for CRC Press: *Safety Analysis of Foods of Animal Origin* and *Sensory Analysis of Foods of Animal Origin*. In 2012, they published the *Handbook of Analysis of Active Compounds in Functional Foods*. In a co-edition with Hamir Rathore, *Handbook of Pesticides: Methods of Pesticides Residues Analysis* was marketed in 2009; *Pesticides: Evaluation of Environmental Pollution* in 2012; *Biopesticides Handbook* in 2015; and *Green Pesticides Handbook: Essential Oils for Pest Control* in 2017. Other finished book projects include *Food Allergens: Analysis, Instrumentation, and Methods* (with A. van Hengel; CRC Press, 2011) and *Analysis of Endocrine Compounds in Food* (Wiley-Blackwell, 2011). Dr. Nollet's recent projects include *Proteomics in Foods* with F. Toldrá (Springer, 2013) and *Transformation Products of Emerging Contaminants in the Environment: Analysis, Processes, Occurrence, Effects, and Risks* with D. Lambropoulou (Wiley, 2014). In the series Food Analysis & Properties, he edited (with C. Ruiz-Capillas) *Flow Injection Analysis of Food Additives* (CRC Press, 2015) and *Marine Microorganisms: Extraction and Analysis of Bioactive Compounds* (CRC Press, 2016). With A.S. Franca, he coedited *Spectroscopic Methods in Food Analysis* (CRC Press, 2017), and with Horacio Heinzen and Amadeo R. Fernandez-Alba, he coedited *Multiresidue Methods for the Analysis of Pesticide Residues in Food* (CRC Press, 2017). Further volumes in the series Food Analysis & Properties are *Phenolic Compounds in Food: Characterization and Analysis* (with Janet Alejandra Gutierrez-Uribe, 2018), *Testing and Analysis of GMO-containing Foods and Feed* (with Salah E. O. Mahgoub, 2018), *Fingerprinting Techniques in Food Authentication and Traceability* (with K.S. Siddiqi, 2018), *Hyperspectral Imaging Analysis and Applications for Food Quality* (with N.C. Basantia and Mohammed Kamruzzaman, 2018), *Ambient Mass Spectroscopy Techniques in Food and the Environment* (with Basil K. Munjanja, 2019), *Food Aroma Evolution: During Food Processing, Cooking, and Aging* (with M. Bordiga, 2019), *Mass Spectrometry Imaging in Food Analysis* (2020), *Proteomics in Food Authentication* (with S. Ötleş, 2020), *Analysis of Nanoplastics and Microplastics in Food* (with K.S. Siddiqi, 2020), *Chiral Organic Pollutants, Monitoring and Characterization in Food and the Environment* (with Edmond Sanganyado and Basil K. Munjanja, 2020), *Sequencing*

Technologies in Microbial Food Safety and Quality (with Devarajan Thangadurai, Saher Islam, Jeyabalan Sangeetha, 2021), and *Nanoemulsions in Food Technology: Development, Characterization, and Applications* (with Javed Ahmad, 2021).

Juliana Bunmi Adetunji is a faculty at the Department of Biochemistry, Osun State University, Osogbo, Nigeria. Her research interest over the years has focused on the nutritional safety of foods and the evaluation of medicinal plants in the management and maintenance of human health. Her work on phytomedicinal potentials of certain medicinal plants and on food safety has made valuable contributions to ongoing research in the use of alternative remedies for disease management in Africa, as well as sustainable food systems for the future. She is a recipient of the Tertiary Educational Fund in Nigeria. She has published articles in several scientific journals and conference proceedings in international and local refereed journals. She is a member of many scientific and professional bodies like the Organization for Women in Science in the Developing World, the Nigerian Society of Biochemistry and Molecular Biology, the Nigerian Society of Experimental Biology, and the Nigeria Bioinformatics and Genetics Network.

Contributors

Charles Oluwaseun Adetunji
Applied Microbiology, Biotechnology, and Nanotechnology Laboratory
Department of Microbiology
Edo University Iyamho
Auchi, Edo State, Nigeria

Juliana Bunmi Adetunji
Nutrition and Toxicology Research Laboratory
Department of Biochemistry
Faculty of Basic and Applied Sciences
Osun State University
Osogbo, Nigeria

Malika Arora
Multidisciplinary Research Unit (Indian Council of Medical Research)
G.G.S. Medical College
Faridkot, India

Sumit Arora
Dairy Chemistry Division
ICAR-National Dairy Research Institute, Karnal
Haryana, India

Umar Farooq Alahmad
Institute of Food Science and Nutrition
University of Sargodha
Sargodha, Pakistan

Rita Carneiro Alves
Department of Chemical Sciences
Faculty of Pharmacy
REQUIMTE/LAQV
University of Porto
Porto, Portugal

Parveen Bansal
University Centre of Excellence in Research
Baba Farid University of Health Sciences
Faridkot, India

Renu Bansal
Department of Microbiology
Government Medical College
Patiala, India

Mahamuda Begum
PG and Research Department of Biotechnology
Marudhar Kesari Jain College for Women, Vaniyambadi
Tamil Nadu, India

Fernanda de Sousa Bezerra
Laboratory of Biotechnology, Food, and Nutrition Graduate Program (PPGAN)
Federal University of the State of Rio de Janeiro (UNIRIO)
Rio de Janeiro, Brazil

Khanita Suman Chinnanai
Sana Hospital and Healthcare
Muslimpur, Vaniyambadi
Tamil Nadu, India

Ramachandran Chelliah
Department of Food Science and Biotechnology
College of Agriculture and Life Sciences
Kangwon National University
Chuncheon
Gangwon-do, Korea

Carolina Thomaz dos Santos D'Almeida
Laboratory of Bioactives (LABBIO), PPGAN

and

Center of Innovation in Mass Spectrometry
Laboratory of Protein Biochemistry (LBP-IMasS)
Rio de Janeiro, Brazil

Ticiane Carvalho Farias
Laboratory of Biotechnology, Food, and Nutrition Graduate Program (PPGAN)
Federal University of the State of Rio de Janeiro (UNIRIO)
Rio de Janeiro, Brazil

Mariana Simões Larraz Ferreira
Laboratory of Bioactives (LABBIO), PPGAN, UNIRIO
Center of Innovation in Mass Spectrometry
Laboratory of Protein Biochemistry (LBP-IMasS)
Rio de Janeiro, Brazil

Shin-Yee Fung
Medicinal Mushroom Research Group (MMRG)
Department of Molecular Medicine
Faculty of Medicine
Centre for Natural Products Research and Drug Discovery (CENAR)
University of Malaya

and

University of Malaya Centre for Proteomics Research (UMCPR)
Kuala Lumpar, Malaysia

Saher Islam
Department of Biotechnology
Lahore College for Women University
Lahore, Pakistan

Srinivasan Kameswaran
Department of Botany
Vikrama Simhapuri University PG Centre, Kavali
Andhra Pradesh, India

Prathap Reddy Kallamadi
National Institute of Nutrition, Tarnaka
Hyderabad, Telangana, India

Maria Gabriela Bello Koblitz
Laboratory of Biotechnology, Food, and Nutrition Graduate Program (PPGAN)
Federal University of the State of Rio de Janeiro (UNIRIO)
Rio de Janeiro, Brazil

Andrea Furtado Macedo
Integrated Laboratory of Plant Biology (LIBV)
Department of Botany
Institute of Biosciences
Rio de Janeiro, Brazil

Inamul Hasan Madar
Department of Biotechnology
School of Biotechnology and Genetic Engineering
Bharathidasan University, Tiruchirappalli

and

Sana Hospital and Healthcare, Muslimpur, Vaniyambadi
Tamil Nadu, India

Talita Pimenta do Nascimento
Laboratory of Bioactives (LABBIO), PPGAN, UNIRIO
Center of Innovation in Mass Spectrometry
Laboratory of Protein Biochemistry (LBP-IMasS)A
Rio de Janeiro, Brazil

Maria Antónia da Mota Nunes
Department of Chemical Sciences
Faculty of Pharmacy
REQUIMTE/LAQV
University of Porto
Porto, Portugal

Deog-Hwan Oh
Department of Food Science and Biotechnology
College of Agriculture and Life Sciences
Kangwon National University, Chuncheon
Gangwon-do, Korea

Maria Beatriz Prior Pinto Oliveira
Department of Chemical Sciences
Faculty of Pharmacy
REQUIMTE/LAQV
University of Porto
Porto, Portugal

Gopikrishna Pitchika
Department of Zoology, Vikrama Simhapuri
University PG Centre, Kavali
Andhra Pradesh, India

Bandana Pahi
Department of Bioinformatics
Sambalpur University, Jyoti Vihar, Burla
Sambalpur, Odisha, India

Ravali Parvartam
Dairy Chemistry Division
ICAR-National Dairy Research Institute, Karnal
Haryana, India

Bellemkonda Ramesh
Department of Food Technology
Vikrama Simhapuri University, Nellore
Andhra Pradesh, India

Asish K. Saha
Inflammation Research Foundation
Peabody, MA

Barry Sears
Inflammation Research Foundation
Peabody, MA

Richa Singh
Dairy Chemistry Division
ICAR-National Dairy Research Institute, Karnal
Haryana, India

M. Srinivasulu
Department of Biotechnology
Yogi Vemana University, Kadapa
Andhra Pradesh, India

M. Subhosh
Chandra Department of Microbiology
Yogi Vemana University, Kadapa
Andhra Pradesh, India

Thaiza Serrano de Souza
Laboratory of Biotechnology, Food, and Nutrition Graduate Program (PPGAN)
Federal University of the State of Rio de Janeiro (UNIRIO)
Rio de Janeiro, Brazil

G. Sudhakara
Department of Biochemistry
Sri Krishnadevaraya University
Anantapur, India

Ghazala Sultan
Department of Computer Science
Faculty of Science
Aligarh Muslim University
Uttar Pradesh, India

Devarajan Thangadurai
Department of Botany
Karnatak University, Dharwad
Karnataka, India

Pravitha Kasu Sivanandan
Department of Bioinformatics
School of Biosciences
Sri Krishna Arts and Science College, Coimbatore
Tamil Nadu, India

Roberta Nogueira Pereira da Silva
Laboratory of Biotechnology, Food, and Nutrition Graduate Program (PPGAN)
Federal University of the State of Rio de Janeiro (UNIRIO)
Rio de Janeiro, Brazil

Iftikhar Aslam Tayubi
Faculty of Computing and Information Technology
Rabigh, King Abdulaziz University
Jeddah, Kingdom of Saudi Arabia

Ch. Venkatrayulu
Department of Marine Biology
Vikrama Simhapuri University, Nellore
Andhra Pradesh, India

Yeannie Hui-Yeng Yap
Department of Oral Biology and Biomedical Sciences
Faculty of Dentistry
MAHSA University
Selangor, Malaysia

Syeda Mahvish Zahra
Department of Environmental Design and Nutritional Sciences
Allama Iqbal Open University
Islamabad, Pakistan

and

Institute of Food Science and Nutrition
University of Sargodha
Sargodha, Pakistan

1 Traditional and Advanced Molecular Approaches in Nutrition Research

*Parveen Bansal, Renu Bansal, and Malika Arora**

CONTENTS

1.1 INTRODUCTION

Ayurveda is a traditional medicinal system that believes in regulating the diet for a healthy body and mind. Traditional Ayurvedic literature illustrates how an individual can recuperate by establishing the connection between elements of life, food, and body. According to Ayurvedic concepts, food is responsible for different aspects of

* Corresponding author email: maliksmonu@gmail.com

DOI: 10.1201/9781003142195-1

an individual, including physical, temperamental, and mental states. To stay healthy, maintaining a stable, healthy diet routinely is essential. The body absorbs the nutrients as a result of digestion. However, Ayurveda states that the food first converts into *rasa* (plasma) and is then followed by successive conversion into blood, muscle, fat, bone marrow, reproductive elements, and body fluids (Ramaswamy 2018). Inappropriate diets create an imbalance of the body's organ systems, the mind, and the spirit, followed by various diseases. The Ayurvedic system explains various treatments for various diseases that are established and are being used consistently over a period. Multiple therapeutic approaches are being used for cleansing the body, which further purifies the body and soul by eliminating various toxins. Traditional Indian foods have been prepared for many years, and preparation varies across the country. Traditional knowledge about the processing of food, its preservation techniques, and its therapeutic effects has been recognized for many generations in India. A variety of foods available in our system can deliver numerous biological functions through nutritional components in the human body. Indian traditional foods are a good example of a variety of natural health components, such as body-healing chemicals, antioxidants, dietary fibers, and probiotics. These functional molecules help the body in a variety of ways, such as weight management, blood sugar level balance, and generation of immunity. The functional properties of foods are further enhanced by processing techniques, such as sprouting, malting, and fermentation (Singh et al. 2015). The most commonly used process is fermentation, and a variety of fermented food products are being consumed in everyday life, which provides a good amount of friendly and healthy bacteria to our bodies. Traditional fermented foods are a rich source of lactic acid bacteria and other good bacteria required for the gut; however, today, these are defined under the category of probiotics. Probiotics are defined as live microorganisms that, when administered in adequate amounts, confer a health benefit on the host, per FAO/WHO. Although these probiotics were defined only in 2002 for the first time, these have been consumed for thousands of years. Present research is inclined toward unfolding the scientific evidence for the traditional probiotic-based fermented foods. Volumes can be written on traditional approaches to nutrition research and development; however, this chapter intends to focus on probiotic-based fermented food to highlight various fermented foods and various nutritional approaches that are being used to unfold their potential by screening, identifying, and evaluating various friendly bacteria in foods.

1.2 TRADITIONAL FOODS

Various unique, indigenous foods, such as vegetables, fruits, cereals, and milk, are produced across the globe and are considered staple food meals in India and other continents, like Asia and Africa (Prajapati and Nair 2003). The optimum health and nutrition of individuals are dependent on a regular supply of food and intake of a balanced diet. When diets are suboptimal, the individual's capacity to work with optimum efficiency is greatly reduced. The most vulnerable groups are women, children, and infants. Non-availability of food, dietary restrictions and taboos, misconceptions, and limited time available for feeding or eating aggravate poor nutritional status.

Traditional foods, being rich sources of almost all nutrients, help in improving the nutritional status of people to a larger extent. Several traditional foods have been endowed with different kinds of medicinal benefits. Indian traditional food has a lot of grains, such as *bajra*, *nachni*, *jowar*, wheat, and different varieties of rice grains. In addition, various cereals are grown in abundance in India and are being used since ancient times for preparing different recipes for breakfast, lunch, and dinner (Manoharlal et al. 2021). Combinations like *khichadi*, dal rice, and *rajma* rice have been popular in India for ages. These combinations are perfect protein meals, with all the essential amino acids, and hence, such traditional Indian foods are wholesome, tasty, and healthy. In the traditional Indian *thali*, each bowl in the *thali* has a small size. It includes two to three varieties of dal, *sabzi*, and some rice or roti or both. The *thali* also includes a small amount of a sweet dish. This *thali* makes for a complete meal, including all essential nutrients in the right proportion (Payyappallimana and Venkatasubramanian 2016). Various cooking oils are also part of the food system, particularly mustard oil, peanut oil, coconut oil, and groundnut oil.

The Indian curry, if cooked with the right ingredients, such as various kitchen spices and herbs, along with proper amounts of oil, is good for immunity (Sarkar et al. 2015). It can help in reducing inflammation, which is the root cause of diseases like diabetes, high blood pressure, and heart diseases. Prepared with curry leaves, tomato, onion, black pepper, garlic, turmeric, and various other spices, the Indian curry has many health benefits. The traditional Indian curry can also help in reducing inflammation.

Pickles, when made with the right quality of salt (rock salt) and oil, prove to be one of the best probiotic foods that anybody can have. Made with ground leafy greens and seeds, the traditional Indian *chutney* is very nutritious (Behera et al. 2020).

Fermentation causes changes in the food quality index, including texture, flavor, appearance, nutrition, and safety. Hence one-third of the diet throughout the world is made up of fermented foods and cereals. Due to rapidly increasing uses of probiotic products throughout the world, countries like Japan, Europe, and India are manufacturing more probiotic-based products and hence fulfilling increased demand for different probiotic products (Arora et al. 2019). Fermenting foods can make poorly digested, reactive foods into health-giving foods. The process of fermentation destroys many of the harmful microorganisms and chemicals in foods and adds beneficial bacteria. These bacteria produce new enzymes to assist in digestion. Foods that benefit from fermentation are soy products, dairy products, grains, and some vegetables (Hasan et al. 2014). The fermented foods exert various health and nutritional benefits, which are as follows.

1.2.1 Probiotics

Probiotics are defined as live microorganisms that, when administered in adequate amounts, confer a health benefit on the host (Hasan et al. 2014). Probiotics may be consumed either as food components or as non-food preparations. Probiotic organisms are sold mainly in fermented foods as starter organisms, and dairy products play a predominant role as carriers of probiotics (Mokoena et al. 2016). These foods are well suited in promoting the positive health impact in lactose intolerance, urinary

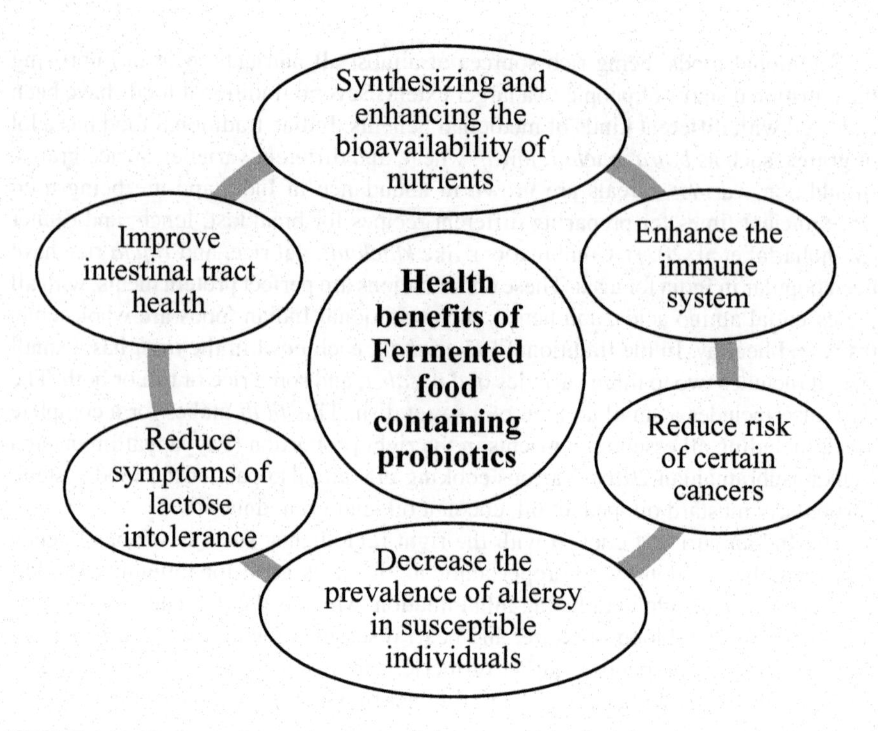

FIGURE 1.1 Health benefits of fermented foods containing probiotics.

tract infections in women, gut function, traveler's diarrhea, infantile diarrhea, antibiotic-associated diarrhea, *Helicobacter pylori* gastritis, inflammatory bowel disease (IBD), irritable bowel syndrome (IBS), colorectal cancer (CRC), immune function, infant health, atopic disease, and atopic dermatitis (Kopp-Hoolihan 2001). Various health benefits of probiotics are shown in Figure 1.1.

When probiotics are added to fermented foods, several factors must be considered that may influence the ability of the probiotics to survive in the product and become active during their entry into the consumer's gastrointestinal tract. These factors include the physiologic state of the probiotic organisms added (whether the cells are from the logarithmic or the stationary growth phase), the physical conditions of product storage (e.g., temperature), the chemical composition of the product to which the probiotics are added (e.g., acidity, available carbohydrate content, nitrogen sources, mineral content, water activity, and oxygen content), and possible interactions of the probiotics with the starter cultures (e.g., bacteriocin production, antagonism, and synergism). The commonly used probiotic bacteria today in commercial products are mainly members of the genera *Lactobacillus* and *Bifidobacterium*. *Lactobacillus* species from which probiotic strains have been isolated include *L. acidophilus*, *L. johnsonii*, *L. casei*, *L. rhamnosus*, *L. gasseri*, and *L. reuteri*. *Bifidobacterium* strains include *B. bifidum*, *B. longum*, and *B. infantis*. Different yeast species of probiotics are *Saccharomyces cerevisiae*, *Debaryomyces hansenii*, *Torulaspora delbrueckii*, and *Kluyveromyces lactis*, *K. marxianus*, and *K. lodderae* (Sales-Campos et al. 2019).

1.2.2 Preservation

Preservation of foods by fermentation has been widely practiced since ancient times (Caplice and Fitzgerald 1999). Fermentation not only ensures increased shelf life and microbiological safety of food but also makes some foods more digestible and, in the case of cassava fermentation, reduces the toxicity of the substrate. Although many fermentation processes are traditionally dependent on inoculation from a previous batch, starter cultures are available for many commercial processes, such as cheese manufacturing, thus ensuring consistency of process and product quality (Tamang et al. 2020). It is anticipated that the contribution of the advances in lactic acid bacteria and certain yeast research toward the improvement of strains for use in food fermentation will benefit both the consumer and the producer (Caplice and Fitzgerald 1999).

1.2.3 Flavor Enhancement

Fermentation makes the food palatable by enhancing its aroma and flavor. These organoleptic properties make fermented foods more popular than unfermented ones in terms of consumer acceptance. However, the specific mechanisms by which flavor is generated are still subject to investigation (Chelule et al. 2010a, 2010b).

1.2.4 Improvement of Nutritional Quality

Fermented foods can be more nutritious than their unfermented counterparts. This can come about in at least three different ways. Not only are microorganisms catabolic, breaking down more complex compounds, but they are also anabolic and synthesize several complex vitamins and other growth factors (Kampen 2014). The second important way in which fermented foods can be improved nutritionally has to do with the liberation of nutrients locked into plant structures and cells by indigestible materials. This is especially true in the case of certain grains and seeds (Sharma et al. 2020). The milling process does much to release nutrients from such items by physically rupturing cellulosic and hemicellulosic structures surrounding the endosperm, which is rich in digestible carbohydrates and proteins. Crude milling, however, practiced in many less-developed regions, often is inadequate to release the full nutritional value of such plant products; even after cooking, some of the entrapped nutrients may remain unavailable to the digestive process of humans (Hasan et al. 2014). Fermentation, especially by certain bacteria, yeasts, and molds, breaks down indigestible coatings and cell walls both chemically and physically. A third mechanism by which fermentation can enhance nutritional value, especially of plant materials, involves the enzymatic splitting of cellulose, hemicellulose, and related polymers that are not digestible by humans into simpler sugars and sugar derivatives. Cellulosic materials in fermented foods can be nutritionally improved for humans by the action of microbial enzymes. A number of foods, especially cereals, are poor in nutritional value, and they constitute the main staple diet of the low-income populations. However, lactic acid bacteria and yeast fermentation have been shown to improve the nutritional value and digestibility of these foods (Admassie 2018). The acidic nature of the fermentation products enhances the activity of microbial enzymes at a temperature range of 22–25°C (Chelule et al. 2010a, 2010b). The enzymes, which include amylases, proteases, phytases, and lipases, modify the primary food products through hydrolysis of polysaccharides, proteins, phytates, and lipids, respectively. Thus, in addition to enhancing the activity of enzymes, fermentation also reduces the levels of antinutrients, such as phytic acid and tannins in food, leading to increased bioavailability of minerals, such as iron, protein, and simple sugars (Chelule et al. 2010a, 2010b).

1.2.5 Alleviation of Lactose Intolerance

The inability to digest lactose, or milk sugar, in lactase-deficient individuals is prevalent worldwide (Swagerty et al. 2002). Consumption of lactose by those lacking adequate levels of lactase produced in the small intestine can result in symptoms of diarrhea, bloating, abdominal pain, and flatulence. Milk with cells of *L. acidophilus* aids digestion of lactose by such persons. It has been documented that many lactose-intolerant individuals are better able to consume fermented dairy foods, such as yogurt, with fewer symptoms than the same amount of unfermented counterparts. Fermented yogurt is found to be helpful in the digestion of lactose because the lactic acid bacteria used to make yogurt produce lactase and digest the lactose (Martini et al. 1991).

1.2.6 Improvement of Immunity System

The immune system acts to protect the host from infectious agents and a variety of noxious agents existing in the environment (Calder 2007). In principle, the immune system has two functional divisions: innate and acquired. Both components involve various blood-borne factors (complement, antibodies, and cytokines) and cells (Delves and Roitt 2000). A variety of secondary plant metabolites, including polyphenols produced from fermented food, may also contribute to the beneficial effects. Polyphenols are prominent in the resulting macerate, and published data have shown the antioxidative and immune-modulating potential in vitro. Several in vitro and in vivo studies have shown that polyphenols such as flavonoids have antioxidative and immunomodulatory actions. The high content of polyphenols might therefore be responsible for the bioactive effects of Regulat (Nakayama et al. 1992). The trial was to identify a suitable marker that could be used to obtain significant insight into the complex network of immune function, inflammation, and the redox state and the impact of Regulat and fermented foods in healthy subjects (Bell et al. 2017). There are several studies indicating the stimulation of the host cell immunity, both innate and adaptive immunity, by *S. cerevisiae* var. *boulardii* in response to pathogen infections. Few of the most used traditional fermented food and their health benefits are shown in Table 1.1.

TABLE 1.1
Few of the Most Used Traditional Fermented Food and Their Health Benefits*

Fermented food	Health/Nutritional benefits
Curd	Makes teeth and bones stronger, improves immunity, home remedy to get fair skin and great hair, improves digestion, good for the heart, helps lose weight, removes dandruff, improves vaginal health
Kanji	Good for gut and improves digestion
Lassi	Helps smoothen digestion, rich in calcium, source of probiotics, prevents bloating
Yogurt	High in protein, calcium, vitamins, and live culture, or probiotics; enhances the gut microbiota; offers protection for bones and teeth and helps prevent digestive problems; low-fat yogurt can be a useful source of protein on a weight-loss diet; may boost the immune system
Kefir	Fantastic source of many nutrients, more powerful probiotic than yogurt, potent antibacterial properties, can improve bone health and lower the risk of osteoporosis, may be protective against cancer
Ice cream	Source of vitamins, provides energy, source of minerals, stimulates the brain

* Shah 2006; Cruz et al. 2009; Balamurugan et al. 2014; Thakkar et al. 2015; Rosa et al. 2017; Behera et al. 2020.

1.3 BACTERIAL/FUNGAL/YEAST-BASED FOOD

The Indian system relies upon various traditional foods that possess various good bacteria and fungal strains that are proved to provide health benefits when consumed by humans, as shown in Table 1.2.

1.4 MOLECULAR NUTRIGENOMIC APPROACH FOR IDENTIFICATION/SCREENING

Nutrigenomics is one of the upcoming sciences that have the potential to open up a new arena toward health and disease management (Hag et al. 2020). Earlier generalized approach toward health and disease management was employed in the health sector in which human genetics and its respective environment were taken into account; nevertheless, in this contemporary approach, nutrition and its interaction with the human genome hold a focal position (Zmora et al. 2016). Regarding nutrition and human genomics and their interaction, nutrigenetics and nutrigenomics are employed, but both of these terms are either distant or closely related, depending upon the context (Ordovas and Corella 2004). Various different research studies conducted on the subject revealed that nutrients have the potential of influencing genes and their expression. Nutrients do serve as qualifying agents that can affect

TABLE 1.2
Traditionally Used Fermented Food Products and Their Associated Microorganisms*

Traditionally used food products	Associated microorganisms
Fermented vegetables and fruits	
Mesu, kanji, kimchi, garlic chilli pickle, sauerkraut, *dua muoi, eup, poi,* mango pickle, *khalpi*	*Pediococcus pentosaceus, Lactobacillus, Leuconostoc, Weissella, L. helveticus, L. plantarum, Leuconostoc mesenteroide, L. fermentum, L. pentos, Lactobacillus lactis, Lactobacillus* sp., *L. ceasi, L. brevis*
Cereal-based fermented foods	
Koozu, rabdi, kllappan, bhatura, boga, oat-based products, malt extract drink	*L. fermentum, W. paramesenteroids, Bacillus* sp., *Micrococcous, L. plantarum, Leuconostoc mesentorids, L. acidophilus, L. Lactis, L. reuteri, L. acidophilus, Bifidobacterium bifidum*
Meat-based fermented foods	
Yak satchu, arjia, meat products	*P. pentosaceous, E. faecium, E. hiras, Lactobacillus* species
Fermented milk products	
Dahi, khadi, kefir, shrikhand	*P. pentosaceous, W. cibara, Lactobacillus* spp., *Pedicoccus* sp., *Lactobacillus* sp.
Legume-based fermented products	
Wadi, kinema, tungrymobai	*Leuconostoc mesentroids, L. fermentum, E. faecium*

* Settanni and Corsetti (2007).

the overall functioning of genes at all levels. In order to uncover the various aspects and to deepen our comprehension of the subject, various different approaches, more precisely *omics* sciences, are employed. Transcriptomics, proteomics, metabolomics, and epigenomics greatly serve the purpose. Nutrigenomics has been anticipated as a revolutionary scientific approach that will provide us with a more customized, tailor-made, and individual-specific approach toward health and disease management (Hag et al. 2020).

Probiotic bacterial identification is the process of tagging a new isolate with probiotic potential that belongs to one of the established, named taxa, whereas classification is the arrangement of organisms into taxonomic groups (taxa) on the basis of similarities or relationships (Felis and Dellaglio 2007). There are two methods for the identification of bacteria/yeasts or fungi present in fermented food: (1) phenotypic identification and (2) genotypic identification.

1.5 PHENOTYPIC IDENTIFICATION

The first and foremost prerequisite while using bacteria as probiotics or as food is its identification, more specifically up to the strain level, as reported in the evaluation guidelines by FAO/WHO joint association (Arora and Baldi 2017). The very first step

TABLE 1.3
Phenotypic Identification Techniques Showing Different Discrimination Levels

Identification technique	Characters identified	Level of identification
Microscopic examination by staining	Shape, size, color, growth pattern, surface, margins, consistency	Genus, Gram+ or gram−
Growth on selective media	Growth of desirable bacteria promoted	Species level
Phenotypic and biochemical tests	Substrate utilization, fermentation pattern, presence or absence of certain enzymes, antibiotic resistivity, antimicrobial activity	Species level

to opt for the same is the identification by phenotypic characteristics consisting of careful microscopic examination of bacterial histology and the growth pattern of a particular microbe on media, based on cell morphology (colony, color, shape, etc.) in culture media, either solid or broth. Other methods include analysis of fermentation product, associated enzyme activity, and the ability to utilize various carbohydrate substrates (Franco-Duarte et al. 2019). The various identification steps needed are as follows:

1. Isolation of bacteria.
2. Microscopic examination of bacteria, which includes shape, size, color, growth pattern, surface, margins, and consistency.
3. Growth on selective media, which includes shape, size, color, growth pattern, surface, margins, and consistency of the colonies on the media.

Various identification steps, along with the level of discrimination achieved at each step, are shown in Table 1.3. Various limitations of the phenotypic identification are as follows:

- Microorganisms can be only broadly identified as bacteria, yeast, or fungus.
- Strain-level identification is not possible.
- The process is time-consuming.
- The results are not 100% reliable.
- In bacterial identification in food, one can't proceed further based on the results of phenotypic identification as bacteria sharing similar phenotypic characters may be harmful or beneficial but cannot be differentiated.

1.6 GENOTYPIC IDENTIFICATION

Satisfactory identification up to strain level cannot be achieved only by phenotypic identification, and hence, a number of advanced, rapid, and more specific molecular techniques are employed for the purpose of identification. Molecular techniques involve nucleic acids, which are not influenced by culture conditions (Siqueira Jr. and Rôças 2005). These high-throughput approaches, including techniques such as DNA-DNA hybridization (DDH), PFGE (pulsed-field gel electrophoresis), and 16S rRNA analysis, are increasingly applied to strains of lactic acid bacteria and *Bifidobacteria* that provide health benefits and are marketed as probiotic bacteria. Various genotypic identification techniques for probiotic microbes with their discrimination level are given in Table 1.4.

Identification of probiotic bacteria in fermented food is one of the major and necessary approaches to determine the nutritional value of food. Satisfactory identification up to strain level cannot be achieved only by phenotypic identification, and hence, a number of advanced, rapid, and more specific molecular techniques are employed for the purpose of identification. Molecular techniques involve nucleic acids, which are not influenced by culture conditions. These high-throughput approaches, including techniques such as DNA-DNA hybridization, RFLP, AFLP, RAPD, and SDS-PAGE, are increasingly applied to strains of lactic acid bacteria and *Bifidobacteria* that provide health benefits and are marketed as probiotic bacteria. Recent advances have led to more reliable techniques like representational differential analysis (RDA) and fluorescent in situ hybridization (FISH). Few techniques used for the molecular identification of microbes in fermented food are discussed below.

1.6.1 DNA-DNA Hybridization and G+C Content Determination

It is a technique used for measurement of the degree of genetic similarity between two species between various DNA sequences to carry out molecular systematics by which species can be arranged in a phylogenetic tree (Meier-Kolthoff et al. 2014). The technique of DNA-DNA hybridization involves immobilization of the target DNA onto a nitrocellulose filter membrane or nylon fibers, then treating it with NaOH and drying and baking it in a vacuum oven at 80°C for two hours. After this, radioactive labeling of the DNA takes place, which is used as a probe, and for the determination of G+C content, dissolution of purified DNA in 0.1X SSC is to be done, which is dialyzed against 0.1X SSC overnight. DNA equivalent to 25 μg in

TABLE 1.4
Most Used and Most Accurate Genotypic Identification Techniques Showing Different Discrimination Level

Identification technique	Characters identified	Level of identification
DNA-DNA hybridization and G+C content determination	Separation on the basis of size and then relatedness between species on the basis of sequence identification	Strain level
RFLP-PFGE, 16S ARDRA ribotyping, RAPD	Difference in variable sequences	Strain level
16S ribotyping	Difference in variable sequences	Strain level

TABLE 1.5
DNA-DNA Hybridization Technique Used for Generating Nutrition Scientific Evidence for Fermented Foods*

Studies	Findings
Identification and classification of *Croceivirga thetidis* sp. nov., a marine *Flavobacteriaceae* isolated from the hard coral *Acropora*	Identification of a new strain of *Croceivirga thetidis* sp. nov. was reported and confirmed using digital DNA-DNA hybridization (dDDH) and G+C content determination.
Identification and classification for the *Lactobacillus casei* group	It was observed that a number of strains of *Lactobacillus casei* group can be identified using DNA-DNA hybridization and G+C content determination.
Large-scale phylogenomics of the *Lactobacillus casei* group highlights taxonomic inconsistencies and reveals novel clade-associated features	Three taxonomic clades (clade A: *L. paracasei*, clade B: *L. casei*, and clade C: *L. rhamnosus*) were identified in the *L. casei* group based on a core genome phylogenetic tree and DNA G+C content analysis. G+C content and DNA-DNA hybridization analysis were performed, which revealed that strain 19 was a novel species, *Anoxybacillus flavithermus* sp. nov.
Molecular typing and probiotic attributes of a new strain of *Bacillus coagulans* – unique IS-2: a potential biotherapeutic agent	Identification of a new strain of *B. coagulans* unique IS2 was reported by using a mole % G+C content of DNA of the *Bacillus* isolate and 16S rRNA gene analysis of the *B. coagulans* DNA-DNA hybridization of the isolate with the other three reference strains, such as *B. coagulans* (NCIM 2030), *B. coagulans* (MTCC 492 and ATCC 7050), and *B. subtilis*.
Notes on the characterization of prokaryote strains for taxonomic purposes	DNA-DNA hybridization plays a key role in polyphasic taxonomy and is required for the classification of novel species, which share greater than 97% 16S rRNA gene sequence similarity with known species.
Genomic diversity of *Vibrio* associated with the Brazilian coral *Mussismilia hispida* and its sympatric zoanthids (*Palythoa caribaeorum*, *Palythoa variabilis*, and *Zoanthus solanderi*)	DNA-DNA hybridization is required for the identification of strains that belong to complex taxonomic groups (e.g., the *Vibrio* species core group).

* Thompson et al. 2009; Sudha et al. 2010; Tindall et al. 2010; Wuyts et al. 2017; Huang et al. 2018; Khalil et al. 2018; Yoon et al. 2021.

0.1X SSC is used for the determination of the % G+C content. Some of the examples of DNA-DNA hybridization are shown in Table 1.5.

For determining the hybridization patterns, DNA is required to undergo spectrophotometric analysis. Later for the comparisons, the DNA of one is labeled and compared against unlabeled DNA (Rosselló-Móra 2006). Mixtures need to withstand for the purpose of incubation in which sequences with high similarity will bind firmly and hence requires more energy to separate them. When this mixture is heated at a higher temperature, the DNA with dissimilar sequences will be separated from each other, and this process is known as DNA melting. The temperature, which is sufficient to make them separate, reflects the amount of similarity between sequences, hence the *Tm* value used to calculate the G+C content (mole %) according to the equation of Schildkraut and Leifson (Schildkraut and Lifson 1965).

1.6.2 16S rRNA Sequencing and PCR-Based Methodologies

The technique called 16S rRNA region amplification by using species-specific primers is the technique of choice for the identification of *Lactobacillus* species. Discrimination of species has been carried out for *Lactobacillus* species isolated from *kargi tulum* cheese, including *L. paracasei, L. plantarum, Enterococcus durans, Streptococcus thermophilus*, and *L. brevis* (Kunduhoglu et al. 2012). With the increasing availability and declining cost of high-throughput sequencing operations, the determination of 16S rRNA gene nucleotide sequences in variable regions V1–V3 has emerged as a technique of choice for strain and phylogenetic analysis (Vandamme et al. 1996). However, one of the limitations of this approach is that as the evolutionary distance decreases, insufficiency generates in the diversity level in the 16S rRNA, and genetic relationships of closely related species cannot be accurately defined on the basis of the 16S rRNA gene sequence. The intergenic spacer region between 16S and 23S rRNA genes containing a variable number of tRNA genes can also be a suitable target for sequencing, and this may also be a possible alternative (Gürtler and Stanisich 1996). Some of the examples of 16S rRNA sequencing and PCR-based methodologies are shown in Table 1.6.

1.6.3 PFGE-DNA Profiling

Pulsed-field gel electrophoresis (PFGE) has been considered as the gold standard among molecular typing methods for various potentially probiotic bacteria, per FAO guidelines. PFGE is being used as a primary typing tool to analyze various bacterial species for the last many years (Herbel et al. 2013). Moreover, this technique is inexpensive and valuable due to its excellent typeability and reproducibility. It may help to establish international fingerprinting databases, which will allow fast detection and monitoring of the pathogenic bacterial strains.

To perform PFGE, a highly purified genomic DNA sample is cleaved with a restriction endonuclease that recognizes restriction sites in the genome of the bacteria species. The resulting restriction fragments can be separated on an agarose gel by pulsed-field electrophoresis, in which the orientation of the electric field across the gel is changed periodically. The separated DNA fragments can be visualized on the gel as bands, which form a particular pattern on the gel, the PFGE pattern. For most bacteria, PFGE can resolve DNA fragments with sizes ranging from about 30 KB to over 1 MB. For making the analysis easier, large restriction fragments are thus separated in a size-dependent manner, and hence, the method yields relatively few bands on the gel. Another advantage of the PFGE method is that it addresses a large portion of an investigated genome (>90%) (Linhardt et al. 1992). Some of the examples of PFGE are shown in Table 1.7.

TABLE 1.6
16S rRNA Sequencing and PCR-Based Methodologies Used for Generating Nutrition Scientific Evidence for Fermented Foods*

Studies	Findings
Bacterial community diversity of fermented pepper in Brazzaville revealed by Illumina Miseq of 16S rRNA gene	The objective of the study was to find bacterial diversity in three fermented foods using the Illumina Miseq technique targeting the 16S rRNA gene. The results showed that EB3 and EB2 samples were more diverse than EB1. *Proteobacteria*, *Firmicutes*, and *Actinobacteria* were the dominant phyla in all three samples. *Lactobacillus* was dominant in the EB1 sample, *Clostridium* sensu stricto in EB2, and *Fructobacillus* in EB3.
Bacterial compositions of indigenous Lanna (Northern Thai) fermented foods and their potential functional properties	The 16S rRNA gene from the fermented food samples is analyzed using 454-pyrosequencing resulted in 113,844 sequences after quality evaluation. Most of the sequences showed similarity with lactic acid bacteria, which is also known as probiotics. The final results showed that traditional Thai fermented food products are rich sources of beneficial bacteria and can potentially be functional/probiotic foods.
Diversity of lactic acid bacteria isolated from Indonesian traditional fermented foods	The identification of 16S rRNA showed that the majority of the strains isolated were *Lactobacillus plantarum*, *Lactobacillus fermentum*, and *Pediococcus pentosaceus*.
Analysis of bacterial communities of traditional fermented West African cereal foods using culture-independent methods	Molecular profiling using 16S rRNA analysis of *kunu zaki* and *ogi* indicated diverse bacterial communities in them. Bacteria identified were mainly members of *Lactobacillaceae* or *Streptococcaceae* families.
Bacterial diversity in traditional Korean fermented soybean foods (*doenjang* and *ganjang*) by 16S rRNA gene sequence analysis	Sequences from 16S rRNA were amplified and cloned from two different fermented soybean foods, such as *doenjang* (soybean paste) and *ganjang* (soybean sauce). The following species were identified in the paste and sauce: *Staphylococcus equorum* (60.6%), *Tetragenococcus halophila* (21.2%), *Leuconostoc mesenteroides* (9.1%), *Lactobacillus sakei* (6.1%), and *Bacillus subtilis* (3.0%) in soybean paste samples and *Halanaerobium* sp. (37.5%), *Halanaerobium fermentans* (37.5%), *T. halophila* (12.5%), *Staphylococcus* sp. (6.3%), *S. equorum* (3.1%) in soybean sauce samples.
Lactobacillus casei, *Lactobacillus rhamnosus*, and *Lactobacillus zeae* isolates identified by sequence signature and immunoblot phenotype	Comparative sequence analysis of V1–V3 regions of 16S rRNA was done for *L. casei, L. paracasei, L. rhamnosus,* and *L. zeae*. Single-locus analyses and genomic DNA profiling for *L. acidophilus*, *L. animalis*, *L. brevis* subsp. *gravesensis*, *L. buchneri*, and *L. fermentum* was performed, and identification at the species level was achieved with BLASTn sequence analyses of the 16S rRNA gene with the exception of *L. reuteri* ATCC 53609 and *L. plantarum* ATCC 49445; all reference strains were found to be most similar to their species designations.

* Dobson et al. 2004; Cho and Seo 2007; Oguntoyinbo et al. 2011; Mustopa and Fatimah 2014; Pakwan et al. 2020; Boumba et al. 2021.

TABLE 1.7
Pulsed-Field Gel Electrophoresis Used for Generating Nutrition Scientific Evidence for Fermented Foods*

Studies	Findings
Molecular investigation of an outbreak associated with total parenteral nutrition contaminated with NDM-producing *Leclercia adecarboxylata*	Clonal diversity was performed using PFGE. The genetic relationships of 31 strains isolated indicated one main lineage highly related to the outbreak with three restriction patterns detected: A (83.9%, 26/31), A1 (12.9%, 4/31), and A2 (2.2%, 1/31), with a percentage of similarity ranging from 90 to 100%.
Tracing of *Listeria monocytogenes* contamination routes in fermented sausage production chain by PFGE typing	The source of contamination was identified using PFGE. The same PFGE profiles of *L. monocytogenes* were found in both semi-dry and fermented sausage mixtures, which indicated that the cross-contamination was probably due to the practice of processing the same raw material (a swab from a bag of frozen beef positive for pathogen) that led to the contact of both mixtures in the production equipment.
Molecular tracing to find the source of the protracted invasive listeriosis outbreak, southern Germany, 2012–2016	The outbreak investigation revealed 26 isolates from food with the 13a/54 PFGE pattern: 24 isolates either originating from or associated with food products from the suspected outbreak source assigned to the cluster type 1248 and two isolates not epidemiologically linked to the suspected outbreak source that differed from cluster type 1248 by >32 alleles.
Molecular typing of foodborne *Staphylococcus aureus* by PFGE in Yunnan Province	Eighty-nine PFGE types were obtained among the 113 strains through cluster analysis. The similarity coefficients of the PFGE atlas were in the range of 56.67 to 100%. The diversity of the PFGE database of foodborne *Staphylococcus aureus* was found to be of great significance for the diagnosis and derivation of the food poisoning caused by *Staphylococcus aureus*.
Safety assessment and molecular genetic profiling by PFGE and PCR-based techniques of *Enterococcus faecium* strains of food origin	The genetic relatedness of *Enterococci* present in food was determined by PFGE. The absence of well-known enterococcal virulence markers in a collection of *E. faecium* strains from food proved them safe to be used in the food industry or as probiotics in animal production.
Antimicrobial resistance and PFGE analyses of *Salmonella senftenberg* from food of animal origins in Shanghai, China	PFGE was used for molecular typing. The molecular typing of 15 *Salmonella senftenberg* isolates resulted in ten unique patterns, among which three (X3, X4, X5) were grouped together at a high similarity index of 88.2%, suggesting that these isolates of different origins may be relevant in the epidemiology.

* Kuang et al. 2015; Guo et al. 2017; Kleta et al. 2017; Muñoz-Atienza et al. 2017; Pažin et al. 2018; Garza-González et al. 2021.

1.7 MOLECULAR APPROACH IN NUTRITION RESEARCH

In spite of the fact that life expectancy has increased markedly during the last few centuries, all populations may benefit from optimized nutrition to reduce the incidence of obesity, type 2 diabetes mellitus (T2D), cardiovascular diseases, and several types of cancers and infectious diseases. Nutritional science should be focused on preventing the development of diseases and supporting the repair processes important for curing already fully developed diseases. Traditional nutrition research has contributed significantly to modern biomedicine and obviously promoted prolonged life expectancy (Norheim et al. 2012). However, it is still a large potential for improving diet and health for many groups in economically developing and developed countries. This potential can be exploited by designing good studies and applying new and advanced techniques, mostly based on molecular methods and advanced biostatistics.

1.7.1 Transcriptomics and Nutrition

Transcriptomics refers to the complete collection of gene transcripts in a cell or a tissue at a given time and may be used to study gene transcription in response to dietary changes (Lowe et al. 2017). The nuclear hormone receptor superfamily of transcription factors is probably the most important group of nutrient sensors, which influence gene expression. Numerous nuclear hormone receptors, such as RXR, PPARs, and liver X receptors (LXRs), bind nutrients and undergo a conformational change that results in the coordinated dissociation of co-repressors and the recruitment of co-activator proteins to enable transcription activation. RNA microarray technologies and sequencing can be used to evaluate the interactions between diet and genes measured as changes in genetic expression (Lockhart and Winzeler 2000). When applied together with traditional biochemical methods, transcriptomics provides more extensive information about the nutrition status and metabolic responses to diet. Transcriptomics is mainly used for three different purposes in nutrition research: first, it can provide information about the mechanism underlying the effects of a certain nutrient or diet; second, it can help identify genes, proteins, or metabolites that are altered in the pre-disease state and might act as molecular biomarkers; third, it can help identify and characterize pathways regulated by nutrients. Human dietary intervention studies have successfully used transcriptomics to show that diet induces alterations in gene expression (Boss et al. 2016). However, an important challenge in human transcriptomic studies is the inaccessibility of human tissues. Blood, subcutaneous adipose tissue, and skeletal muscle are among the tissues, which can be relatively easily collected. Thus, animal studies can be good supplements to human studies to understand how nutrients affect gene regulation in a variety of tissues.

1.7.2 Proteomics

Proteomics represents the large-scale study of the entire set of proteins expressed in a given cell, tissue, or organism at a defined time point. Most biological functions are transmitted via proteins, like enzymes, receptors, and structural components. Studying proteins directly is necessary because gene expression levels do not always correspond to protein abundance because protein levels are determined by regulatory input from synthesis to degradation. Second, pre-mRNA transcripts might give rise to several proteins because of alternative splicing. Third, subcellular localization is important for biological effects. In addition, post-translational modifications and interactions with other proteins or RNA affect protein action and activity. Diet can induce post-translational modifications of proteins. One example is the study of Henze and colleagues showing that protein-energy malnutrition leads both to changes in transthyretin concentration in the blood and post-translational modifications of the protein (Henze et al. 2008). Several review articles on the use of proteomics in nutrition research have been published (Kussmann et al. 2010; Moore and Weeks 2011; Romagnolo and Milner 2012). The focus has been on identifying new health biomarkers and bioactive peptides in foods. Among the potential approaches for studying the proteome on a large scale, chromatography, combined with mass spectrometry (MS), has become a leading method. Other techniques include one- and two-dimensional gel electrophoresis and antibody-based assays, such as protein microarrays (Rabilloud 2002).

1.7.3 Metabolomics

Metabolomics refers to the types and concentrations of all metabolites in a biological sample. Biological metabolites are specific products of genomic, transcriptomic, and proteomic processes of the host or external organisms, as well as the intrinsic and extrinsic influence on these. The characteristics and concentrations of all small molecules, water- and lipid-soluble, provide a potential for measuring flux through all the important biological pathways and thereby allow a detailed understanding of how metabolites interact with tissue components of functional importance (Patti et al. 2012). Metabolomics can also be used to identify biomarkers for the intake of specific nutrients and health. For example, it has recently been shown in a meta-analysis that blood concentrations of carotenoids, a biomarker for fruit and vegetable intake, are strongly associated with reduced breast cancer risk, as assessed by dietary questionnaires (Aune et al. 2012). Ideally, metabolomics should have the ability to provide a detailed snapshot of biological processes at any particular point in time. In nutritional research, such an approach may provide an opportunity to identify changes in metabolic pathways induced by nutrients or other lifestyle factors, to explore relationships between environmental factors, health, and disease, and to discover novel biomarkers (Gibney et al. 2005; Lodge 2010). However, due to the diverse chemical nature of low-molecular metabolites, including lipids, amino acids, peptides, nucleic acids, organic acids, vitamins, thiols, and carbohydrates, the global, untargeted analysis represents a tough challenge. Although the development of analytical platforms enables separation, detection, characterization, and quantification of a large number of metabolites from only minor amounts of biological samples (Zhang et al. 2012), targeted metabolomics is most often used (Griffiths et al. 2010). Targeted analysis, where a pre-defined set of metabolites are monitored, may be used for assessment of single nutrients or metabolites (Karlsen et al. 2011) and the determination of subsets of metabolites, including lipids (German et al. 2007), inflammatory markers (Karlsen et al. 2007; Karlsen et al. 2010), or oxidative damage. The profiling of lipids has developed into its own field of lipidomics, and as adversely altered lipid metabolism is an underlying factor in a number of human chronic diseases, lipidomics has become an important tool to identify potential novel therapeutic targets (Brevik et al. 2011).

1.8 CONCLUSION

Traditional knowledge about the processing, preservation, and therapeutic effects of traditional foods has been recognized for many generations in India. As demonstrated in this chapter, a variety of foods available in our system can deliver numerous biological functions through nutritional components in the human body. Molecular approaches have been implied in nutritional research; however, the application of the same is still limited in traditional foods. The major important point here is the development of standard operating procedures for the standardization and quality control of these traditional foods so that these foods can be used safely by the public all over the world for therapeutic and prophylactic purposes.

REFERENCES

Admassie, M. 2018. A review on food fermentation and the biotechnology of lactic acid bacteria. *World Journal of Food Science and Technology* 2(1):19–24.

Arora, M., and Baldi, A. 2017. Selective identification and characterization of potential probiotic strains: A review on comprehensive polyphasic approach. *Applied Clinical Research, Clinical Trials and Regulatory Affairs* 4(1):60–76.

Arora, M., Kaur, N., Bansal, P., and Baldi, A. 2019. Emergence of traditionally used foods as today's probiotics long journey. *Current Traditional Medicine* 5(2):114–25.

Aune, D., Chan, D. S., Vieira, A. R., et al. 2012. Dietary compared with blood concentrations of carotenoids and breast cancer risk: A systematic review and meta-analysis of prospective studies. *American Journal of Clinical Nutrition* 96(2):356–73.

Balamurugan, R., Chandragunasekaran, A. S., Chellappan, G., Rajaram, K., Ramamoorthi, G., and Ramakrishna, B. S. 2014. Probiotic potential of lactic acid bacteria present in home made curd in southern India. *Indian Journal of Medical Research* 140(3):345.

Behera, S. S., El Sheikha, A. F., Hammami, R., and Kumar, A. 2020. Traditionally fermented pickles: How the microbial diversity associated with their nutritional and health benefits?. *Journal of Functional Foods* 70:103971.

Bell, V., Ferrão, J., and Fernandes, T. 2017. Nutritional guidelines and fermented food frameworks. *Foods* 6(8):65.

Boss, A., Kao, C. H. J., Murray, P. M., Marlow, G., Barnett, M. P., and Ferguson, L. R. 2016. Human intervention study to assess the effects of supplementation with olive leaf extract on peripheral blood mononuclear cell gene expression. *International Journal of Molecular Sciences* 17(12):2019.

Boumba, A. E. L., Lebonguy, A. A., Goma-Tchimbakala, J., Nzaou, S. A. E., Polo, C. P. L., and Moukala, M. B. 2021. Bacterial community diversity of fermented pepper in Brazzaville revealed by Illumina Miseq of 16S rRNA gene. *Food and Nutrition Sciences* 12(01):37.

Brevik, A., Karlsen, A., Azqueta, A., Estaban, A. T., Blomhoff, R., and Collins, A. 2011. Both base excision repair and nucleotide excision repair in humans are influenced by nutritional factors. *Cell Biochemistry and Function* 29(1):36–42.

Calder, P. C. 2007. Immunological parameters: What do they mean? *Journal of Nutrition* 137(3):773S-80S.

Caplice, E., and Fitzgerald, G. F. 1999. Food fermentations: Role of microorganisms in food production and preservation. *International Journal of Food Microbiology* 50(1–2):131–49.

Chelule, P. K., Mbongwa, H. P., Carries, S., and Gqaleni, N. 2010a. Lactic acid fermentation improves the quality of amahewu, a traditional South African maize-based porridge. *Food Chemistry* 122(3):656–61.

Chelule, P. K., Mokoena, M. P., and Gqaleni, N. 2010b. Advantages of traditional lactic acid bacteria fermentation of food in Africa. *Current Research, Technology and Education Topics in Applied Microbiology and Microbial Biotechnology* 2:1160–7.

Cho, K. M., and Seo, W. T. 2007. Bacterial diversity in a Korean traditional soybean fermented foods (doenjang and ganjang) by 16S rRNA gene sequence analysis. *Food Science and Biotechnology* 16(2):320–4.

Cruz, A. G., Antunes, A. E., Sousa, A. L. O., Faria, J. A., and Saad, S. M. 2009. Ice-cream as a probiotic food carrier. *Food Research International* 42(9):1233–9.

Delves, P. J., and Roitt, I. M. 2000. The immune system. *New England Journal of Medicine* 343(1):37–49.

Dobson, C. M., Chaban, B., Deneer, H., and Ziola, B. 2004. *Lactobacillus casei*, *Lactobacillus rhamnosus*, and *Lactobacillus zeae* isolates identified by sequence signature and immunoblot phenotype. *Canadian Journal of Microbiology* 50(7):482–8.

Felis, G. E., and Dellaglio, F. 2007. Taxonomy of lactobacilli and bifidobacteria. *Current Issues in Intestinal Microbiology* 8(2):44.

Franco-Duarte, R., Černáková, L., Kadam, S., et al. 2019. Advances in chemical and biological methods to identify microorganisms – from past to present. *Microorganisms* 7(5):130.

Garza-González, E., Bocanegra-Ibarias, P., Rodríguez-Noriega, E., et al. 2021. Molecular investigation of an outbreak associated with total parenteral nutrition contaminated with NDM-producing *Leclercia Adecarboxylata*. *BMC Infectious Diseases* 21(1):1–8.

German, J. B., Gillies, L. A., Smilowitz, J. T., Zivkovic, A. M., and Watkins, S. M. 2007. Lipidomics and lipid profiling in metabolomics. *Current Opinion in Lipidology* 18(1):66–71.

Gibney, M. J., Walsh, M., Brennan, L., Roche, H. M., German, B., and Van Ommen, B. 2005. Metabolomics in human nutrition: Opportunities and challenges. *American Journal of Clinical Nutrition* 82(3):497–503.

Griffiths, W. J., Koal, T., Wang, Y., Kohl, M., Enot, D. P., and Deigner, H. P. 2010. Targeted metabolomics for biomarker discovery. *Angewandte Chemie International Edition* 49(32):5426–45.

Guo, Y., Yang, Z., and Gu, W. 2017. Molecular typing of foodborne *Staphylococcus aureus* by pulsed-field gel electrophoresis in Yunnan province. *Journal of Food Safety and Quality* 8(10):3826–30.

Gürtler, V., and Stanisich, V. A. 1996. New approaches to typing and identification of bacteria using the 16S-23S rDNA spacer region. *Microbiology* 142(1):3–16.

Hag, S. N., Siddique, R., Altay, V., et al. 2020. Nutrigenomics – An emerging field of science and technology unrevealing inter-relationships between nutrients and human genome using modern tools such as transcriptomics, metabolomics, epigenomics and proteomics. *Biyolojik Çeşitlilik ve Koruma* 13(3):372–80.

Hasan, M. N., Sultan, M. Z., and Mar-E-Um, M. 2014. Significance of fermented food in nutrition and food science. *Journal of Scientific Research* 6(2):373–86.

Henze, A., Rohn, S., Gericke, B., Raila, J., and Schweigert, F. J. 2008. Structural modifications of serum transthyretin in rats during protein-energy malnutrition. *Rapid Communications in Mass Spectrometry* 22(20):3270–4.

Herbel, S. R., Vahjen, W., Wieler, L. H., and Guenther, S. 2013. Timely approaches to identify probiotic species of the genus *Lactobacillus*. *Gut Pathogens* 5(1):1–13.

Huang, C. H., Li, S. W., Huang, L., and Watanabe, K. 2018. Identification and classification for the *Lactobacillus casei* group. *Frontiers in Microbiology* 9, 22(1974):1–13.

Kampen, W. H. 2014. Nutritional requirements in fermentation processes. In *Fermentation and Biochemical Engineering Handbook*, 37–57. William Andrew Publishing, Norwich, NY.

Karlsen, A., Paur, I., Bøhn, S. K., et al. 2010. Bilberry juice modulates plasma concentration of NF-κB related inflammatory markers in subjects at increased risk of CVD. *European Journal of Nutrition* 49(6):345–55.

Karlsen, A., Retterstøl, L., Laake, P., et al. 2007. Anthocyanins inhibit nuclear factor-κ B activation in monocytes and reduce plasma concentrations of pro-inflammatory mediators in healthy adults. *Journal of Nutrition* 137(8):1951–4.

Karlsen, A., Svendsen, M., Seljeflot, I., et al. 2011. Compliance, tolerability and safety of two antioxidant-rich diets: A randomised controlled trial in male smokers. *British Journal of Nutrition* 106(4):557–71.

Khalil, A., Sivakumar, N., Arslan, M., and Qarawi, S. 2018. Novel *Anoxybacillus flavithermus* AK1: A thermophile isolated from a hot spring in Saudi Arabia. *Arabian Journal for Science and Engineering* 43(1):73–81.

Kleta, S., Hammerl, J. A., Dieckmann, R., et al. 2017. Molecular tracing to find source of protracted invasive listeriosis outbreak, southern Germany, 2012–2016. *Emerging Infectious Diseases* 23(10):1680.

Kopp-Hoolihan, L. 2001. Prophylactic and therapeutic uses of probiotics: A review. *Journal of the American Dietetic Association* 101(2):229–41.

Kuang, D., Xu, X., Zhang, J., et al. 2015. Antimicrobial resistance and pulse field gel electrophoresis analyses of *Salmonella senftenberg* from food of animal origins in Shanghai, China. *Journal of South China Agricultural University* 36(1):113–6.

Kunduhoglu, B., Elcioglu, O., Gezginc, Y., Akyol, I., Pilatin, S., and Cetinkaya, A. 2012. Genotypic identification and technological characterization of lactic acid bacteria isolated from traditional Turkish Kargi tulum cheese. *African Journal of Biotechnology* 11(28):7218–26.

Kussmann, M., Panchaud, A., and Affolter, M. 2010. Proteomics in nutrition: Status quo and outlook for biomarkers and bioactives. *Journal of Proteome Research* 9(10): 4876–87.

Linhardt, F., Ziebuhr, W., Meyer, P., Witte, W., and Hacker, J. 1992. Pulsed-field gel electrophoresis of genomic restriction fragments as a tool for the epidemiological analysis of *Staphylococcus aureus* and coagulase-negative staphylococci. *FEMS Microbiology Letters* 95(2–3):181–5.

Lockhart, D. J., and Winzeler, E. A. 2000. Genomics, gene expression and DNA arrays. *Nature* 405(6788):827–36.

Lodge, J. K. 2010. Symposium 2: Modern approaches to nutritional research challenges. Targeted and non-targeted approaches for metabolite profiling in nutritional research: Conference on "Over-and undernutrition: Challenges and approaches." *Proceedings of the Nutrition Society* 69(1):95–102.

Lowe, R., Shirley, N., Bleackley, M., Dolan, S., and Shafee, T. 2017. Transcriptomics technologies. *PLoS Computational Biology* 13(5):e1005457.

Manoharlal, R., Saiprasad, G. V. S., and Madhavakrishna, K. 2021. Evaluation of mono-, di-and oligo-saccharides of staple Indian grain flours. *Journal of Microbiology, Biotechnology and Food Sciences* 2021:799–804.

Martini, M. C., Lerebours, E. C., Lin, W. J., et al. 1991. Strains and species of lactic acid bacteria in fermented milks (yogurts): Effect on in vivo lactose digestion. *American Journal of Clinical Nutrition* 54(6):1041–6.

Meier-Kolthoff, J. P., Klenk, H. P., and Göker, M. 2014. Taxonomic use of DNA G+C content and DNA-DNA hybridization in the genomic age. *International Journal of Systematic and Evolutionary Microbiology* 64:352–6.

Mokoena, M. P., Mutanda, T., and Olaniran, A. O. 2016. Perspectives on the probiotic potential of lactic acid bacteria from African traditional fermented foods and beverages. *Food and Nutrition Research* 60(1):29630.
Moore, J. B., and Weeks, M. E. 2011. Proteomics and systems biology: Current and future applications in the nutritional sciences. *Advances in Nutrition* 2(4):355–64.
Muñoz-Atienza, E., et al. 2017. Generation and characterisation of Porphyromonas gingivalis mutant lacking peptidylarginine deiminase activity. *Journal of Oral Microbiology* 9(sup1):1325258.
Mustopa, A. Z., and Fatimah, F. 2014. Diversity of lactic acid bacteria isolated from Indonesian traditional fermented foods. *Microbiology Indonesia* 8(2):2.
Nakayama, I., Kobayashi, M., Kamiya, Y., Abe, H., and Sakurai, A. 1992. Effects of a plant-growth regulat or, prohexadione-calcium (BX-112), on the endogenous levels of gibberellins in rice. *Plant and Cell Physiology* 33(1):59–62.
Norheim, F., Gjelstad, I. M., Hjorth, M., et al. 2012. Molecular nutrition research – the modern way of performing nutritional science. *Nutrients* 4(12):1898–944.
Oguntoyinbo, F. A., Tourlomousis, P., Gasson, M. J., and Narbad, A. 2011. Analysis of bacterial communities of traditional fermented West African cereal foods using culture independent methods. *International Journal of Food Microbiology* 145(1):205–10.
Ordovas, J. M., and Corella, D. 2004. Nutritional genomics. *Annual Review of Genomics and Human Genetics* 5:71–118.
Pakwan, C., Chitov, T., Chantawannakul, P., Manasam, M., Bovonsombut, S., and Disayathanoowat, T. 2020. Bacterial compositions of indigenous Lanna (Northern Thai) fermented foods and their potential functional properties. *PLoS One* 15(11):e0242560.
Patti, G. J., Yanes, O., and Siuzdak, G. 2012. Metabolomics: The apogee of the omics trilogy. *Nature Reviews Molecular Cell Biology* 13(4):263–9.
Payyappallimana, U., and Venkatasubramanian, P. 2016. Exploring Ayurvedic knowledge on food and health for providing innovative solutions to contemporary healthcare. *Frontiers in Public Health* 4:57.
Pažin, V., Jankuloski, D., Kozačinski, L., et al. 2018. Tracing of *Listeria monocytogenes* contamination routes in fermented sausage production chain by pulsed-field gel electrophoresis typing. *Foods* 7(12):198.
Prajapati, Jashbhai B., and Nair, Baboo M. 2003. The history of fermented foods. In *Fermented Functional Foods*, 1–25. CRC Press, Boca Raton, New York, London, Washington DC.
Rabilloud, T. 2002. Two-dimensional gel electrophoresis in proteomics: Old, old fashioned, but it still climbs up the mountains. *Proteomics* 2(1):3–10.
Ramaswamy, S. 2018. Reflections on current Ayurveda research. *Journal of Ayurveda and Integrative Medicine* 9(4):250–1.
Romagnolo, D. F., and Milner, J. A. 2012. Opportunities and challenges for nutritional proteomics in cancer prevention. *Journal of Nutrition* 142(7):1360S–9S.
Rosa, D. D., Dias, M. M., Grześkowiak, Ł. M., Reis, S. A., Conceição, L. L., and Maria do Carmo, G. P. 2017. Milk kefir: Nutritional, microbiological and health benefits. *Nutrition Research Reviews* 30(1):82–96.
Rosselló-Móra, R. 2006. DNA-DNA reassociation methods applied to microbial taxonomy and their critical evaluation. In *Molecular Identification, Systematics, and Population Structure of Prokaryotes*, 23–50. Springer, Berlin, Heidelberg.
Sales-Campos, H., Soares, S. C., and Oliveira, C. J. F. 2019. An introduction of the role of probiotics in human infections and autoimmune diseases. *Critical Reviews in Microbiology* 45(4):413–32.
Sarkar, P., DH, L. K., Dhumal, C., Panigrahi, S. S., and Choudhary, R. 2015. Traditional and ayurvedic foods of Indian origin. *Journal of Ethnic Foods* 2(3):97–109.
Schildkraut, C., and Lifson, S. 1965. Dependence of the melting temperature of DNA on salt concentration. *Biopolymers: Original Research on Biomolecules* 3(2):195–208.

Settanni, L., and Corsetti, A. 2007. The use of multiplex PCR to detect and differentiate food and beverage-associated microorganisms: A review. *Journal of Microbiological Methods* 69(1):1–22.

Shah, N. P. 2006. Health benefits of yogurt and fermented milks. *Manufacturing Yogurt and Fermented Milks* 327.

Sharma, R., Garg, P., Kumar, P., Bhatia, S. K., and Kulshrestha, S. 2020. Microbial fermentation and its role in quality improvement of fermented foods. *Fermentation* 6(4):106.

Singh, A. K., Rehal, J., Kaur, A., and Jyot, G. 2015. Enhancement of attributes of cereals by germination and fermentation: A review. *Critical Reviews in Food Science and Nutrition* 55(11):1575–89.

Siqueira Jr., J. F., and Rôças, I. N. 2005. Exploiting molecular methods to explore endodontic infections: Part 1 – Current molecular technologies for microbiological diagnosis. *Journal of Endodontics* 31(6):411–23.

Sudha, R., Chauhan, P., Dixit, K., Babu, S. M., and Jamil, K. 2010. Molecular typing and probiotic attributes of a new strain of *Bacillus coagulans* unique IS-2: A potential biotherapeutic agent. *Genetic Engineering and Biotechnology Journal* 7:1–20.

Swagerty Jr, D. L., Walling, A., and Klein, R. M. 2002. Lactose intolerance. *American Family Physician* 65(9):1845.

Tamang, J. P., Cotter, P. D., Endo, A., et al. 2020. Fermented foods in a global age: East meets West. *Comprehensive Reviews in Food Science and Food Safety* 19(1):184–217.

Thakkar, P., Modi, H. A., and Prajapati, J. B. 2015. Isolation, characterization and safety assessment of lactic acid bacterial isolates from fermented food products. *International Journal of Current Microbiology and Applied Sciences* 4(4):713–25.

Thompson, C. C., Vicente, A. C. P., and Souza, R. C. 2009. Genomic taxonomy of *Vibrios*. *BMC Evolutionary Biology* 9(1):1–16.

Tindall, B. J., Rosselló-Móra, R., Busse, H. J., Ludwig, W., and Kämpfer, P. 2010. Notes on the characterization of prokaryote strains for taxonomic purposes. *International Journal of Systematic and Evolutionary Microbiology* 60(1):249–66.

Vandamme, P., Pot, B., Gillis, M., De Vos, P., Kersters, K., and Swings, J. 1996. Polyphasic taxonomy, a consensus approach to bacterial systematics. *Microbiological Reviews* 60(2):407–38.

Wuyts, S., Wittouck, S., De Boeck, I., et al. 2017. Large-scale phylogenomics of the *Lactobacillus casei* group highlights taxonomic inconsistencies and reveals novel clade-associated features. *mSystems* 2(4):e00061–17.

Yoon, J., Yasumoto-Hirose, M., and Kasai, H. 2021. Identification and classification of *Croceivirga thetidis* sp. nov., a marine Flavobacteriaceae isolated from the hard coral Acropora. *Antonie van Leeuwenhoek* 1–10.

Zhang, A., Sun, H., Wang, P., Han, Y., and Wang, X. 2012. Modern analytical techniques in metabolomics analysis. *Analyst* 137(2):293–300.

Zmora, N., Zeevi, D., Korem, T., Segal, E., and Elinav, E. 2016. Taking it personally: Personalized utilization of the human microbiome in health and disease. *Cell Host and Microbe* 19(1):12–20.

Sechi, L. [illegible] and Ca[illegible], S. 2004. The use of multiplex PCR to detect and differentiate [illegible] and [illegible] associated [illegible]: A review. [illegible] 60(1):1–2[illegible].

S[illegible], [illegible] 2015. [illegible] [illegible] and [illegible] and [illegible] [illegible].

[illegible], [illegible], Ga[illegible], P., [illegible], P., Bhatia, S. K. and [illegible] S. 2020. Microbial [illegible] [illegible] and its role in quality improvement of fermented foods. [illegible] 6(4):106.

Singh, A. K., Rehal, J., Kaur, A. and Jyot, G. 2015. Enhancement of [illegible] by [illegible] and [illegible]: A review. Critical Reviews in Food Science and Nutrition 55(11):1575–89.

[illegible], [illegible] and [illegible], N. 2005. Exploiting [illegible] [illegible] to explore [illegible] [illegible]. Part I: [illegible] molecular techniques [illegible]. Journal of [illegible] [illegible] 1–3[illegible].

Sethi, R., Rajbhar, P., Dhar, K., [illegible], S. [illegible] and [illegible], [illegible] 2010. Molecular typing and probiotic [illegible] of a new strain of [illegible] [illegible] [illegible]: A potential [illegible]. [illegible] [illegible] [illegible].

S[illegible], J. D., Walt[illegible], A. and Kl[illegible], M. 2016. [illegible] [illegible] [illegible] [illegible] [illegible]. [illegible] [illegible] 2:16048.

[illegible], J., Crane, [illegible], [illegible] [illegible] [illegible]. [illegible] of [illegible] on a global [illegible] [illegible]. [illegible] [illegible] [illegible].

[illegible], R., [illegible], [illegible] A. and [illegible], [illegible]. [illegible] [illegible] formation and [illegible] [illegible] [illegible] [illegible] [illegible]. [illegible] [illegible].

[illegible]

[illegible], [illegible], [illegible], [illegible], [illegible] [illegible] [illegible]. [illegible] [illegible] [illegible] [illegible] [illegible].

[illegible], P., [illegible], [illegible], [illegible]. [illegible] taxonomy, a [illegible] approach [illegible]. [illegible] Microbiology Reviews 60(2):407–38.

Wyplo[illegible], [illegible], [illegible], S., [illegible] [illegible] 2012. [illegible] [illegible] [illegible] [illegible] [illegible] [illegible] [illegible].

Yang, [illegible], [illegible] M. [illegible]. [illegible] [illegible] [illegible] and [illegible] of [illegible] [illegible] [illegible] [illegible] 1–11.

Zhang, A., Sun, H., Wang, P., Han, Y. and Wang, X. 2012. Modern analytical techniques in metabolomics analysis. Analyst 137(2):293–300.

Zhang, N., [illegible], [illegible], [illegible], [illegible] and [illegible] 2016. [illegible] [illegible] [illegible] [illegible] of the [illegible] [illegible] and [illegible] [illegible]. [illegible] 13(1):12–20.

2 Traditional Nutritional Approaches and Nutriomics Evidence

Nutrition from Inception to Evidence

*Parveen Bansal, Renu Bansal, and Malika Arora**

CONTENTS

2.1 INTRODUCTION

Food is a physical necessity for leading a healthy lifestyle and has unquestionable cultural and ethical value (Corvo 2016). The selection of foods and the way we choose food generally depict who we are and the values we represent. Moreover,

* Corresponding author email: maliksmonu@gmail.com

DOI: 10.1201/9781003142195-2

the selection of food is the source of inspiration and motivation that fulfills one's body and confirms one's deepest identity. In today's scenario, the food industry is going through an interesting time that has inculcated multiple intersecting trends to work upon how and what to eat. There is no denying that health-and-wellness-oriented eating is becoming a big trend in the food space. The traditional therapies are stepping into deep research to explore their own foundational theories and their connection with modern science. In the current scenario, modern biology is partnered with technology that further involves a better understanding of the genome for predicting its roles in the human body. The omics era of research has provided significant information regarding the genetic and biochemical variability of individuals (Sumantran and Tillu 2013). The main objective of research in nutrigenomics is to explore the influence of nutrients on gene and protein expression. It is also conducted to know why this expression varies between individuals. It is well-known that even though individuals were to eat similarly, a few will still develop obesity and others will express cardiovascular diseases, diabetes, allergies, and so on (Jenzer and Sadeghi-Reeves 2020). Diet and the genome may influence various aspects of health through a variety of intertwined/interconnected intermediate perturbations that can be measured through omics technologies, including RNA expression (transcriptome), epigenetic modifications (epigenome), metabolites (metabolome), lipids (lipidome), proteins (proteome), and resident microbial communities (microbiome) (Yang 2016). The present-day nutrition, lifestyle, and the environment are drastically changed from ancient times. Traditional foods are being used since ancient times, and the preparation of these foods varies across the world. Multiple traditional techniques have been developed over generations of time regarding the processing and preservation of food and its therapeutic value (Hotz and Gibson 2007). It has been demonstrated that traditional foods are also known as functional foods due to the fact that foods consist of various functional components that deliver numerous biological functions. These functional molecules involve various components, such as body-building materials, antioxidants, healing components, dietary fibers, and probiotics (Hotz and Gibson 2007). Moreover, the functional and therapeutic qualities of these functional foods are further enhanced by various techniques, such as sprouting, malting, and fermentation (Sarkar et al. 2015). It has been observed that the human body and its constitution change over time, and hence, eating habits also change for the sustainability of normal physiological functions. Traditional ancestors' wisdom has claimed different foods for different stages of life that are found to be nutritionally rich. In addition, it also has been observed that every community has a spate and clear belief system regarding the selection of food items, and most of the food beliefs are influenced by Aryan beliefs and practices. According to Aryan belief, food is considered a source of strength and a gift from God (Achaya 1994). Ayurveda is the traditional Indian medicine system that clearly depicts that the regulation of diet is crucial and important to establish the connection between elements of life, food, and body. According to Ayurvedic concepts, food maintains the overall health by maintaining physical, temperamental, and mental states (Ravishankar and Shukla 2007). A similar pattern has been observed in Ayurvedic dietetics and traditional foods. These days it has been observed that globalization and tremendously increasing nutritional research have made the citizens much more conscious with respect to food selections. Although people are following the advice of dieticians, the strategies followed in ancient times are returning due to growing scientific evidence. The growing nutriomic evidence around the globe will benefit the wealth of knowledge that has already been documented years and years ago. Evolution, globalization, and internationalization of nutritional habits make genetic impacts slowly disappear by genetic recombination and/or by adaption. Epidemiologic assessments are more and more difficult to interpret since, at least in Western countries, mixed populations lead to the recombination of genetic codes (Jenzer and Sadeghi-Reeves 2020). This chapter highlights various nutriomic-based facts related to the traditional Indian foods that have been used since ancient times.

2.2 TRADITIONAL FOODS

The foods that are being used through generations and passed to the next generations due to their historical precedent are known as traditional foods (Sen 2004). Traditional foods and dishes are traditional in nature, and in Indian cuisine, a variety of regional and traditional foods are available. Most of the traditional foods/cuisines, such as spices, herbs, vegetables, and fruits, are locally available, but these are being used differently per their regional uses. Dating back to Vedic times, the Vedas (an important class of religious texts) holds significant importance in describing various grains and millets being used in day-to-day life along with their importance in our daily life (Burrow and Emeneau 1984; Dubey 2010). Moreover, per the ancient literature, foods have been classified into various classes, as shown in Figure 2.1.

Traditional foods are further classified according to their nature:

- Grain-based traditional foods
- Fruit- and vegetable-based traditional foods
- Milk-based traditional foods
- Miscellaneous food items

2.2.1 Grain-Based Traditional Foods

Grains are considered to be the primary staple food in India and other countries. Grains are nutritionally rich and deliver various nutrients and advantages to the body. In different civilizations, various grains are being consumed, particularly grains derived from starchy sources and protein-rich grains with good calorific value. The four Vedas, namely Rigveda, Samaveda, Yajurveda, and Atharvaveda, describe different cereal grains and their use in our daily life (Egounlety and Aworh 2003; Nikgudkar 2014). Some of the traditional grain-based fermented and complementing health foods with their functional and health benefits are discussed below.

2.2.1.1 *Khichdi*

Khichdi is an ancient food product that has been used for many generations. It is the oldest food that is prepared by the combination of rice and lentils or dal, and it is

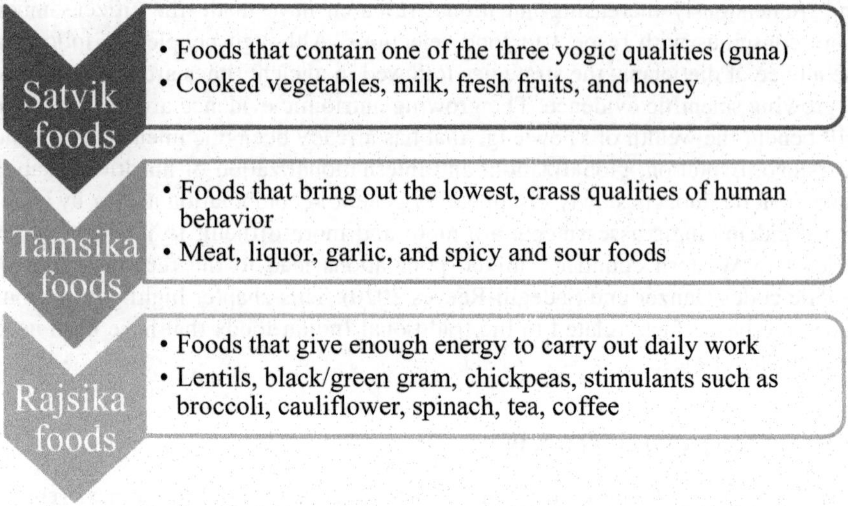

Satvik foods
- Foods that contain one of the three yogic qualities (guna)
- Cooked vegetables, milk, fresh fruits, and honey

Tamsika foods
- Foods that bring out the lowest, crass qualities of human behavior
- Meat, liquor, garlic, and spicy and sour foods

Rajsika foods
- Foods that give enough energy to carry out daily work
- Lentils, black/green gram, chickpeas, stimulants such as broccoli, cauliflower, spinach, tea, coffee

FIGURE 2.1 Classification of a variety of foods per ancient literature.

supposed to be highly nutritious (Chhabra and Kaur 2021). Per the belief system of Aryans, it was supposed that lentils and rice are going to make a healthy combination due to the complementation of nutritional elements. According to nutritional research, it has been revealed that *khichdi* is a great example of protein complementation that ensures the availability of all the amino acids by combining two or more protein sources instead of consuming one of them at a time. *Khichdi* is being used as a staple food for more than 1,000 years since the Aryan times, whereas amino acid discovery and amino acid complementation were established in 19th century and in 20th century, respectively.

2.2.1.2 *Idli, Dosa,* and *Sambhar*

Idli is a well-known fermented food that is prepared by mixing rice and black gram (Agrawal et al. 2002). A ratio of 1:2 of black gram and rice is used for batter preparation, followed by the fermentation of the mixture. It has been observed that a mixed microflora is needed for the fermentation that is being produced by the combination of rice and dal. Moreover, black gram is the source of natural microflora due to its primary ingredient. *Phaseolus mungo* L. acts as the substrate for fermentation of the mixture of rice and black gram. Fermentation of the mixture of dal and rice together improves the nutritional value and amino acid efficiency (Reddy et al. 1982). In addition to the fermentation, leavening is another important process in *idli* formation, which involves major microorganisms (Radhakrishnamurty et al. 1961), such as the heterofermentative lactic acid bacterium *Lactobacillus mesenteroides*. However, the homofermentative lactic acid bacterium *Streptococcus faecalis* plays a significant role in acidity regulation. Microorganisms such as *Lactobacillus plantarum* and *Lactobacillus lactis* are available in the batter, which can produce vitamin B12 and β-galactosidase enzyme, which enhances the probiotic activity and promotes health (Mukherjee et al. 1965). Since *idli* is a fermented steamed food, it is considered to be easily digestible and can be used in any season. In addition, it is a good source of healthy/friendly bacteria and a good quantity of protein, and it is recommended for all age groups (Iyer et al. 2013; Sarkar et al. 2015).

Dosa is another common fermented food similar to *idli*. On a similar line to *idli*, *dosa* is also prepared from similar ingredients – rice and the black gram as primary ingredients (Palanisamy et al. 2012). To improve the nutritional efficiency of *dosa*, other millets/grains are being used these days in the preparation of the *dosa* batter. It has been indicated that after fermentation, the volume of *dosa* batter doubles, and as the time of fermentation increases, the protein content is also increased in it (Soni et al. 1985). In different areas, the ingredient used for the preparation of *dosa* is variable as in some of the places parboiled rice is used, whereas in other places grinding boiled red rice with aniseed and palm jaggery are used. The preparation of the *dosa* batter is similar to *idli*, yet the cooking protocol of both dishes varies significantly (Sarkar et al. 2015). *Dosa* is a type of pancake that is cooked with a variety of seasonings and spices in the *dosa* pan and can be served with a variety of stuffing in it (Roy et al. 2007). It has been documented that the dish is nutritionally dense due to the availability of healthy/friendly bacteria and due to the presence of good quality and quantity of proteins. It is a digestible dish and hence recommended for all age groups. Its multiple nutritional benefits have been observed in lactating mothers as it is helpful in the purification of lactating women's blood (Hegde et al. 2013). *Sambhar* is a very popular South Indian dish/curry that is commonly used with the abovementioned dishes and with boiled rice. The version of *sambhar* varies from region to region, yet the preparation of *sambhar* involves coriander seeds, fenugreek seeds, turmeric rhizomes, black pepper, curry leaves, cumin seeds, and asafoetida, in combination with *toor dal*. *Sambhar* is being used with *idli, dosa*, and rice for many generations, yet its health benefits are unfolded only later due to development in nutritional research. It has been observed that in most of the areas, *sambhar* is a combination of *toor dal*, a mixture of vegetables, and a variety of spices. Hence, it is considered to be healthy as it adds lots of fiber to the diet and is helpful in the colon, cleansing and detoxifying it. In addition, the anticancer potential of *sambhar* against colon cancer also has been observed (Prasad et al. 2016). In these preparations also, the basic point is the complementation of amino acids from dal and rice to give good-quality protein, and fermentation gives friendly bacterial strains to the gut.

2.2.1.3 *Saag* and *Makki Ki Roti*

Sarson ka saag and *makki ki roti* are famous foods of India specifically used in the state of Punjab. *Sarson ka saag* is a coarse puree of mustard leaves, spinach, and chenopodium (optional) that is further fried using a variety of oils, chopped onion, tomatoes, garlic, ginger, and spices. This puree is usually eaten with a famous Indian bread made up of corn flour. The combination is known to be scientific and medically correct because *sarson* is abundant in winter, and its pungency, enhanced with spices, ginger, and garlic, is a perfect combination of thermogenic foods, that is, foods that increase body warmth. *Sarson* is a common green leafy vegetable that is packed with vitamins and minerals. It is a good source of fiber and, when sautéed with mustard oil or ghee, becomes much healthier as ghee enhances its calorific value, which further acts as a great winter warmer. In addition, *makki ki roti* is a source of complex carbohydrates that can provide sustainable energy throughout the day in sluggish and cold winters. The body uses the energy as fuel as these whole grains are rich sources of various vitamins and minerals, such as vitamins A, C, and K, beta-carotene, and so on. The combination is helpful in dealing with skin, hair, heart, brain, and digestion issues (Anushree Gupta 2020). In addition, it is a good alternative for gluten-sensitive individuals and is helpful in providing antioxidants and essential micronutrients, primarily iron. In these preparations also, the basic point is the complementation of amino acids from *dal* and rice to give good-quality protein. The flour from *makki* has more thermogenic value and hence is preferred in cold climates and winter season (Amit 2014).

2.2.1.4 *Dhokla*

Dhokla is a probiotic-based breakfast commonly used in the state of Gujarat and those from this state all over the world. This preparation is not limited to Gujarat only; rather, it is widely used all over the country due to its lower fat content and good protein value. It is prepared from the fermentation of *chana dal* or a mixture of rice and Bengal gram. Sometimes a mixture of *chana dal* is mixed with semolina for its preparation. The process is fermentation, almost similar to *idli*, but it is prepared in steam in an open dish (Steinkraus 1995). Fermentation of *dhokla* adds lactic acid bacteria to the mixture that regulates the acidity of the mixture and enhances the flavor of the dish (Kanekar and Joshi 1993; Evans et al. 2002). Most of the time, yeast is also used for the fermentation and to add a spongy texture to the food and increase the batter volume by increasing the aeration capacity. In addition, the antioxidant potential of fermented batter is much more than the unfermented mixture. Intake of fatty acids helps cure age-related issues and manage oxidative-stress-induced diseases (Moktan et al. 2011). Hence *dhokla* is considered a good food item for diabetic patients.

2.2.2 Fruit- and Vegetable-Based Traditional Foods

In early Indian culture, people used to eat natural and easily available food from nature. Fruits are considered to be a good source of flavonoids, minerals, vitamins, carotenoids, electrolytes, and other bioactive compounds that provide beneficial health effects to the human body. Some of the traditional fruits and vegetables and their health impact are discussed below in Table 2.1.

2.2.3 Kitchen Spices and Herbs

Per the general routine of humans, everyone has been ingesting a cocktail of thousands of phytochemicals in the form of spices and other food additives for a long

TABLE 2.1
Traditional Fruits/Vegetables along with Their Nutriomic Evidence, Reported as Active Ingredients and Health Benefits*

Fruit/ Vegetable source	Compounds reported for benefits	Health benefits in various diseases
Grapes	Resveratrol	Diabetes mellitus, cardiovascular disease, metabolic syndrome, obesity, inflammatory, neurodegenerative, and age-related diseases
Citrus fruits	Limonene	Anti-inflammatory, antioxidant, antinociceptive, anticancer, antidiabetic, antihyperalgesic, antiviral, and gastroprotective effects
Pineapple	Bromelain	Angina pectoris, bronchitis, sinusitis, surgical trauma, and thrombophlebitis, and debridement of wounds
Mango	Lupeol	Antioxidant, anti-inflammatory, anti-hyperglycemic, anti-dyslipidemic, and anti-mutagenic
Pomegranate	Anthocyanin/ delphinidin	Coronary heart disease, cerebrovascular disease, peripheral artery disease, rheumatic heart disease, congenital heart disease, deep vein thrombosis, and pulmonary embolism
Almond	Morin	Diabetes, arthritis, heart disease, stroke, cancer, and chronic respiratory problems
Guava	Gallic acid	Gastrointestinal diseases, metabolic diseases, miscellaneous diseases, neuropsychological diseases, radiation-induced toxicity, and urogenital issues
Black raspberries	Cynidin glycosides	Natural antioxidant
Mulberry	Sanggenon- C	Antioxidant, anti-inflammatory, and antitumor
Banana	Gallic acid, catechin, epicatechin, tannins	Antioxidant, diabetic, gastric problems, and anemia
Jackfruit	Carotenoids, phenolic compounds	Antioxidant, anticarcinogenic, antimicrobial, antifungal, anti-inflammatory, wound healing, and hypoglycemic effects
Papaya	Glucosinolates	Anticancer, anti-inflammatory, immunomodulatory, antibacterial, and antiviral
Saag	Iron	Antioxidant, hypertension, and heart problems
Cruciferous vegetables	Brassinin, isothicyanates, sulphoraphane	Anticancer and also treats other neural disorders
Karela	Momorcharaside B	Antidiabetic
Garlic	Ajoein, allicin, Alliumin, Allixin	Antibacterial activity and helps in cardiovascular disease
Onion	Organo-sulfur compounds	Osteoporosis; prevents sore throat, fever, dropsy, catarrh, and chronic bronchitis; reduces the risk of head and neck cancers

(Continued)

TABLE 2.1 (CONTINUED)
Traditional Fruits/Vegetables along with Their Nutriomic Evidence, Reported as Active Ingredients and Health Benefits*

Fruit/ Vegetable source	Compounds reported for benefits	Health benefits in various diseases
Artichoke	Silymarin, silibinin	Anti-hepatocellular carcinoma
Lettuce	Apigenin	Antiallergic, antidermatitic, antiestrogenic, antiherpetic, antihistaminic, anti-inflammatory, antimutagenic, and anticancer
Soyabean	Genistein	Cancer chemopreventive agent, phytoestrogen, and helps in cardiovascular disease
Tomato	Lycopene, lutein	Helps in Alzheimer's disease and cardiovascular disease
Carrots	Beta-carotenes	Antidiabetic, lowers cholesterol and helps in cardiovascular disease, antihypertensive, hepatoprotective, renoprotective, and wound healing
Aloe vera	Acemannan, emodin	Skin injuries (burns, cuts, insect bites, and eczemas) and digestive problems because of its anti-inflammatory and antimicrobial properties, and wound healing

* Arab and Steck 2000; Duke Ja 2000; Dixon and Ferreira 2002; Acquaviva et al. 2003; Mohapatra et al. 2010; Wallace 2011; Pavan et al. 2012; Pereira et al. 2013; Min and Min 2014; Prati et al. 2014; Sinha et al. 2016; Tsai et al. 2016; Koushki et al. 2018; Vieira et al. 2018; Wang et al. 2018; Kahkeshani et al. 2019; Ranasinghe et al. 2019; Sánchez et al. 2020; Singh et al. 2020.

time. However, most of the population is unaware of their biochemical, physiological, and pharmacological therapeutic effects. Per literature, chemoprevention by the use of naturally occurring dietary substances has been reported as a practical approach to reducing the ever-increasing incidence of a variety of cancers. Various examples of nutriomic evidence showing cell cycle arrest/apoptosis at various stages due to kitchen spice phytochemicals and herbs having anticancer potential are compiled in Table 2.2.

2.2.4 Milk-Based Health Foods

The animals were an integral part of Vedic culture. Since ancient times, milk from cows, buffalo, and goats is being used either in raw form or after boiling (Sarkar et al. 2015). Ayurvedic literature has described various benefits and distinct qualities of various milks, such as cow milk and human milk. Most commonly used food products include curd, *lassi,* ghee, butter, and cheese, which have been used for so many years. Although milk and milk products have been used for many years, with time various discoveries, such as the presence of colostrum and the availability and role of probiotics in milk, have been described the milk products in a better way. Per Ayurvedic literature, milk is a unique food that can provide various nutritional health benefits. Some of the common milk-based health products are as follows.

TABLE 2.2
Nutriomic Evidence Showing Cell Cycle Arrest/Apoptosis at Various Stages due to Kitchen Spice Phytochemicals and Herbs Having Anticancer Potential*

Name of spices/Herbs	Active component	Changes in cell cycle arrest/Apoptosis
Kitchen herbs/spices used in various homemade drinks		
Mulethi (*Glycerrhiza glabra*)	Glycyrrhetic acid, glycyrrhetinic acid, glycyrrhizin	Inhibits the proliferation, cytotoxic, release of cytochrome C from mitochondria, activation of caspases, mitochondrial membrane potential, inhibit NF-kB activation pathway
Tulasi (*Ocimum sanctum*)	Orientin, vicenin	DNA fragmentation, shrunken cytoplasm
Black tea (*Camelia sinensis*)	Theaflavins	Inhibits matrix metalloproteinases, inhibits NF-kB activation pathway
Green tea (*Camelia sinensis*)	Epigallocatechin gallate	Activates TRAIL-induced apoptosis, activation of Fas, inhibition of Bcl2, mitochondrial membrane potential
Coffee (*Theobroma cacao*)	Caffeine	Changes in p53, inhibits NF-kB activation pathway
Fennel (*Foeniculum vulgare*)	Anethol	Inhibits NF-kB activation pathway
Clove (*Syzigium aromaticum*)	Eugenol	Activation of caspases-3, downregulation of Bcl-2
Cardamom (*Elettarria cardamomum*)	Limonene	Inhibits NF-kB activation pathway
Cinnamon	Polyphenols	G2M cell cycle arrest
Honey (*Apis mellifera*)	Caffeic acid	Activation of caspases and Fas, induction of p53
Kitchen spice phytochemicals used in various homemade drinks		
—	Luteolin, fertinin, ferutidin	Sensitizes TRAIL-induced apoptosis, inhibit cell proliferation at level of DNA synthesis (S- phase)
—	Curcumin	Activation of caspases, TRAIL induction, release of cytochrome C from mitochondria, arrest G2M phase, downregulates expression of cyclin D1, upregulation of Cdk inhibitors
—	Capsaicin	Mitochondrial membrane potential, caspases- 3
—	Piperine	Inhibit NF-kB activation pathway
—	Gingerol, 6-shogaol	Mitochondrial membrane potential, release of cytochrome C from mitochondria, activation of caspases, increase in Bax

(Continued)

TABLE 2.2 (CONTINUED)
Nutriomic Evidence Showing Cell Cycle Arrest/Apoptosis at Various Stages due to Kitchen Spice Phytochemicals and Herbs Having Anticancer Potential*

Name of spices/Herbs	Active component	Changes in cell cycle arrest/Apoptosis
—	Linalool	Inhibit NF-kB activation pathway
—	Garcinol	Release of cytochrome C from mitochondria, activation of caspases
—	Secoiridoid, tyrosol	Inhibit cell proliferation
—	Proanthocyanidins	Release of cytochrome C from mitochondria, activation of caspases, Induction of Apaf-1, change in Bax/Bcl2 ratio

* Ahmad et al. 1997; Huang et al. 1997; Cao and Cao 1999; Lou et al. 1999; Ye et al. 1999; Chainy et al. 2000; Yang et al. 2001; Pan et al. 2001; Choudhuri et al. 2002; Fabiani et al. 2002; Lu et al. 2002; Park et al. 2002; Brusselmans et al. 2003; Mittal et al. 2003; Miyoshi et al. 2003; Roy et al. 2003; Watabe et al. 2004; Babich et al. 2005; Bhattacharyya et al. 2005; Devrajan et al. 2005; Gao et al. 2005; Hastak et al. 2005; Horinaka et al. 2005; Kundu et al. 2005; Nayak and Devi 2005; Oh et al. 2005; Poli et al. 2005; Qanungo et al. 2005; Schoene et al. 2005; Shi et al. 2005; Banerjee et al. 2006; Fabiani et al. 2006; Hong et al. 2006; Juan et al. 2006; Mantena et al. 2006; Mori et al. 2006; Nishikawa et al. 2006; Sanchez et al. 2006; Sartippour et al. 2006; Selvendiran et al. 2006; Siddiqui et al. 2006; Stuart et al. 2006; Bisht et al. 2007; Chen et al. 2007; Kim et al. 2007; Ko et al. 2007; Kunnumakkara et al. 2007; Lee et al. 2007; Lu et al. 2007; Nonn et al. 2007; Shankar and Srivastava 2007; Weir et al. 2007; Bansal et al. 2012.

2.2.4.1 *Dahi*

Dahi is the oldest traditional fermented milk product manufactured using boiled cow or buffalo milk and soured using mixed lactic cultures (Agarwal and Bhasin 2002; Sarkar et al. 2015). *Dahi* is used in daily life and is considered a potential source of vitamin B complex, folic acid, riboflavin, and so on. The dish is a rich source of friendly microbiota, which are beneficial for the maintenance of gut health, controlling diarrhea, treating irritable bowel syndrome, and so on. Moreover, bioactive compounds produced by various probiotic bacteria, such as diacetyl, hydrogen peroxide, and reuterin, suppress the normal growth of undesirable flora, especially *E. coli, Bacillus subtilis*, and *Staphylococcus aureus* (Sharma and Lal 1997; Sarkar and Misra 2001).

2.2.4.2 *Lassi*

Lassi is a traditional milk beverage that is also known as a probiotic drink due to the presence of *L. acidophilus* and *S. thermophiles* as active cultures. The drink is used in the summer season as it provides refreshment (Patidar and Prajapati 1998). For the preparation of *lassi, dahi* is blended with water, sugar, salt, and spices, such as cumin seeds and coriander leaves. The presence of spices decreases thirst and helps in relieving digestive problems, skin-related problems, fever, and sunstroke (Backes 2014).

2.2.4.3 *Sandesh*

Sandesh is a milk product that is rich in protein prepared by heating milk and using acid coagulation techniques. After coagulation, the final ingredient of the recipe is called *chenna*. *Chhena* is kneaded and mixed with sugar, followed by cooking over low flame and cooled (Aneja et al. 2002). Studies are being conducted to improve the nutritional value of traditional *sandesh* by incorporating herbs that add to the antioxidant value of the product (Bandyopadhyay et al. 2007). This dish has a unique aroma and is found to be a rich source of vitamins A and D.

2.3 FERMENTED FOODS AND PROBIOTICS

Earlier, food was considered to satisfy hunger and provide necessary nutrients, but nowadays, per modern nutritional concepts, consumers are inclined to consume foods that decrease the development and consequences of diseases and improve the quality of life instead of consuming food for the taste (Menrad 2003; Kaushik and Kaushik 2010). Today, novel food products, which particularly include various foods or phytochemical compounds from edible plants and live microorganisms, are coming into the picture to put a stop to nutrition-based diseases and to enhance the physical and mental well-being of people. These types of food items are considered functional foods and were introduced first in Japan in the early 1980s. Rapidly increasing acceptance and demand of these healthier functional foods and dietary supplements has aggravated the commercialization of these products on a large scale since the last decade. It is pertinent to mention that the concept of functional foods has been originated in the 21st century, yet their nutritional claims were claimed years ago. In recent years, scientific evidence is being originated for various traditional foods, such as *lassi*, *dahi*, and *sandesh*. Sharma et al. 2016 have demonstrated the presence of two potential bacterial isolates, *Pediococcus acidilactici* and *Lactobacillus casei* KL14, isolated from traditional fermented dairy products (Sharma et al. 2016). It has been observed that these potential probiotic strains are exhibiting different desirable traits (e.g., low pH tolerance, bile tolerance, autoaggregation, co-aggregation with pathogenic bacteria, cell surface hydrophobicity against O-xylene, antimicrobial activity against challenging foodborne pathogens, and antibiotic sensitivity). Even in the present scenario, the need to maintain higher immunity and health status has been recommended due to the emergence of the COVID-19 pandemic (Kumar et al. 2021). Emphasis has also been made to use natural/traditional/functional foods to enhance the immunity of human beings. A report by WHO (2020) highlighted that the virus is stable at 4°C and might remain active for about two years at –20°C (World Health Organization, "COVID-19 and food safety: guidance for food businesses: interim guidance", 2020). On the other hand, the activity of the virus has been reported to decrease as the pH of the system was reduced, and complete inactivation was observed at pH <3 (Darnell et al. 2004). Due to the availability of various nutritional research approaches, it has been indicated that among the different food products, fermented dairy products are relatively less susceptible to act as coronavirus carriers because of their lower pH. The present research highlights their use on the basis of their scientifically supported health/nutritional benefits.

Fermented products have long been consumed since time immemorial for improving well-being, and it has been observed that their benefits are further enhanced by the addition of different functional ingredients or by supplementing with probiotics. In addition, it also has been observed that probiotic-based foods are reported to possess activity against various viral infections (Galanakis et al. 2020). Moreover, it also has been reported that *Lactobacillus gasseri* SBT2055 (LG2055) is involved in reducing viral respiratory infection by increasing the expression of IFN-β and IFN-γ genes (Wink 2020). Probiotic-based dairy products are also reported to possess a number of health benefits: they have antimicrobial, antimutagenic, anticarcinogenic, and antihypertensive attributes (Roobab et al. 2020). Probiotic food products hold a new position in the human dietary portfolio. The market for various probiotic foods that are supposed to promote health further instead of just providing basic nourishment is thriving at a rapid pace. In the early 1900s, live microbial ingredients were made, with a positive effect on human health. This concept has grabbed the major focus of scientists only due to their promising health benefits. In addition to it, their applications offer an innovative move toward the advancement of probiotic-based products. Due to outweighed health benefits of probiotics and rapidly increasing market value, novel probiotic-based products are constantly being reported. Major health benefits offered by probiotic microorganisms are listed in Table 2.3.

TABLE 2.3
Health Benefits of Probiotics

Reported facts in various ailments	References
Use of probiotics in clinical improvement of atopic dermatitis	Climent et al. 2021
Use of probiotics in reducing the number of mutants of streptococci in saliva, periodontal inflammation, oral candida, and halitosis	Karbalaei et al. 2021
Use of probiotic bacteria in weight reduction and obesity control due to their short-chain fatty-acid production and low-grade inflammation	Mullish et al. 2021
Production of lactic acid by probiotic bacteria that increase gut pH and improve calcium absorption	Arnold et al. 2021
Immunomodulatory effect and a significant role in fighting SARS-CoV-2 infection	Bottari et al. 2021; Santacroce et al. 2021
Delayed progression of human immunodeficiency virus type 1 (HIV-1) infection and improved growth in infants suffering from congenital AIDS	Geng et al. 2020
Immunomodulation by *L. acidophilus* is strain-specific, may stimulate other macrophages directly or indirectly	Ren et al. 2020; Engevik et al. 2021
Improved lipid profiles in hypercholesterolemic rats by *Lactobacillus rhamnosus* GG and *Aloe vera* gel in combination	Chiu et al. 2021; Liang et al. 2021
Significantly delayed glucose intolerance hyperglycemia, hyperinsulinemia, dyslipidemia, and oxidative stress observed after supplementing with a fermented probiotic product with *L. acidophilus* and *L. casei*	Liang et al. 2021

2.4 DIETARY MICROBIOTA AND GUT HEALTH

Every human being has a wide variety of bacteria, viruses, fungi, and other single-celled species, somewhere between 10–100 trillion microbial cells, in a symbiotic relationship. Usually, the gut microbiota of each individual is unique and maintains a symbiotic relationship for the benefit of humans, as it has been observed that these microbes are key contributors to various vital metabolic requirements and others. There is significant variability in individual microbiota composition, which is influenced particularly by external factors, such as diet (Sun et al. 2020). In healthy individuals, there is a balance between different classes of bacteria, including symbionts (health promoters), commensals (which promote no benefit or harm to the host), and pathogens (Martínez et al. 2015). According to Lagier et al. (2015), it has been observed that 2,172 species have been identified that reside in the human gut, which are further classified into 12 different phyla, including Proteobacteria, Firmicutes, Actinobacteria, and Bacteroidetes. In addition, it has been observed that a total of 93.5% belonged to these phyla. Moreover, it also has been observed that more than 300 species strictly belong to the anaerobic group and are found to be present in the oral cavity and gastrointestinal tract (Lagier et al. 2015). It has been observed that the small-intestinal microbial community is largely dominated by Lactobacillaceae, which includes a dense and diverse community of bacteria, mainly anaerobes with the ability to utilize complex carbohydrates that are undigested in the small intestine. Moreover, per today's scenario, these beneficial microbes (i.e., probiotics) are becoming a potential source of novel diagnostic and therapeutic modalities. Undeniably, it is due to the fact that the research in the field of microbiome and metagenomics is revolutionary. Moreover, the general role of microbes in different body parts and their role in disease generation are being targeted by various scientists to link them with potential diseases, risks, or even clear onsets of clinical symptoms. The gastrointestinal tract in humans provides a complex and dynamic environment for sheltering a variety of various microorganisms to reside in the gut or intestine. Recently, various scientists have focused on the role of permanent microbiota, specifically the probiotic species, as these hold an important role in health and disease (Green and Cellier 2007; Krishnareddy 2019). Although probiotic/friendly bacteria are involved in various diseases, yet a very good example of the role of probiotic microbiota has been explored in celiac disease (CD) (Caminero and Verdu 2019). CD is an autoimmune intestinal enteropathy activated by the ingestion of gluten and other associated prolamins in genetically susceptible individuals. Gliadin peptides have HLA-DQ2 (a major class II histocompatibility complex) specific amino-acid sequences, which make them resistant to gastrointestinal enzymes, and hence, they exert damaging effects in the gastrointestinal tract. Gliadins also have preferred glutamine residues for tissue transglutaminase (tTG)-mediated deamidation, which leads to activated immune responses to dietary products (Barker and Liu 2008). They bind to the CXCR3 receptor present in the intestinal epithelium of genetically predisposed individuals, and in response, zonulin release is triggered, which affects intestinal permeability. Genetic predisposition of CD is mainly associated with HLA, MYO9B, exogenous factor (gluten), proactive autoimmune genetic background, tissue damage, viral infections, early termination of breastfeeding, and gender. As reported in earlier studies, various infectious agents, such as adenovirus type 12, hepatitis C virus, *Campylobacter jejuni*, *Giardia lamblia*, rotavirus, and enterovirus, may also play a role in the development of CD, other than gluten. The timing of gluten ingestion and cessation of breastfeeding may also be involved in the pathogenesis of CD. In addition to genetic and environmental factors, a large number of studies have evidenced the role of various pathogenic/non-pathogenic bacterial species in disease generation and microbial modulation of gluten-induced immune responses (Cristofori et al. 2018). Bacterial species such as *Escherichia coli*, *Bacteroides fragilis*, and *Staphylococcus epidermidis* clones isolated from CD patients were observed to have increased pathogenic genes (Wacklin et al. 2014). Moreover, a number of in vitro and in vivo studies were performed to check the effect of CD-associated bacteria on gluten-induced immune responses. *E. coli*, *Shigella*, *Salmonella*, and so on enhanced gluten-induced pro-inflammatory immune responses and intestinal barrier dysfunction in epithelial and peripheral blood mononuclear cell (PBMC) cultures (D'Argenio et al. 2016; Giron Fernández-Crehuet et al. 2016; Quagliariello et al. 2016), whereas *Bifidobacterium/Lactobacillus* altered gluten-induced barrier dysfunction and modified immune responses in in vitro and in vivo (Guandalini and Assiri 2014; Sanz 2015; Quagliariello et al. 2016; Tian et al. 2017). These studies suggest that a variety of microbes are involved in the modulation of immune responses to gluten, as shown in Figure 2.2.

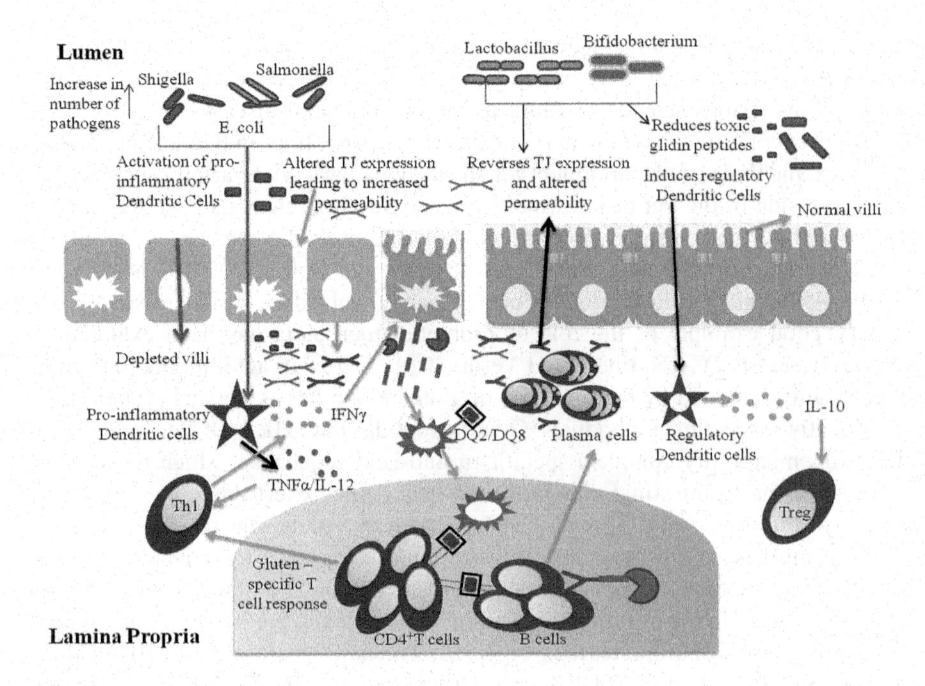

FIGURE 2.2 Pathogenic and protective role of microbiota in regulation of CD.

Pathogenic bacteria are reported to promote pro-inflammatory anti-gluten immune responses. Increased virulence has been observed due to the *E. coli* strains isolated from CD patients. *E. coli*, *Shigella,* and *Salmonella* can induce the maturation of dendritic cells (DCs), leading to the production of pro-inflammatory cytokines (IL-12 [interleukin 12], TNFα [tumor necrosis factor α]) after stimulation of gliadin in vitro. They can also increase intestinal permeability by altering intestinal tight junction (TJ) protein expression. On the other hand, probiotic bacteria such as *Bifidobacteria* and *Lactobacillus* may reverse these gluten-induced pathogenic responses. They can reverse the altered TJ expression and gluten-induced increased permeability leading to increased production of IL-10 from DCs in vitro.

2.5 PERSONALIZED MEDICINE AND NUTRIGENOMIC APPROACHES

The present era is the era of personalized medicines based on disease prevention and wellness individually on a person-to-person basis. Ayurveda has always emphasized individual and personalized medicine since its foundation thousands of years ago, considering a person's inherent individuality. On the contrary part, it has been observed that allopathy lacks the concept of recognizing pertaining to *prakriti* and inherent qualities of a person, such as *doshas, vata, pitta,* and *kapha*, ultimately neglecting the individual behavior, physiology, and predisposition to illnesses for each person (Coffin et al. 2019). Although the concept of personalized medicine is new to modern medicine, it is a well-established concept in Ayurveda, the traditional system of Indian medicine that is still being practiced. Personalized medicine aims to design specific drugs for individual patients or similar subtypes of patients that contraindicates the concept of "one drug fits all" approach (Chatterjee and Pancholi 2011). The Ayurvedic system has documented the concept of personalized medicine approach since 1500 B.C. for the management of health and disease. According to this system, every individual is born with his or her own basic constitution, termed *prakriti*, which to a great extent determines inter-individual variability in susceptibility to diseases and response to the external environment, diet, and drugs. Nutrigenomics has become a significant tool in designing predictive, preventive, and individual-based personalized medicines. The days are not too far in the future when there would be a paradigm shift in the practice of medicine from a generalized symptomatic approach to an individualized approach based on a person's genetic makeup. Scientists are consistently putting their efforts into unfolding the genetic variations that are responsible for susceptibility to diseases and differential response to drugs. The integration of Ayurveda and genomics have given birth to a new branch (i.e., ayurogenomics) that may be helpful to fill the gap between the genetic pattern and differential responses to disease generation and drug response. There are multiple studies that indicate that healthy individuals of contrasting *prakriti* types (i.e., *vata*, *pitta*, and *kapha*) identified on the basis of Ayurveda exhibit striking differences at the biochemical and genome-wide gene expression level. Therefore, a number of studies are available that particularly demonstrate the need to study gene expression differences and identify a genetic marker that is associated with specific diseases.

TABLE 2.4
Nutrigenomic Evidence Supporting Personalized Medicines*

Analysis and concept	Conclusion from present studies
Genome-wide SNP (single-nucleotide polymorphism) analysis (Affymetrix, 6.0) of 262 well-classified male individuals (after screening 3,416 subjects) belonging to three *prakritis* have been performed	*PGM1* correlates with the phenotype of *pitta* as described in the ancient text of *Caraka Samhita*, suggesting that the phenotypic classification of India's traditional medicine has a genetic basis, and its *prakriti*-based practice in vogue for many centuries resonates with personalized medicine.
Analysis of the role of *prakriti* variations on dysbiosis of the gut microbiome and concomitantly its effect on human health	*Prakriti* phenotyping can function as a potential stratifier of the gut microbiome in a given population and may provide evidence for the conceptual framework of personalized medicine in the Ayurvedic system of medicine.
Correlation of genotypes with *parkriti* have shown a wide range of utilities of *prakriti* assessment in therapeutics – that is, from the prediction of disease susceptibility of an individual, prevention of impending diseases, early diagnosis through screening of the high risk, rational drug designing, customization of therapy (drug, diet, and lifestyle), and health maintenance	Ayurvedic *prakriti*-based treatment resonates with PM and pharmacogenomics and holds potential and promise for future predictive or preventive medicine.
The yield of ROS and total cell damage were significantly higher in the diabetic *vata* ($p < 0.001$) group compared with other *prakriti*. Decreased DNA content and increased DNA damage were observed in T2D patients who belonged to *vata* ($p < 0.01$) *prakriti*. DNA of *vata prakriti* was more prone to lead and arsenic.	The diabetic *vata prakriti* is a genetically susceptible group as it has a tendency to get affected by increased DNA damage, which could help in creating personalized management of diabetes among individual *prakriti*.
Hyperbaric medicine is personalized as the parameters of hyperbaric oxygen application can be adjusted depending on the response to initial treatment. Other supporting measures, such as nutrition and physical exercise, can be personalized.	Ayurveda, a personalized healthcare system, has a holistic approach aimed to cure disease, but therapy is customized to the individual's constitution – an ancient counterpart of genotype. Acupuncture needs to be tailored to each patient's symptoms and responsiveness, and it is generally recognized that the individualization of acupuncture treatment enhances its effectiveness.

* Govindaraj et al. 2015; Jnana et al. 2020; Sharma and Prajapati 2020; Banerjee et al. 2021; Jain 2021.

The integration of these fields may generate gene expression differences and specific genetic markers for predictive and personalized medicine. Some of the studies focusing on personalized medicine are compiled in Table 2.4.

2.6 CONCLUSION

For ages, Ayurveda has been focused on regulating the body with the help of an appropriate diet as it has been considered that the etiology of all diseases is a collection of toxic (excretory) products in the body. Moreover, it also has been described in ancient literature that diet is an essential factor for the formation of our body, and irregular diets will lead to disease, as explained under the heading *Astaaharvidha vishesayatana*. In addition, an ancient Ayurvedic proverb (i.e., Lolimbaraja) describes that "when diet is wrong medicine is of no use and when diet is correct medicine is of no need". It has been observed that ancient literature has highlighted various aspects of life that are being used long ago yet introduced into the modern world with the latest supporting evidence. It is pertinent to mention that literature published years ago has been compiled by the enlightened people who support today's scientific facts and figures before their actions were investigated on scientific lines. Scientific minds are satisfied only after the rational justifications rather than believing empirical facts. The current interdisciplinary study of Ayurveda incorporating genetic, epigenetic, biochemical, and microbiome factors can help us discover novel paradigms that may lead us to healthy habits and personalized medicines. To date, there are many gray areas that need a substantial amount of work. Moreover, it is clear from the facts that a holistic approach is required to alleviate the diseases by the combination of modern scientific knowledge and traditional folk knowledge. Thus, the time has come to take stock of our previous literature, prospects, and further potential in this field to strengthen and revitalize health by the judicious use of food and medicines.

REFERENCES

Achaya, K. T. 1994. *Indian Food: A Historical Companion*. Oxford University Press; 2nd edition (July 30, 1998), Oxford.

Acquaviva, R., Russo, A., Galvano, F., et al. 2003. Cyanidin and cyanidin 3-O-β-D-glucoside as DNA cleavage protectors and antioxidants. *Cell Biology and Toxicology* 19(4):243–52.

Agarwal, K. N., and Bhasin, S. K. 2002. Feasibility studies to control acute diarrhoea in children by feeding fermented milk preparations Actimel and Indian Dahi. *European Journal of Clinical Nutrition* 56(4):S56–9.

Agrawal, R., Rati, E. R., Vijayendra, S. V. N., Varadaraj, M. C., Prasad, M. S., and Nand, K. 2000. Flavour profile of idli batter prepared from defined microbial starter cultures. *World Journal of Microbiology and Biotechnology* 16(7):687–90.

Ahmad, N., Feyes, D. K., Agarwal, R., Mukhtar, H., and Nieminen, A. L. 1997. Green tea constituent epigallocatechin-3-gallate and induction of apoptosis and cell cycle arrest in human carcinoma cells. *Journal of the National Cancer Institute* 89(24):1881–6.

Amit, D. 2014. Sarson ka saag. Available from: www.vegrecipesofindia.com/sarson-ka-saag/.

Aneja, R. P., Mathur, B. N., Chandan, R. C., and Banerjee, A. K. 2002. *Technology of Indian Milk Products: Handbook on Process Technology Modernization for Professionals, Entrepreneurs and Scientists*. Dairy India Yearbook, New Delhi.

Anushree Gupta. 2020. Makki Roti: What are the health benefits of the fibre-rich, winter-favourite flatbread? *News, Health News*. Available from: www.timesnownews.com/health/article/makki-roti-what-are-the-health-benefits-of-the-fibre-rich-winter-favourite-flatbread/690486

Arab, L., and Steck, S. 2000. Lycopene and cardiovascular disease. *American Journal of Clinical Nutrition* 71(6):1691S–5S.

Arnold, M., Rajagukguk, Y. V., and Gramza-Michałowska, A. 2021. Functional food for elderly high in antioxidant and chicken eggshell calcium to reduce the risk of osteoporosis – a narrative review. *Foods* 10(3):656.

Babich, H., Krupka, M. E., Nissim, H. A., and Zuckerbraun, H. L. 2005. Differential in vitro cytotoxicity of (–)-epicatechin gallate (ECG) to cancer and normal cells from the human oral cavity. *Toxicology in Vitro* 19(2):231–42.

Backes, M. 2014. *Cannabis Pharmacy: The Practical Guide to Medical Marijuana*. Hachette, Paris, France.

Bandyopadhyay, M., Chakraborty, R., and Raychaudhuri, U. 2007. Incorporation of herbs into Sandesh, an Indian sweet dairy product, as a source of natural antioxidants. *International Journal of Dairy Technology* 60(3):228–33.

Banerjee, S., Biswas, T. K., Chattopadhyay, K., Arzoo, S. H., and Chattopadhyay, B. 2021. An approach to screen genotoxic-susceptible diabetic population of various prakriti groups for personalized disease management. *Journal of Alternative and Complementary Medicine* 27(1):80–7.

Banerjee, S., Panda, C. K., and Das, S. 2006. Clove (*Syzygium aromaticum* L.), a potential chemopreventive agent for lung cancer. *Carcinogenesis* 27(8):1645–54.

Bansal, P., Bansal, R., and Sapra, R. 2012. Dietary phytochemicals in cell cycle arrest and apoptosis-an insight. *Journal of Drug Delivery and Therapeutics* 2(2).

Barker, J. M., and Liu, E. 2008. Celiac disease: Pathophysiology, clinical manifestations, and associated autoimmune conditions. *Advances in Pediatrics* 55(1):349–65.

Bhattacharyya, A., Lahiry, L., Mandal, D., Sa, G., and Das, T. 2005. Black tea induces tumor cell apoptosis by Bax translocation, loss in mitochondrial transmembrane potential, cytochrome c release and caspase activation. *International Journal of Cancer* 117(2):308–15.

Bisht, S., Feldmann, G., Soni, S., Ravi, R., Karikar, C., Maitra, A., and Maitra, A. 2007. Polymeric nanoparticle-encapsulated curcumin ("nanocurcumin"): A novel strategy for human cancer therapy. *Journal of Nanobiotechnology* 5(1):1–18.

Bottari, B., Castellone, V., and Neviani, E. 2021. Probiotics and covid-19. *International Journal of Food Sciences and Nutrition* 72(3):293–9.

Brusselmans, K., De Schrijver, E., Heyns, W., Verhoeven, G., and Swinnen, J. V. 2003. Epigallocatechin-3-gallate is a potent natural inhibitor of fatty acid synthase in intact cells and selectively induces apoptosis in prostate cancer cells. *International Journal of Cancer* 106(6):856–62.

Burrow, T., and Emeneau, M. B. 1984. *A Dravidian Etymological Dictionary*. 2nd ed., Clarendon Press, Oxford [Oxfordshire].

Caminero, A., and Verdu, E. F. 2019. Celiac disease: Should we care about microbes? *American Journal of Physiology-Gastrointestinal and Liver Physiology* 317(2):G161–70.

Cao, Y., and Cao, R. 1999. Angiogenesis inhibited by drinking tea. *Nature* 398(6726):381.

Chainy, G. B., Manna, S. K., Chaturvedi, M. M., and Aggarwal, B. B. 2000. Anethole blocks both early and late cellular responses transduced by tumor necrosis factor: Effect on NF-κB, AP-1, JNK, MAPKK and apoptosis. *Oncogene* 19(25):2943–50.

Chatterjee, B., and Pancholi, J. 2011. Prakriti-based medicine: A step towards personalized medicine. *AYU* 32(2):141.

Chen, C. Y., Liu, T. Z., Liu, Y. W., et al. 2007.6-shagaol (alkanone from ginger) induces apoptotic cell death of human Hepatoma p53 mutant Mahlavu subline via an oxidative stress mediated caspases dependent mechanism. *Journal of Agricultural and Food Chemistry* 55(3):948–54.

Chhabra, I., and Kaur, A. 2021. Development of a convenient, nutritious ready to cook packaged product using millets with a batch scale process development for a small-scale enterprise. *Journal of Food Science and Technology* 1–10.

Chiu, H. F., Fang, C. Y., Shen, Y. C., Venkatakrishnan, K., and Wang, C. K. 2021. Efficacy of probiotic milk formula on blood lipid and intestinal function in mild hypercholesterolemic volunteers: A placebo-control, randomized clinical trial. *Probiotics and Antimicrobial Proteins* 13(3):624–32.

Choudhuri, T., Pal, S., Agwarwal, M. L., Das, T., and Sa, G. 2002. Curcumin induces apoptosis in human breast cancer cells through p53-dependent Bax induction. *FEBS Letters* 512(1–3):334–40.

Climent, E., Martinez-Blanch, J. F., Llobregat, L., et al. 2021. Changes in gut microbiota correlates with response to treatment with probiotics in patients with atopic dermatitis. A post hoc analysis of a clinical trial. *Microorganisms* 9(4):854.

Coffin, J. D., Rao, R., and Lurie, D. I. 2019. Translational potential of Ayurveda Prakriti: Concepts in the area of personalized medicine. In: *Translational Ayurveda*, 21–32. Springer, Singapore.

Corvo, P. 2016. *Food Culture, Consumption and Society.* Springer, Berlin Germany.

Cristofori, F., Indrio, F., Miniello, V. L., De Angelis, M., and Francavilla, R. 2018. Probiotics in celiac disease. *Nutrients* 10(12):1824.

D'Argenio, V., Casaburi, G., Precone, V., et al. 2016. Metagenomics reveals dysbiosis and a potentially pathogenic, *N. flavescens* strain in duodenum of adult celiac patients. *American Journal of Gastroenterology* 111:879–90.

Darnell, M. E., Subbarao, K., Feinstone, S. M., and Taylor, D. R. 2004. Inactivation of the coronavirus that induces severe acute respiratory syndrome, SARS-CoV. *Journal of Virological Methods* 121(1):85–91.

Della Ragione, F., Cucciolla, V., Borriello, A., et al. 2000. Hydroxytyrosol, a natural molecule occurring in olive oil, induces cytochrome c-dependent apoptosis. *Biochemical and Biophysical Research Communications* 278(3):733–9.

Devrajan, K., Ramachandran, R., and Santosh, K. 2005. Involvement of Bax in the regulation of curcumin-induced apoptosis. *Indian Journal of Medical Research* 121:4–31.

Dixon, R. A., and Ferreira, D. 2002. Genistein. *Phytochemistry* 60(3):205–11.

Dubey, K. G. 2010. *The Indian Cuisine.* PHI Learning Pvt. Ltd, New Delhi.

Duke, J. A. 2000. Wild lettuce: A bitter herb of biblical proportions. *Journal of Medicinal Food* 3(3):153–4.

Egounlety, M., and Aworh, O. C. 2003. Effect of soaking, dehulling, cooking and fermentation with *Rhizopus oligosporus* on the oligosaccharides, trypsin inhibitor, phytic acid and tannins of soybean (*Glycine max* Merr.), cowpea (*Vigna unguiculata* L. Walp) and groundbean (*Macrotyloma geocarpa* Harms). *Journal of Food Engineering* 56(2–3):249–54.

Engevik, M. A., Ruan, W., Esparza, M., et al. 2021. Immunomodulation of dendritic cells by *Lactobacillus reuteri* surface components and metabolites. *Physiological Reports* 9(2):e14719.

Evans, J. L., Goldfine, I. D., Maddux, B. A., and Grodsky, G. M. 2002. Oxidative stress and stress-activated signaling pathways: A unifying hypothesis of type 2 diabetes. *Endocrine Reviews* 23(5):599–622.

Fabiani, R., Barteolomeo, A. D., Rosignoli, P., et al. 2002. Cancer chemoprevention by hydroxy tyrosol from virgin olive oil through G1 cell cycle arrest and apoptosis. *European Journal of Cancer Prevention* 11:351–8.

Fabiani, R., De Bartolomeo, A., Rosignoli, P., et al. 2006. Virgin olive oil phenols inhibit proliferation of human promyelocytic leukemia cells (HL60) by inducing apoptosis and differentiation. *Journal of Nutrition* 136(3):614–9.

Fernández-Crehuet, F. G., Tapia-Paniagua, S., Morinigo-Gutiérrez, M. A., et al. 2016. The duodenal microbiota composition in children with active coeliac disease is influenced by the degree of enteropathy. *Anales de Pediatría (English Edition)* 84(4):224–30.

Galanakis, C. M., Aldawoud, T., Rizou, M., Rowan, N. J., and Ibrahim, S. A. 2020. Food ingredients and active compounds against the coronavirus disease (COVID-19) pandemic: A comprehensive review. *Foods* 9(11):1701.

Gao, X., Deeb, D., Jiang, H., Liu, Y. B., Dulchavsky, S. A., and Gautam, S. C. 2005. Curcumin differentially sensitizes malignant glioma cells to TRAIL/Apo2L-mediated apoptosis through activation of procaspases and release of cytochrome c from mitochondria. *Journal of Experimental Therapeutics and Oncology* 5(1).

Geng, S. T., Zhang, Z. Y., Wang, Y. X., et al. 2020. Regulation of gut microbiota on immune reconstitution in patients with acquired immunodeficiency syndrome. *Frontiers in Microbiology* 11.

Govindaraj, P., Nizamuddin, S., Sharath, A., et al. 2015. Genome-wide analysis correlates Ayurveda Prakriti. *Scientific Reports* 5(1):1–12.

Green, P. H., and Cellier, C. 2007. Celiac disease. *New England Journal of Medicine* 357(17):1731–43.

Guandalini, S., and Assiri, A. 2014. Celiac disease: A review. *JAMA Pediatrics* 168(3):272–8.

Hastak, K., Agarwal, M. K., Mukhtar, H., and Agarwal, M. L. 2005. Ablation of either p21 or Bax prevents p53-dependent apoptosis induced by green tea polyphenol epigallocatechin-3-gallate. *FASEB Journal* 19(7):1–19.

Hegde, S., Yenagi, N. B., and Kasturiba, B. 2013. Indigenous knowledge of the traditional and qualified Ayurveda practitioners on the nutritional significance and use of red rice in medications.

Hong, J., Sang, S., Park, H. J., et al. 2006. Modulation of arachidonic acid metabolism and nitric oxide synthesis by garcinol and its derivatives. *Carcinogenesis* 27(2):278–86.

Horinaka, M., Yoshida, T., Shiraishi, T., et al. 2005. Luteolin induces apoptosis via death receptor 5 upregulation in human malignant tumor cells. *Oncogene* 24(48):7180–9.

Hotz, C., and Gibson, R. S. 2007. Traditional food-processing and preparation practices to enhance the bioavailability of micronutrients in plant-based diets. *Journal of Nutrition* 137(4):1097–100.

Huang, M. T., Xie, J. G., Wang, Z. Y., et al. 1997. Effects of tea, decaffeinated tea, and caffeine on UVB light-induced complete carcinogenesis in SKH-1 mice: Demonstration of caffeine as a biologically important constituent of tea. *Cancer Research* 57(13):2623–9.

Iyer, B. K., Singhal, R. S., and Ananthanarayan, L. 2013. Characterization and in vitro probiotic evaluation of lactic acid bacteria isolated from idli batter. *Journal of Food Science and Technology* 50(6):1114–21.

Jain, K. K. 2021. Personalized complementary and alternative therapies. In *Textbook of Personalized Medicine*, 203–12. Springer, Cham.

Jenzer, H., and Sadeghi-Reeves, L. 2020. Nutrigenomics-associated impacts of nutrients on genes and enzymes with special consideration of aromatase. *Frontiers in Nutrition* 7:37.

Jnana, A., Murali, T. S., Guruprasad, K. P., and Satyamoorthy, K. 2020. Prakriti phenotypes as a stratifier of gut microbiome: A new frontier in personalized medicine? *Journal of Ayurveda and Integrative Medicine* 11(3):360–5.

Juan, M. E., Wenzel, U., Ruiz-Gutierrez, V., Daniel, H., and Planas, J. M. 2006. Olive fruit extracts inhibit proliferation and induce apoptosis in HT-29 human colon cancer cells. *Journal of Nutrition* 136(10):2553–7.

Kahkeshani, N., Farzaei, F., Fotouhi, M., et al. 2019. Pharmacological effects of gallic acid in health and diseases: A mechanistic review. *Iranian Journal of Basic Medical Sciences* 22(3):225.

Kanekar, P., and Joshi, N. 1993. *Lactobacillus fermentum*, *Leuconostoc mesenteroides* and *Hansenula silvicola* contributing to acetoin and folic acid during dhokla' fermentation. *Indian Journal of Microbiology* 33(2):111–7.

Karbalaei, M., Keikha, M., Kobyliak, N. M., Khatibzadeh, Z., Yousefi, B., and Eslami, M. 2021. Alleviation of halitosis by use of probiotics and their protective mechanisms in the oral cavity. *New Microbes and New Infections* 100887.

Karthikeyan, K., Gunasekaran, P., Ramamurthy, N., and Govindasamy, S. 1999. Anticancer activity of *Ocimum sanctum. Pharmaceutical Biology* 37(4):285–290.

Kaushik, N., and Kaushik, D. 2010. Functional foods: Overview and global regulation. *International Journal of Pharm Recent Research* 2(2):47–52.

Khan, N., Afaq, F., Saleem, M., Ahmad, N., and Mukhtar, H. 2006. Targeting multiple signaling pathways by green tea polyphenol (–)-epigallocatechin-3-gallate. *Cancer Research* 66(5):2500–5.

Kim, J. K., Kim, Y., Na, K. M., Surh, Y. J., and Kim, T. Y. 2007. [6]-Gingerol prevents UVB-induced ROS production and COX-2 expression in vitro and in vivo. *Free Radical Research* 41(5):603–14.

Ko, S. Y., Chang, K. W., Lin, S. C., Hsu, H. C., and Liu, T. Y. 2007. The repressive effect of green tea ingredients on amyloid precursor protein (APP) expression in oral carcinoma cells in vitro and in vivo. *Cancer Letters* 245(1–2):81–9.

Koushki, M., Amiri-Dashatan, N., Ahmadi, N., Abbaszadeh, H. A., and Rezaei-Tavirani, M. 2018. Resveratrol: A miraculous natural compound for diseases treatment. *Food Science and Nutrition* 6(8):2473–90.

Krishnareddy, S. 2019. The microbiome in celiac disease. *Gastroenterology Clinics* 48(1):115–26.

Kumar, A., Hussain, S. A., Prasad, W., Singh, A. K., and Singh, R. R. B. 2021. Effect of oxygen tolerant probiotic strain, stabilizers and copper addition on the storage stability of *Aloe vera* supplemented synbiotic lassi. *Future Foods* 3:100021.

Kumar, D. S., Sharathnath, K. V., Yogeswaran, P., et al. 2010. A medicinal potency of *Momordica charantia. International Journal of Pharmaceutical Sciences Review and Research* 1(2):95–9.

Kundu, T., Dey, S., Roy, M., Siddiqi, M., and Bhattacharya, R. K. 2005. Induction of apoptosis in human leukemia cells by black tea and its polyphenol theaflavin. *Cancer Letters* 230(1):111–21.

Kunnumakkara, A. B., Guha, S., Krishnan, S., Diagaradjane, P., Gelovani, J., and Aggarwal, B. B. 2007. Curcumin potentiates antitumor activity of gemcitabine in an orthotopic model of pancreatic cancer through suppression of proliferation, angiogenesis, and inhibition of nuclear factor-κB – regulated gene products. *Cancer Research* 67(8):3853–61.

Lagier, J. C., Hugon, P., Khelaifia, S., Fournier, P. E., La Scola, B., and Raoult, D. 2015. The rebirth of culture in microbiology through the example of culturomics to study human gut microbiota. *Clinical Microbiology Reviews* 28(1):237–64.

Lee, C. S., Kim, Y. J., and Han, E. S. 2007. Glycyrrhizin protection against 3-morpholinosydnonime-induced mitochondrial dysfunction and cell death in lung epithelial cells. *Life Sciences* 80(19):1759–67.

Liang, T., Wu, L., Xi, Y., et al. 2021. Probiotics supplementation improves hyperglycemia, hypercholesterolemia, and hypertension in type 2 diabetes mellitus: An update of meta-analysis. *Critical Reviews in Food Science and Nutrition* 16(10):1670–88.

Lou, Y. R., Lu, Y. P., Xie, J. G., Huang, M. T., and Conney, A. H. 1999. Effects of oral administration of tea, decaffeinated tea, and caffeine on the formation and growth of tumors in high-risk SKH-1 mice previously treated with ultraviolet B light. *Nutrition and Cancer* 33(2):146–53.

Lu, Y. P., Lou, Y. R., Li, X. H., Xie, J. G., Lin, Y., Shih, W. J., and Conney, A. H. 2002. Stimulatory effect of topical application of caffeine on UVB-induced apoptosis in mouse skin. *Oncology Research Featuring Preclinical and Clinical Cancer Therapeutics* 13(2):61–70.

Lu, Y. P., Lou, Y. R., Xie, J. G., et al. 2007. Caffeine and caffeine sodium benzoate have a sunscreen effect, enhance UVB-induced apoptosis, and inhibit UVB-induced skin carcinogenesis in SKH-1 mice. *Carcinogenesis* 28(1):199–206.

Mantena, S. K., Baliga, M. S., and Katiyar, S. K. 2006. Grape seed proanthocyanidins induce apoptosis and inhibit metastasis of highly metastatic breast carcinoma cells. *Carcinogenesis* 27(8):1682–91.

Martínez, I., Stegen, J. C., Maldonado-Gómez, M. X., et al. 2015. The gut microbiota of rural Papua New Guineans: Composition, diversity patterns, and ecological processes. *Cell Reports* 11(4):527–38.

Menrad, K. 2003. Market and marketing of functional food in Europe. *Journal of Food Engineering* 56(2–3):181–8.

Min, J. Y., and Min, K. B. 2014. Serum lycopene, lutein and zeaxanthin, and the risk of Alzheimer's disease mortality in older adults. *Dementia and Geriatric Cognitive Disorders* 37(3–4):246–56.

Mittal, A., Elmets, C. A., and Katiyar, S. K. 2003. Dietary feeding of proanthocyanidins from grape seeds prevents photocarcinogenesis in SKH-1 hairless mice: Relationship to decreased fat and lipid peroxidation. *Carcinogenesis* 24(8):1379–88.

Miyoshi, N., Nakamura, Y., Ueda, Y., et al. 2003. Dietary ginger constituents, galanals A and B, are potent apoptosis inducers in Human T lymphoma Jurkat cells. *Cancer Letters* 199(2):113–9.

Mohapatra, D., Mishra, S., and Sutar, N. 2010. Banana and its by-product utilisation: An overview. *Journal of Scientific and Industrial Research* 69:323–9.

Moktan, B., Roy, A., and Sarkar, P. K. 2011. Antioxidant activities of cereal-legume mixed batters as influenced by process parameters during preparation of dhokla and idli, traditional steamed pancakes. *International Journal of Food Sciences and Nutrition* 62(4):360–9.

Mori, A., Lehmann, S., O'Kelly, J., et al. 2006. Capsaicin, a component of red peppers, inhibits the growth of androgen-independent, p53 mutant prostate cancer cells. *Cancer Research* 66(6):3222–9.

Mukherjee, S. K., Albury, M. N., Pederson, C. S., Van Veen, A. G., and Steinkraus, K. H. 1965. Role of *Leuconostoc mesenteroides* in leavening the batter of idli, a fermented food of India. *Applied Microbiology* 13(2):227–31.

Mullish, B. H., Marchesi, J. R., McDonald, J. A., et al. 2021. Probiotics reduce self-reported symptoms of upper respiratory tract infection in overweight and obese adults: Should we be considering probiotics during viral pandemics? *Gut Microbes* 13(1):1–9.

Nanda, D. K., Singh, R., Tomar, S. K., et al. 2013. Indian Chilika curd – A potential dairy product for Geographical Indication registration. *Indian Journal of Traditional Knowledge* 12(4):707–13.

Nayak, V., and Devi, P. U. 2005. Protection of mouse bone marrow against radiation-induced chromosome damage and stem cell death by the ocimum flavonoids orientin and vicenin. *Radiation Research* 163(2):165–71.

Nikgudkar, M. R. 2014. Estimation of resistant starch content of selected routinely consumed Indian food preparations. *Current Research in Nutrition and Food Science Journal* 2(2):73–83.

Nishikawa, T., Nakajima, T., Moriguchi, M., et al. 2006. A green tea polyphenol, epigalocatechin-3-gallate, induces apoptosis of human hepatocellular carcinoma, possibly through inhibition of Bcl-2 family proteins. *Journal of Hepatology* 44(6):1074–82.

Nonn, L., Duong, D., and Peehl, D. M. 2007. Chemopreventive anti-inflammatory activities of curcumin and other phytochemicals mediated by MAP kinase phosphatase-5 in prostate cells. *Carcinogenesis* 28(6):1188–96.

Oh, J. I., Chun, K. H., Joo, S. H., Oh, Y. T., and Lee, S. K. 2005. Chemopreventive properties of ethanol extracts of Chinese licorice root induction of apoptosis and G1 cell cycle arrest in MCF-7 human breast cancer cells. *Cancer Letters* 230(2):228–38.

Palanisamy, B. D., Rajendran, V., Sathyaseelan, S., Bhat, R., and Venkatesan, B. P. 2012. Enhancement of nutritional value of finger millet-based food (Indian dosa) by co-fermentation with horse gram flour. *International Journal of Food Sciences and Nutrition* 63(1):5–15.

Pan, M. H., Chang, W. L., Lin-Shiau, S. Y., Ho, C. T., and Lin, J. K. 2001. Induction of apoptosis by garcinol and curcumin through cytochrome c release and activation of caspases in human leukemia HL-60 cells. *Journal of Agricultural and Food Chemistry* 49(3):1464–74.

Pareek, S., Sagar, N. A., Sharma, S., and Kumar, V. 2017. Onion (*Allium cepa* L.). Fruit and vegetable phytochemicals: *Chemistry and Human Health* 2:1145–62.

Park, M. J., Kim, E. H., Park, I. C., et al. 2002. Curcumin inhibits cell cycle progression of immortalized human umbilical vein endothelial (ECV304) cells by up-regulating cyclin-dependent kinase inhibitor, p21WAF1/CIP1, p27KIP1 and p53. *International Journal of Oncology* 21(2):379–83.

Patidar, S. K., and Prajapati, J. B. 1998. Standardisation and evaluation of lassi prepared using *Lactobacillus acidophilus* and *Streptococcus thermophilus*. *Journal of Food Science and Technology (Mysore)* 35(5):428–31.

Pavan, R., Jain, S., and Kumar, A. 2012. Properties and therapeutic application of bromelain: A review. *Biotechnology Research International* 2012.

Pereira, C., Calhelha, R. C., Barros, L., and Ferreira, I. C. 2013. Antioxidant properties, anti-hepatocellular carcinoma activity and hepatotoxicity of artichoke, milk thistle and borututu. *Industrial Crops and Products* 49:61–5.

Poli, F., Appendino, G., Sacchetti, G., Ballero, M., Maggiano, N., and Ranelletti, F. O. 2005. Antiproliferative effects of daucane esters from *Ferula communis* and *F. arrigonii* on human colon cancer cell lines. *Phytotherapy Research* 19(2):152–7.

Prasad, V. G., Reddy, N., Francis, A., et al. 2016. Sambar, an Indian dish prevents the development of dimethyl hydrazine-induced colon cancer: A preclinical study. *Pharmacognosy Magazine* 12(Suppl. 4):S441.

Prati, P., Henrique, C. M., Souza, A. S. D., Silva, V. S. N. D., and Pacheco, M. T. B. 2014. Evaluation of allicin stability in processed garlic of different cultivars. *Food Science and Technology* 34:623–8.

Qanungo, S., Das, M., Haldar, S., and Basu, A. 2005. Epigallocatechin-3-gallate induces mitochondrial membrane depolarization and caspase-dependent apoptosis in pancreatic cancer cells. *Carcinogenesis* 26(5):958–67.

Quagliariello, A., Aloisio, I., Bozzi Cionci, N., et al. 2016. Effect of *Bifidobacterium breve* on the intestinal microbiota of coeliac children on a gluten free diet: A pilot study. *Nutrients* 8:660.

Radhakrishnamurty, R., Desikachar, H. S., Srinivasan, M., and Subrahmanyan, V. 1961. Studies on Idli fermentation. II. Relative participation of black gram flour and rice semolina in the fermentation. *Journal of Scientific and Industrial Research. C Biological Sciences* 20:342–5.

Ranasinghe, R. A. S. N., Maduwanthi, S. D. T., and Marapana, R. A. U. J. 2019. Nutritional and health benefits of jackfruit (*Artocarpus heterophyllus* Lam.): A review. *International Journal of Food Science* 2019.

Ravishankar, B., and Shukla, V. J. 2007. Indian systems of medicine: A brief profile. *African Journal of Traditional, Complementary and Alternative Medicines* 4(3):319–37.

Reddy, N. R., Sathe, S. K., Pierson, M. D., and Salunkhe, D. K. 1982. Idli, an Indian fermented food: A review. *Journal of Food Quality* 5(2):89–101.

Ren, C., Cheng, L., Sun, Y., et al. 2020. Lactic acid bacteria secrete toll like receptor 2 stimulating and macrophage immunomodulating bioactive factors. *Journal of Functional Foods* 66:103783.

Roobab, U., Batool, Z., Manzoor, M. F., Shabbir, M. A., Khan, M. R., and Aadil, R. M. 2020. Sources, formulations, advanced delivery and health benefits of probiotics. *Current Opinion in Food Science* 32:17–28.

Roy, A., Moktan, B., and Sarkar, P. K. 2007. Traditional technology in preparing legume-based fermented foods of Orissa. *Indian Journal of Traditional Knowledge* 6(1):12–16.

Roy, M., Chakrabarty, S., Sinha, D., Bhattacharya, R. K., and Siddiqi, M. 2003. Anticlastogenic, antigenotoxic and apoptotic activity of epigallocatechin gallate: A green tea polyphenol. *Mutation Research/Fundamental and Molecular Mechanisms of Mutagenesis* 523:33–41.

Sánchez, A. M., González-Burgos, E., Iglesias, I., and Gómez-Serranillos, M. P. 2020. Pharmacological update properties of Aloe vera and its major active constituents. *Molecules* 25(6):1324.

Sánchez, A. M., Sanchez, M. G., Malagarie-Cazenave, S., Olea, N., and Diaz-Laviada, I. 2006. Induction of apoptosis in prostate tumor PC-3 cells and inhibition of xenograft prostate tumor growth by the vanilloid capsaicin. *Apoptosis* 11(1):89–99.

Santacroce, L., Inchingolo, F., Topi, S., Del Prete, R., Di Cosola, M., Charitos, I. A., and Montagnani, M. 2021. Potential beneficial role of probiotics on the outcome of COVID-19 patients: An evolving perspective. *Diabetes and Metabolic Syndrome: Clinical Research and Reviews* 15(1):295–301.

Sanz, Y. 2015. Microbiome and gluten. *Annals of Nutrition and Metabolism* 67(Suppl. 2):27–42.

Sarkar, P., Dhumal, C., Panigrahi, S. S., and Choudhary, R. 2015. Traditional and ayurvedic foods of Indian origin. *Journal of Ethnic Foods* 2(3):97–109.

Sarkar, S., and Misra, A. K. 2001. Bio-preservation of milk and milk products. *Indian Food Industry* 20(4):74–7.

Sartippour, M. R., Pietras, R., Marquez-Garban, D. C., et al. 2006. The combination of green tea and tamoxifen is effective against breast cancer. *Carcinogenesis* 27(12):2424–33.

Schoene, N. W., Kelly, M. A., Polansky, M. M., and Anderson, R. A. 2005. Water-soluble polymeric polyphenols from cinnamon inhibit proliferation and alter cell cycle distribution patterns of hematologic tumor cell lines. *Cancer Letters* 230(1):134–40.

Selvendiran, K., Koga, H., Ueno, T., et al. 2006. Luteolin promotes degradation in signal transducer and activator of transcription 3 in human hepatoma cells: An implication for the antitumor potential of flavonoids. *Cancer Research* 66(9):4826–34.

Sen, C. T. 2004. *Food Culture in India*. Greenwood Publishing Group, Westport, Connecticut.

Shankar, S., and Srivastava, R. K. 2007. Bax and Bak genes are essential for maximum apoptotic response by curcumin, a polyphenolic compound and cancer chemopreventive agent derived from turmeric, *Curcuma longa*. *Carcinogenesis* 28(6):1277–86.

Sharma, K., Sharma, N., and Sharma, R. 2016. Identification and evaluation of in vitro probiotic attributes of novel and potential strains of lactic acid bacteria isolated from traditional dairy products of North-West Himalayas. *Journal of Clinical Microbiology and Biochemical Technology* 2(1):18–25.

Sharma, R., and Lal, D. 1997. Effect of dahi preparation on some water-soluble vitamins. *Indian Journal of Dairy Science* 50(4):318–20.

Sharma, R., and Prajapati, P. K. 2020. Predictive, preventive and personalized medicine: Leads from Ayurvedic concept of Prakriti (human constitution). *Current Pharmacology Reports* 1–10.

Shi, R. X., Ong, C. N., and Shen, H. M. 2005. Protein kinase c inhibition and x-linked inhibitor of apoptosis protein degradation contribute to the sensitization effect of luteolin on tumor necrosis factor-related apoptosis-inducing ligand-induced apoptosis in cancer cells. *Cancer Research* 65(17):7815–23.

Siddiqui, I. A., Zaman, N., Aziz, M. H., et al. 2006. Inhibition of CWR22Rv1 tumor growth and PSA secretion in athymic nude mice by green and black teas. *Carcinogenesis* 27(4):833–9.

Singh, S. P., Kumar, S., Mathan, S. V., et al. 2020. Therapeutic application of *Carica papaya* leaf extract in the management of human diseases. *DARU Journal of Pharmaceutical Sciences* 1–10.

Sinha, K., Ghosh, J., and Sil, P. C. 2016. Morin and its role in chronic diseases. *Anti-inflammatory Nutraceuticals and Chronic Diseases* 453–471.

Soni, S. K., Sandhu, D. K., and Vilkhu, K. S. 1985. Studies on dosa – an indigenous Indian fermented food: Some biochemical changes accompanying fermentation. *Food Microbiology* 2(3):175–81.

Steinkraus, K. 1995. *Handbook of Indigenous Fermented Foods*. CRC Press, Boca Raton, FL.

Stuart, E. C., Scandlyn, M. J., and Rosengren, R. J. 2006. Role of epigallocatechin gallate (EGCG) in the treatment of breast and prostate cancer. *Life Sciences* 79(25):2329–36.
Sumantran, V. N., and Tillu, G. 2013. Insights on personalized medicine from Ayurveda. *The Journal of Alternative and Complementary Medicine* 19(4):370–5.
Sun, J., Liao, X. P., D'Souza, A. W., et al. 2020. Environmental remodeling of human gut microbiota and antibiotic resistome in livestock farms. *Nature Communications* 11(1):1427.
Tian, N., Faller, L., Leffler, D. A., et al. 2017. Salivary gluten degradation and oral microbial profiles in healthy individuals and celiac disease patients. *Applied and Environmental Microbiology* 83(6):e03330–16.
Tsai, F. S., Lin, L. W., and Wu, C. R. 2016. Lupeol and its role in chronic diseases. *Drug Discovery from Mother Nature*:145–75.
Vieira, A. J., Beserra, F. P., Souza, M. C., Totti, B. M., and Rozza, A. L. 2018. Limonene: Aroma of innovation in health and disease. *Chemico-Biological Interactions* 283:97–106.
Wacklin, P., Laurikka, P., Lindfors, K., et al. 2014. Altered duodenal microbiota composition in celiac disease patients suffering from persistent symptoms on a long-term gluten-free diet. *Official Journal of the American College of Gastroenterology* 109(12):1933–41.
Wallace, T. C. 2011. Anthocyanins in cardiovascular disease. *Advances in Nutrition* 2(1):1–7.
Wang, H., Feng, T., Guo, D., Zhang, M., Chen, L., and Zhou, Y. 2018. Sanggenon C stimulates osteoblastic proliferation and differentiation, inhibits osteoclastic resorption, and ameliorates prednisone-induced osteoporosis in zebrafish model. *Molecules* 23(9):2343.
Watabe, M., Hishikawa, K., Takayanagi, A., Shimizu, N., and Nakaki, T. 2004. Caffeic acid phenethyl ester induces apoptosis by inhibition of NFκB and activation of Fas in human breast cancer MCF-7 cells. *Journal of Biological Chemistry* 279(7):6017–26.
Weir, N. M., Selvendiran, K., Kutala, V. K., et al. 2007. Curcumin induces G2/M arrest and apoptosis in cisplatin-resistant human ovarian cancer cells by modulating Akt and p38 MAPK. *Cancer Biology and Therapy* 6(2):178–84.
Wink, M. 2020. Potential of DNA intercalating alkaloids and other plant secondary metabolites against SARS-CoV-2 causing COVID-19. *Diversity* 12(5):175.
World Health Organization. 2020. *COVID-19 and Food Safety: Guidance for Food Businesses: Interim Guidance*. World Health Organization, Geneva.
Yang, C. S., Landau, J. M., Huang, M. T., and Newmark, H. L. 2001. Inhibition of carcinogenesis by dietary polyphenolic compounds. *Annual Review of Nutrition* 21(1):381–406.
Yang, P. L. 2016. Metabolomics and Lipidomics: Yet more ways your health is influenced by fat. In: *Viral Pathogenesis*, 181–198. Academic Press, Cambridge, Massachusetts, US.
Ye, X., Krohn, R. L., Liu, W., et al. 1999. The cytotoxic effects of a novel IH636 grape seed proanthocyanidin extract on cultured human cancer cells. In: *Stress Adaptation, Prophylaxis and Treatment*, 99–108. Springer, Boston, MA.

3 Nutritional Epigenomics and Disease Prevention

Juliana Bunmi Adetunji, Charles Oluwaseun Adetunji, Saher Islam, and Devarajan Thangadurai*

CONTENTS

3.1 INTRODUCTION

Cellular networks depend mostly on nutrients that are essentially derived from some diets and intermediary metabolites, which could serve as molecular signals that could change the genome role for cellular adaptation. Thus, the direct or indirect influence of nutrition on the gene has a great impact on metabolic pathway alteration and disease predisposition. However, the use of nutrients can be enhanced at the molecular level, which involves some genes in order to prevent the development of diseases and adequately maintain good health in humans. Moreover, there is a need for the optimization of nutrients, which is critical in the sustenance and maintenance of individual well-being so as to curtail the progression or the development

* Corresponding author email: adetunjibj@gmail.com

DOI: 10.1201/9781003142195-3

of diseases at the epigenetic level. Interestingly, it has been observed that epigenetics could frequently provide adequate insight into several factors responsible for the proper regulation of gene expression, which might be independent of the genetic sequence in a biological way. However, it has been observed that diet-gene interactions are paramount in understanding the role of diet in the modification of genes or the whole genome for disease prevention. The impact of diet on the epigenetic architecture of the genome could be transient, reversible, and/or persistence through life, with the potential to be transmitted from one generation to another via germ cells (Stover et al. 2018).

Interestingly, the epigenetic signal strength is conserved during aging, and its effects on tissue-specific gene regulation are found to be related to specific genomic loci, which is subject to epigenetic modification and the extent of the epigenetic modifications on the DNA and histone methylation, among other factors (Jones 2012; Pal and Tyler 2016). Consequently, the effect of diet on the epigenome and the subsequent effect of the epigenome on disease prevention could be determined on various epigenetic molecules like methylation of DNA, histone modifications, and some non-coding RNAs (microRNAs), chromosomal proteins, and long non-coding RNAs.

Therefore, this chapter intends to address the role of nutrigenomic on disorders resulting from metabolic pathways interference, and it also discusses diet as a key factor in altering the structure of chromatin and post-translational histone modification to influence gene transcription.

3.2 EPIGENETICS

Epigenetics gives information on heritable changes that could be useful to gene function in the genome. This might take place without alteration in the sequence or structure of DNA nucleotides (Franks and Ling 2010). It was established that diet portends the capacity to directly influence epigenetic alteration of the human health status and programming level. Haggarty demonstrated that epigenome is extremely dynamic and could be affected by changes and alterations from physical exercise, aging, and nutrient response (Haggarty 2013). Consequently, epigenetics is now becoming a crucial area for the proper understanding of the underlying mechanism governing diet and nutrients influence on the genome, which could lead to modulating gene expression (Siddique et al. 2009).

3.3 NUTRIENT-GENE INTERACTION

The nutrients that humans and animals consume via diet are significant to their well-being. However, this association can be well understood primarily at the level of nutrient-gene relationship, which could either be through genetic variation, direct gene interaction, and epigenetic interactions. Genetic variations like single-nucleotide polymorphisms (SNPs) are nutrient requirement influencers. Meanwhile, Joffe et al. (2013) reported that the stimulation and release of pro-inflammatory factors like cytokines that predispose an individual to inflammation and development of obesity are regulated through functional SNPs present in inflammatory genes, like IL-1, TNF-α, and IL-6, which interact with dietary lipids. The direct interactions are connected to nutrient association with the receptor via transcription factor, which is concerned with modulating gene transcription.

Moreover, it was gathered that nuclear receptors like the liver X receptor (LXR) family, which are stimulated by bile acids and cholesterol, can enhance reverse cholesterol efflux and lipid catabolism (Franks and Ling 2010; Huang 2014), whereas the epigenetic interactions are linked with alteration of DNA structure or histone proteins by nutrients; this will, in turn, frequently alter or affect gene expression. Meanwhile, Haggarty (2013) demonstrated the alteration caused by alcohol, protein, B vitamins, and micronutrients on DNA via DNA methylation with clear changes in epigenetic caused by dietary nutrients that are critical determinants of biological functionality and disease susceptibility of an organism (Perry et al. 2007).

3.4 EPIGENETIC MOLECULES RESPONSIBLE FOR GENE REGULATION

Godfrey et al. (2007) also suggested that future disease risk can be controlled through a mechanism that will alter the gene-regulating epigenetics (Godfrey et al. 2007). However, the process of epigenetic creates a conducive environment for rapid and variable adaptability that could lead to developmental modifications that could be induced or maintained during an organism's lifespan. It was also reported that epigenetic changes without DNA alteration could be inherited during cell division, and this might allow a wide range of control on gene transcriptional states resulting in gene expression or repression.

Moreover, processes in epigenetic include (1) DNA methylation, which occurs mainly on the fifth carbon atom of cytosines and could be followed by guanine; (2) histone modifications, which include acetylation, methylation, ubiquitination, lysine sumoylation serine, and threonine phosphorylation, as well as arginine methylation; (3) other nuclear proteins, which include chromatin effector proteins, remodeling complexes, and some binding proteins; and (4) non-coding RNAs like miRNAs (microRNAs) responsible for binding and regulating multiple mRNAs histone variants, such as H3.3 and H2A.Z (Kim et al. 2009; Sharma et al. 2010), and other chromosomal proteins and non-coding RNAs, such mRNAs.

3.4.1 DNA Methylation (Epigenetic Role of DNA Methylation)

Methylation of the DNA has several genetic functions based on its location. For instance, methylation of DNA around the promoter region could regulate gene transcription (Portela and Esteller 2010), while modification, splicing events, and alternative promoters are found within the gene (Maunakea et al. 2013). The process involves transferring a methyl group to cytosine 5′ carbon to form 5-methylcytosine (Kumar et al. 1994), which occurs within the dinucleotide sequence CpG in mammals when cytosine is instantly fused to the 5′ of guanine. When gene silencing occurs, there is hypermethylation, while gene activation is linked with hypomethylation (Song et al. 2005).

DNA methylation also has the potential to restrict the binding of transcription factors through the mobilization of a myriad of other repressive factors that prevent chromatin modification (Bell and Felsenfeld 2000; Miranda and Jones 2007). However, Patel et al. (1997) observed that histone changes need to access and open the chromatin, which is antagonized by DNA methylation that could eventually lead to the alteration of the nucleosome, hence preventing the binding of transcription factors and polymerase II (pol II) (Patel et al. 1997). The methylation occurring in the de novo system could cause a sporadic increase in the design of actual methylation conserved in different tissues (Li 2002). Furthermore, in the epigenetic study, the loci used often demonstrate interindividual DNA methylation variation, with its stability over time.

3.4.2 Modification of Histones

Histone acetylation is connected with chromatin open-state and transcriptional activity (Grunstein 1997; Struhl 1998) controlled by two groups of enzymes; histone acetyltransferases (HATs) responsible for acetyl transfer to the amino acid (lysine) residues in the histone tails from acetyl-CoA. This could result in the removal of positive charge from the histones, thereby weakening the interaction of the DNA phosphate with the histone. Hence, the chromatin at this stage becomes accessible to the transcription machine due to its less compatibility. The histone deacetylases (HDACs), on the other hand, work as repressors to gene expression because it removes the acetyl groups from lysine residue at the tail of the histone (Ceccacci and Minucci 2016; Harb et al. 2016).

3.4.2.1 Histone Methylation

This process is stimulated by histone methyltransferase (HMTs) together with arginine methyltransferase (ARMTs), lysine methyltransferases (LMTS), and histone demethylases (HDMs) which remove methyl groups. However, the electrostatic bond in DNA is not affected by the methylation of histone arginine or lysine from S-adenosyl-L-methionine but rather influences the binding of regulatory proteins to chromatin (Morera et al. 2016; Kaniskan et al. 2017).

3.4.2.2 Histone Ubiquitination

The ubiquitination of histones helps in the post-translational modification responsible for the regulation of critical cellular functions in most eukaryotic cell signaling pathways. The conjugation of ubiquitin with proteins in the ubiquitin-proteasome system control and stabilize the replication of target proteins (Alhamwe et al. 2018). The enzyme ubiquitin ligases also stimulate ubiquitination, while specific peptidases caused the removal of ubiquitin through a process referred to as deubiquitinating enzymes (Ravid and Hochstrasser 2008; Schwertman et al. 2016).

Alhamwe et al. (2018) documented that DNA damage signaling, protein translocation, and transcriptional regulation play a critical role in linking histone 2A monoubiquitination with gene silencing. Meanwhile, histone H3 monoubiquitination was able to induce acetylation of the same histone (Zhang et al. 2017). Histone 2B monoubiquitination is known to be connected with the activation of transcription.

Protein activation or degradation in some signaling pathways has been marked with polyubiquitination (Weake and Workman 2008; Schwertman et al. 2016).

3.4.2.3 Histone Phosphorylation

In histone phosphorylation, the genes are regulated by two opposing enzymes: kinases add phosphate groups, and phosphatases remove the phosphates, with the two having opposing modes of action (Bannister and Kouzarides 2011; Rossetto et al. 2012). The phosphorylation of histone could occur as damage DNA repair, chromatin association with meiosis and mitosis, and transcriptional activity regulation (Pal and Tyler 2016; Hussey et al. 2017). The histone phosphorylation is in a mutual relationship with other histone modifications. This could result in suppressing the downstream regulation of chromatic status and its adverse consequences (Hussey et al. 2017; Jensen et al. 2018). Meanwhile, H3S10ph phosphorylation can have a direct effect on acetylation levels by inducing transcription through activation of H4K16ac interaction via the same residue amino acids H3K9ac and H3K14ac (Ruegsegger et al. 2017; Jeyapal et al. 2018).

3.4.3 MicroRNA Modifications

RNA modification, which is often referred to as epitranscriptome in epigenetics, was discovered over a decade ago (Helm and Motorin 2017). The epitranscriptome represents a pattern in post-transcriptional modifications of RNA that does not affect the RNA sequence. Moreover, a number of these modifications are recognized in non-coding RNA species, specifically the tRNA and some mRNA modification with m5C (equivalent DNA modification), N6-methyladenosine (m6A), and pseudouridine (Ψ). However, the presence of pseudouridine in RNA has been available for the past ten years with an unclear function. Esteller and Pandolfi (2017) documented that chemically modified nucleosides in RNA are critical in homeostasis because they regulate the amounts of RNA and its activities in a specified species. This is carried out through RNA stability alteration, coding, and non-coding miRNA editing or splicing, and by adding the complex of repertoire controls to the post-transcriptional steps in gene expression.

Consequently, some epitranscriptomic marks could be reversible. This is demonstrated by dynamics in mRNA alteration by enzymatic demethylation complex with the fat mass and obesity-associated protein (Jia et al. 2011), which reveals that nutrition and obesity-related factors could stimulate the epitranscriptome. Interestingly, there is remarkable documentation that RNA modifications are involved in the development of multiple diseases like cancer (Esteller and Pandolfi 2017).

3.4.3.1 Non-Coding RNA

Non-coding RNAs (ncRNAs) are specific epigenetic factors that mediate lots of intracellular processes (Huang et al. 2014). However, the ncRNAs are functional RNA that does not translate into protein but are transcribed from DNA. MicroRNAs (miRNAs) with short single-strand and within 19–24 nucleotides are the best-characterized ncRNAs. The miRNAs also control gene silencing at either transcriptional and/or translational levels of genes protein-coding (Ameres and Zamore 2013). Short and long non-coding RNAs (sncRNAs and lncRNAs) are major parts or components of the regulatory machinery of transcription, which is vital for transcriptional and translational regulation within the cell during the synthesis of protein (Kapranov et al. 2007). Far above 200 nucleotides in length compose lncRNAs, which function as transcriptional and post-transcriptional regulators and chromatin remodelers. Moreover, lots of lncRNA complexes having chromatin-modifying proteins are capable of changing their catalytic activity region to specific genomic sites and, as such, lead to modified chromatin states and influenced gene expression. The lncRNAs participate in many intracellular processes with little or no protein-coding potential (Huang et al. 2014), and it was also documented by Weisbeck and Jansen (2017) that lncRNAs are specifically linked to certain cancers.

Consequently, the small ncRNAs are capable of inducing mRNA catabolism or repress translation after binding a gene-promoter site, stimulate DNA methylation, and/or repress modification of histone and, as such, result in complete repression or transcriptional activities decrease (Kim et al. 2008; Hawkins et al. 2009). However, the large ncRNAs have the potential to coat chromosome regions, thereby developing repressor-domains with many kilobases, which are critical in processes like imprinting and X-inactivation (Reik and Lewis 2005).

3.5 NUTRIENT-GENE INTERACTIONS IN DISEASES

3.5.1 Obesity

In 2012, Milagro and colleagues reported on the significance of diet and epigenetic modification on obesity. It was established that nutritional factors are key to human health, and one of the mechanisms by which the bioactive constituents and nutrients in food affect metabolism is through epigenetics, thereby regulating gene expression. In their findings, they documented several food compounds and nutrients that can alter the epigenetic pattern of various tissue cell lines. This is important to formulate a functional food that will be useful in the prevention of diseases (vel Szic et al. 2010). Moreover, there is a clear difference in preadipocytes and mature adipocytes of human in DNA methylation, this suggests the role played by epigenetics in the adipocyte differentiation process (Zhu et al. 2012). Though some other mechanisms, like histone modification (Okamura et al. 2010), acetylation and deacetylation (Chatterjee et al. 2011), and poly ADP-ribosylation, also played a critical role during adipogenesis. Fujiki et al. (2009) established the involvement of the PPARγ gene (an important transcriptional regulator) in 3T3-L1 hypermethylation during adipogenesis, which in turn was demethylated upon differentiation induction. It was also documented that in obese individuals, methylation alteration in the DNA of blood leukocytes was observed (Wang et al. 2010), while TFAM gene-promoter methylation in the white blood cells was connected to insulin resistance in an individual (Gemma et al. 2010).

However, there are numerous genes with differential methylation status in skeletal muscle, which relates to a tolerance of glucose in diabetic and normal individuals, which serves as a pointer to the role that DNA methylation plays in the development of obesity and its associated disorders.

Milagro and colleagues, in 2013, claimed that the knowledge of epigenetics is a tool to understating the onset of chronic disorders, fetal genetic programming, and differences in monozygotic twin-linked to diet and nutritional processes. Moreover, epigenetics will provide useful information on how some genes carrying identical sequences could respond differently under the same nutrient exposure via chromatin architecture modification, DNA methylation, and small and non-coding RNA processes (Milagro et al. 2013). Consequently, there is a link between high-sugar or high-fat consumption and overweightness in rodents and the modification in DNA methylation regions that affect different gene-promoter regions, like fatty acid synthase (FASN), leptin, pro-opiomelanocortin (POMC), NADH dehydrogenase (ubiquinone) 1 β subcomplex subunit 6 (NDUFB6), and circadian locomotor output cycles kaput (CLOCK) responsible for obesity and energy homeostasis. However, the biomarkers of epigenetics, like aquaporin 9 (AQP9), CD44, ATPase class V type 10A (ATP10A), specific miRNAs, and TNFα, are useful tools in determining the actual body weight. Hence, it was revealed that the results of nutrition-linked diseases, like obesity and diabetes, in different individuals do not rely on the diet and DNA sequence alone but also on the epigenome and nutritional influence that affects the genetic expression and changes the epigenetic marks resulting in covalent histone changes, chromatin folding, DNA methylation, and miRNA regulatory actions (Milagro et al. 2013).

Choi, in his report, claims that diet is responsible for regulating the interactions that exist in gene and diseases following the mechanism of epigenetics. However, epigenetic marks are often affected by aging. It was revealed in a study that Western diet was able to induce 24 differential methylated regions localized to genes that regulate lipid metabolism, cellular and maintenance functions, and cardiovascular diseases in the liver (Choi et al. 2013). Furthermore, Choi and colleagues report that providing substantial and adequate micronutrients to rodents while restricting their energy intake by 20 to 50% was able to retard all age-linked disorders, specifically cancer, thereby prolonging their lifespan (Choi et al. 2013). It is, therefore, clear that the generation of DNA-methylated regions can be achieved in age- and calorie-restricted diet.

Interestingly, the differential methylated regions generated in aging from a calorie-restricted diet are often different from that of normal aging. This clearly indicates that epigenetic modification resulting from aging can be alleviated through a calorie-restricted diet. Meanwhile, the high-fat diets fed to mice could alter the DNA methylation across the adipocyte genome, while the comparison of the high-fat-diet region can induce differential methylation, which can lead to overlap with the adipose tissue DNA methylation from a lean individual in comparison with obese individuals pre- and post-Roux-en-Y gastric bypass surgery (Multhaup et al. 2015).

Also, diet is a key factor that could alter the structure of chromatin and post-translational histones modification to influence gene transcription. In a study by Zheng et al. (2012) that used rats that were fed a high-fat diet to initiate obesity in comparison with obesity-resistant phenotype rats, the induction of aging and senescence pathways was demonstrated in obese rats through p21Cip1 and p16INK4a genes. The authors demonstrated the associated interaction of diet with histone modifications like methylation and acetylation. Meanwhile, the report showed that the offspring of rats maintained on a low-protein diet in the gestation period reduced the cell cycle regulator p21 expression in the mammary gland; this could be linked with histone modification at the promoter of the p21 gene (Zheng et al. 2012). These authors suggest that a maternal protein-restricted diet during pregnancy may alter cell cycle control of offspring, thereby predisposing them to the risk of developing breast cancer.

3.5.2 Diabetes

Epigenetics has been of great importance in understanding the preventive role of diet in ameliorating some metabolic disorders. The report has shown that there are about 44 genes with DNA methylation that are connected to a mitochondrial role in muscle insulin resistance in diabetic individuals in comparison with normal insulin-sensitive groups whose cytosine methylation is greater in a tissue-specific and inducible transcriptional cofactor (peroxisome proliferator-activated receptors c-coactivator 1α [PGC-1α]) promoter region.

However, the PGC-1α is known to regulate nuclear-encoded gene expression and its functions. Barres and colleagues, in 2009, established the fact that changes in methylation were connected to low mRNA PGC-1α and lower densities of mitochondrial and DNA molecules in the muscles of diabetic individuals. Diet has been reported as one major factor that impacted the methylome; meanwhile, changes in methylation of the chromatin could occur reversibly or rapidly in response to a specific exercise, dietary factors, or some physiological conditions. An increase in cytokines and dietary fats has been linked to insulin resistance induction in experimental animals, and these are connected to changes in specific tissues causing gene-expression alterations.

Meanwhile, a sharp alteration in methylation was observed in skeletal muscle cells of normal insulin-sensitive individuals incubated with either TNF-α causing an elevation in non-CpG dinucleotides PGC-1α methylation levels in an insulin-sensitive muscle (Barrès et al. 2009). Also, an in vivo study on exercising individuals' skeletal muscle revealed short-lived and rapid demethylation of some promoter genes, like PPAR-delta, PGC-1α, and PDK4, along with elevated respective mRNA levels (Barrès et al. 2012).

Moreover, instant insulin changes are often observed in obese and insulin-resistant patients going through Roux-en-Y gastric bypass surgery. The whole-body insulin sensitivity changes could be coupled with changes that occur in the methylation levels of PGC-1α and PDK4 promoters in the skeletal muscle (Barres et al. 2013).

3.5.3 Aging

It is evident that the nutrients consumed directly inhibit some epigenetic enzymes like HDAC, DNMT, and HAT or alter the substrate available for some enzymatic reactions. As a result, the expression of some major genes that have the potential for promoting human health and longevity are modified (Davis and Ross 2007; Choi and Friso 2010).

Researchers have also documented that diet has an epigenetic effect on phenotype and human exposure to diseases in a lifetime. In 2009, Kim and colleagues studied the relationship that exists between folate (a component of vitamin B complex and a source of single carbon for the synthesis of AdoMet) metabolism and phenotype alteration in DNA methylation. Also, some nutrients that donate methyl, like choline, have the capability to change the DNA methylation pattern and then influence gene expression (Choi and Friso 2010). In an experiment on maternal diet restriction in animals, it was revealed that the methyl donated by the nutrients before conception altered the offspring's DNA methylation patterns and caused a change (Choi and Friso 2010). It is worth noting here that nutrients that donate methyl to mother during early pregnancy are of high impact on proper fetal growth.

Furthermore, Ford et al. (2011) examine the impact of dietary restriction without major nutrient deprivation on different models. The restriction of calories has been shown to have anti-inflammatory potential via the inhibition of NFkB and some specific genes (Choi and Friso 2010). It was revealed that cross-link existing in DNA methylation and modification of histone suggests that the structure of chromatin could determine DNA methylation (Lillycrop et al. 2014). In the interaction of nutrients with genes, Sirtuin 1, which is NAD^+-dependent HDAC with substrate specificity like histone proteins, was reported to be stimulated via some dietary components like resveratrol. Also, Sirtuin 1 is known to mediate some dietary restriction, which can delay/reverse changes associated with aging by DNA methylation (Ford et al. 2011).

3.5.4 Cancer

Epigenetic active ingredients, like folate and cobalamin, for instance, have been documented to play a critical role in DNA metabolism and maintenance of pattern of DNA methylation through chemical association with methyl product. In a study, the positive intake of dietary folic acid was positively correlated with the p16 gene tumor suppressor, a major cancer-linked gene having a consistent DNA methylation silencer on its promoter (Choi and Friso 2010). Meanwhile, in the p16 gene expressions in aged mouse colons, there is an altered and concurrent decrease in DNMT expression with aging. It was also reported that hypomethylation with increased risk of pancreatic and colorectal cancer is linked with reduced folate consumption (Larsson et al. 2006; Weisbeck and Jansen 2017). Moreover, it is epidemiological proven that folate can modulate anticarcinogenic properties via altered epigenetic because deficiency of folate deficiency decreases DNA methylation potential, which is linked to cancer development.

Bishop and Ferguson (2015) studied the impact of several nutrients derived from vegetables in addition to folate on epigenetic; it was observed that the nutrients have the capability of reducing DNA hypermethylation of critical genes, thereby suppressing tumors. Meanwhile, several dietary constituents have the potential of modulating HDAC and HAT. Plants like broccoli sprouts, which contain sulforaphane and isothiocyanate, and garlic, which contain an organosulfur diallyl disulfide, have been proven to suppress HDAC (Weisbeck and Jansen 2017). Consequently, several dietary components have also been considered to be capable of inhibiting cancer progression via various epigenetic modifications.

Finally, miRNAs could control modifications of histones and DNA methylation while histone acetylation and promoter methylation are capable of modulating miRNA expression. However, dysregulated expression of miRNA is linked with tumor progression of human cancers via altered cell proliferation and apoptosis. Diets deficient in methyl and folate can also lead to abnormal miRNA expression leading to pro-cancer effects (Choi and Friso 2010).

3.6 CONCLUSION

This chapter discussed epigenetics and its efficacy in interacting with diets. Various epigenetic molecules and their key roles in gene regulation were also mentioned. Furthermore, it was observed in the chapter that nutrients consumed have the potential to prevent or inhibit the action of some epigenetic enzymes that could change the DNA structure and, hence, contribute to the development of some disease conditions like obesity, diabetics, cancer, and aging.

REFERENCES

Alhamwe, B. A., Khalaila, R., Wolf, J., et al. 2018. Histone modifications and their role in epigenetics of atopy and allergic diseases. *Allergy, Asthma & Clinical Immunology* 14:39. https://doi.org/10.1186/s13223-018-0259-4

Ameres, S. L., and Zamore, P. D. 2013. Diversifying microRNA sequence and function. *Nature Reviews Molecular Cell Biology* 14:475–88.

Bannister, A. J., and Kouzarides, T. 2011. Regulation of chromatin by histone modifications. *Cell Research* 21(3):381–95. https://doi.org/10.1038/cr.2011.22

Barres, R., Kirchner, H., Rasmussen, M., Yan, J., Kantor, F. R., and Krook, A. 2013. Weight loss after gastric bypass surgery in human obesity remodels promoter methylation. *Cell Reports* 3(4):1020–7. https://doi.org/10.1016/j.celrep.2013.03.018

Barrès, R., Osler, M. E., Yan, J., Rune, A., Fritz, T., and Caidahl, K. 2009. Non-CpG methylation of the PGC-1alpha promoter through DNMT3B controls mitochondrial density. *Cell Metabolism* 10(3):189–98. https://doi.org/10.1016/j.cmet.2009.07.011

Barrès, R., Yan, J., Egan, B., Treebak, J. T., Rasmussen, M., and Fritz, T. 2012. Acute exercise remodels promoter methylation in human skeletal muscle. *Cell Metabolism* 15(3): 405–11. https://doi.org/10.1016/j.cmet.2012.01.001

Bell, A. C., and Felsenfeld, G. 2000. Methylation of a CTCF-dependent boundary controls imprinted expression of the Igf2 gene. *Nature* 405:482–5.

Bishop, K. S., and Ferguson, L. R. 2015. The interaction between epigenetics, nutrition and the development of cancer. *Nutrients* 7(2):922–47. https://doi.org/10.3390/nu7020922

Ceccacci, E., and Minucci, S. 2016. Inhibition of histone deacetylases in cancer therapy: Lessons from leukaemia. *British Journal of Cancer* 114:605–11. https://doi.org/10.1038/bjc.2016.36

Chatterjee, T. K., Idelman, G., Blanco, V., et al. 2011. Histone deacetylase 9 is a negative regulator of adipogenic differentiation. *Journal of Biological Chemistry* 286: 27836–47.

Choi, S. W., Claycombe, K. J., Martinez, J. A., Friso, S., and Schalinske, K. L. 2013. Nutritional epigenomics: A portal to disease prevention. *Advances in Nutrition* 4(5):530–2. https://doi.org/10.3945/an.113.004168.

Choi, S. W., and Friso, S. 2010. Epigenetics: A new bridge between nutrition and health. *Advances in Nutrition* 1:8–16.

Davis, C. D., and Ross, S. A. 2007. Dietary components impact histone modifications and cancer risk. *Nutrition Reviews* 65:88–94.

Esteller, M., and Pandolfi, P. P. 2017. The epitranscriptome of noncoding RNAs in cancer. *Cancer Discovery* 7(4):359–68. https://doi.org/10.1158/2159-8290.CD-16-1292

Ford, D., Ions, L. J., Alatawi, F., and Wakeling, L. A. 2011. The potential role of epigenetic responses to diet in ageing. *The Proceedings of the Nutrition Society* 70(3):374–84. https://doi.org/10.1017/S0029665111000851

Franks, P. W., and Ling, C. 2010. Epigenetics and obesity: The devil is in the details. *BMC Medicine* 8:88.

Fujiki, K., Kano, F., Shiota, K., and Murata, M. 2009. Expression of the peroxisome proliferator activated receptor gamma gene is repressed by DNA methylation in visceral adipose tissue of mouse models of diabetes. *BMC Biology* 7:38.

Gemma, C., Sookoian, S., Dieuzeide, G., García, S. I., Gianotti, T. F., and González, C. D. 2010. Methylation of TFAM gene promoter in peripheral white blood cells is associated with insulin resistance in adolescents. *Molecular Genetics and Metabolism* 100:83–7.

Godfrey, K. M., Lillycrop, K. A., Burdge, G. C., Gluckman, P. D., and Hanson, M. A. 2007. Epigenetic mechanisms and the mismatch concept of the developmental origins of health and disease. *Pediatric Research* 61(5 Pt 2):5R–10R. https://doi.org/10.1203/pdr.0b013e318045bedb.

Grunstein, M. 1997. Histone acetylation in chromatin structure and transcription. *Nature* 389(6649):349–52. https://doi.org/10.1038/38664

Haggarty, P. 2013. Epigenetic consequences of a changing human diet. *Proceedings of the Nutrition Society* 72:363–71.

Harb, H., Alashkar, A. B., Garn, H., Renz, H., and Potaczek, D. P. 2016. Recent developments in epigenetics of pediatric asthma. *Current Opinion in Pediatrics* 28:754–63. https://doi.org/10.1097/MOP.00000 00000 00042

Hawkins, P. G., Santoso, S., Adams, C., Anest, V., and Morris, K. V. 2009. Promoter targeted small RNAs induce long-term transcriptional gene silencing in human cells. *Nucleic Acids Research* 37(9):2984–95. https://doi.org/10.1093/nar/gkp127

Helm, M., and Motorin, Y. 2017. Detecting RNA modifications in the epitranscriptome: Predict and validate. *Nature Reviews Genetics* 18(5):275–291. https://doi.org/10.1038/nrg.2016.169

Huang, B., Jiang, C., and Zhang, R. 2014. Epigenetics: The language of the cell? *Epigenomics* 6:73–88.

Huang, C. 2014. Natural modulators of liver X receptors. *Journal of Integrative Medicine* 12:76–85.

Hussey, B., Lindley, M. R., and Mastana, S. 2017. Epigenetics and epigenomics: The future of nutritional interventions. *Future Science* 3:FSO237.

Jensen, V. S., Hvid, H., Damgaard, J., Nygaard, H., Ingvorsen, C., and Wulff, E. M. 2018. Dietary fat stimulates development of NAFLD more potently than dietary fructose in Sprague – Dawley rats. *Diabetology & Metabolic Syndrome* 10:4.

Jeyapal, S., Kona, S. R., Mullapudi, S. V., Putcha, U. K., Gurumurthy, P., and Ibrahim, A. 2018. Substitution of linoleic acid with α-linolenic acid or long chain n-3 polyunsaturated fatty acid prevents Western diet induced nonalcoholic steatohepatitis. *Scientific Reports* 8:10953.

Jia, G., Fu, Y., Zhao, X., et al. 2011. N6-methyladenosine in nuclear RNA is a major substrate of the obesity-associated FTO. *Nature Chemical Biology* 7(12):885–7. https://doi.org/10.1038/nchembio.687

Joffe, Yael T., Collins, M., and Goedecke, J. H. 2013. The relationship between dietary fatty acids and inflammatory genes on the obese phenotype and serum lipids. *Nutrients* 5(5):1672–1705.

Jones, P. A. 2012. Functions of DNA methylation: Islands, start sites, gene bodies and beyond. *Nature Reviews Genetics* 13:484–92.

Kaniskan, H. Ü., Martini, M. L., and Jin, J. 2017. Inhibitors of protein methyltransferases and demethylases. *Chemical Reviews*. https://doi.org/10.1021/acs.chemrev.6b008 01.

Kapranov, P., Willingham, A. T., and Gingeras, T. R. 2007. Genome-wide transcription and the implications for genomic organization. *Nature Reviews Genetics* 8:413–23.

Kim, D. H., Saetrom, P., Snøve, O., and Rossi Jr, J. J. 2008. MicroRNA-directed transcriptional gene silencing in mammalian cells. *Proceedings of the National Academy of Sciences of the United States of America* 105(42):16230–5. https://doi.org/10.1073/pnas.0808830105

Kim, K. C., Friso, S., and Choi, S. W. 2009. DNA methylation, an epigenetic mechanism connecting folate to healthy embryonic development and aging. *Journal of Nutritional Biochemistry* 20:917–26.

Kumar, S., Cheng, X., Klimasauskas, S., et al. 1994. The DNA (cytosine-5) methyltransferases. *Nucleic Acids Research* 22(1):1–10. https://doi.org/10.1093/nar/22.1.1

Larsson, S. C., Giovannucci, E., and Wolk, A. 2006. Folate intake, MTHFR polymorphisms, and risk of esophageal, gastric, and pancreatic cancer: A meta-analysis. *Gastroenterology* 131:1271–83.

Li, E. 2002. Chromatin modification and epigenetic reprogramming in mammalian development. *Nature Reviews Genetics* 3:662–73.

Lillycrop, K. A., Hoile, S. P., Grenfell, L., and Burdge, G. C. 2014. DNA methylation, ageing and the influence of early life nutrition. *Proceedings of the Nutrition Society* 73:413–21.

Maunakea, A. K., Chepelev, I., Cui, K., and Zhao, K. 2013. Intragenic DNA methylation modulates alternative splicing by recruiting MeCP2 to promote exon recognition. *Cell Research* 23(11):1256–69. https://doi.org/10.1038/cr.2013.110

Milagro, F. I., Mansego, M. L., Miguel, C. D., and Martínez, J. A. 2013. Dietary factors, epigenetic modifications and obesity outcomes: Progresses and perspectives. *Molecular Aspects of Medicine* 34(4):782–812. https://doi.org/10.1016/j.mam.2012.06.010

Miranda, T. B., and Jones, P. A. 2007. DNA methylation: The nuts and bolts of repression. *Journal of Cellular Physiology* 213:384–90.

Morera, L., Lübbert, M., and Jung, M. 2016. Targeting histone methyltransferases and demethylases in clinical trials for cancer therapy. *Clinical Epigenetics* 8:57. https://doi.org/10.1186/s13148-016-0223-4.

Multhaup, M. L., Seldin, M. M., Jaffe, A. E., Lei, X., Kirchner, H., and Mondal, P. 2015. Mouse-human experimental epigenetic analysis unmasks dietary targets and genetic liability for diabetic phenotypes. *Cell Metabolism* 21(1):138–49. https://doi.org/10.1016/j.cmet.2014.12.014

Okamura, M., Inagaki, T., Tanaka, T., and Sakai, J. 2010. Role of histone methylation and demethylation in adipogenesis and obesity. *Organogenesis* 6:24–32.

Pal, S., and Tyler, J. K. 2016. Epigenetics and aging. *Science Advances* 2:e1600584.

Patel, S. A., Graunke, D. M., and Pieper, R. O. 1997. Aberrant silencing of the CpG island-containing human O6-methylguanine DNA methyltransferase gene is associated with the loss of nucleosome-like positioning. *Molecular and Cellular Biology* 17:5813–22.

Perry, G. H., Dominy, N. J., Claw, K. G., Lee, A. S., Fiegler, H., and Redon, R. 2007. Diet and the evolution of human amylase gene copy number variation. *Nature Genetics* 39(10):1256–60. https://doi.org/10.1038/ng2123

Portela, A., and Esteller, M. 2010. Epigenetic modifications and human disease. *Nature Biotechnology* 28:1057–68.

Ravid, T., and Hochstrasser, M. 2008. Diversity of degradation signals in the ubiquitin-proteasome system. *Nature Reviews Molecular Cell Biology* 9:679–90. https://doi.org/10.1038/nrm24 68.

Reik, W., and Lewis, A. 2005. Co-evolution of X-chromosome inactivation and imprinting in mammals. *Nature Reviews Genetics* 6:403–10.

Rossetto, D., Avvakumov, N., and Côté, J. 2012. Histone phosphorylation: A chromatin modification involved in diverse nuclear events. *Epigenetics* 7:1098–108. https://doi.org/10.4161/epi.21975.

Ruegsegger, G. N., Grigsby, K. B., Kelty, T. J., Zidon, T. M., Childs, T. E., and Vieira-Potter, V. J. 2017. Maternal Western diet age-specifically alters female offspring physical activity and dopamine-and leptin-related gene expression. *FASEB Journal* 31:5371–83.

Schwertman, P., Bekker-Jensen, S., and Mailand, N. 2016. Regulation of DNA double strand break repair by ubiquitin and ubiquitin-like modifiers. *Nature Reviews Molecular Cell Biology* 17:379–94. https://doi.org/10.1038/nrm.2016.58.

Sharma, Shikhar, Kelly, Theresa K., and Jones, Peter A. 2010. Epigenetics in cancer. *Carcinogenesis* 31(1):27–36.

Siddique, R. A., Tandon, M., Ambwani, T., Rai, S. N., and Atreja, S. K. 2009. Nutrigenomics: Nutrient-gene interactions. *Food Reviews International* 25:326–45.

Song, F., Smith, J. F., Kimura, M. T., Morrow, A. D., Matsuyama, T., and Nagase, H. 2005. Association of tissue-specific differentially methylated regions (TDMs) with differential gene expression. *Proceedings of the National Academy of Sciences of the United States of America* 102(9):3336–41. https://doi.org/10.1073/pnas.0408436102

Stover, P. J., James, W. P. T., Krook, A., and Garza, C. 2018. Emerging concepts on the role of epigenetics in the relationships between nutrition and health. *Journal of Internal Medicine* 284:37–49.

Struhl, K. 1998. Histone acetylation and transcriptional regulatory mechanisms. *Genes & Development* 12:599–606.

vel Szic, K. S., Ndlovu, M. N., Haegeman, G., Haegeman, G., and Vanden Berghe, W. 2010. Nature or nurture: Let food be your epigenetic medicine in chronic inflammatory disorders. *Biochemical Pharmacology* 80:1816–32.

Wang, X., Zhu, H., Snieder, H., Su, S., Munn, D., and Harshfield, G. 2010. Obesity related methylation changes in DNA of peripheral blood leukocytes. *BMC Medicine* 8:87.

Weake, V. M., and Workman, J. L. 2008. Histone ubiquitination: Triggering gene activity. *Molecular Cell* 29:653–63. https://doi.org/10.1016/j.molce l.2008.02.014.45–48.

Weisbeck, A., and Jansen, R. J. 2017. Nutrients and the pancreas: An epigenetic perspective. *Nutrients* 9:283.

Zhang, X., Li, B., Rezaeian, A. H., Xu, X., Chou, P. C., and Jin, G. 2017. H3 ubiquitination by NEDD4 regulates H3 acetylation and tumorigenesis. *Nature Communications* 8:14799. https://doi.org/10.1038/ncomms14799

Zheng, S., Rollet, M., Yang, K., and Pan, Y. X. 2012. A gestational low-protein diet represses p21(WAF1/Cip1) expression in the mammary gland of offspring rats through promoter histone modifications. *British Journal of Nutrition* 108:998–1007.

Zhu, J. G., Xia, L., Ji, C. B., Zhang, C. M., Zhu, G. Z., and Shi, C. M. 2012. Differential DNA methylation status between human preadipocytes and mature adipocytes. *Cell Biochemistry and Biophysics* 63:1–15.

4 Potential Applications of Proteomics for Nutritional Safety and Healthcare

Srinivasan Kameswaran, Bellemkonda Ramesh, M. Subhosh Chandra, and Gopikrishna Pitchika*

CONTENTS

* Corresponding author email: kambharath@gmail.com

DOI: 10.1201/9781003142195-4

4.1 INTRODUCTION

In an ever-changing state, a growing population has accumulated a demand for food, which underlines the event of advanced production technologies and food processes. The increased need for food science research focuses on improving the nutritional quality of foods and food safety. New techniques are introduced to characterize food quality and safety. One such approach is research based on omics, which is especially important for understanding a fundamental phenomenon in food science called foodomics (Herrero et al. 2012). Foodomics is defined as a study of food through the application of advanced omics approaches. Foodomics include genomics, transcription, epigenetics, proteomics, peptidomics, and/or metabolomics to check food safety, food quality, food traceability, and the creation of new bioactive ingredients in food. Marc Wilkins coined the term "proteomics" at the Siena conference in 1994, and the word "proteome" is abbreviated from "protein complement of the genome", meaning the complete set of proteins that a cell expresses (Wilkins et al. 1996). Protein science can be described as a "large-scale analysis of proteins" (Pandey and Mann 2000). "Proteomics also assist in determining their location, interactions, modifications, activities ultimately, and, their function" (Fields 2001).

4.2 BRANCHES OF PROTEOMICS

4.2.1 Protein Separation

All proteomic technologies are based on the ability to separate a complex mixture so that individual proteins are processed more easily with other techniques.

4.2.2 Protein Identification

Known methods include low-throughput sequencing through Edman degradation. High-throughput proteomic technologies rely on MS, typically peptide mass fingerprints on simpler tools or de novo detection sequences replicated on instruments capable of more than one round of MS. Antibody-based assays can also be used, but they are unique to a single sequence motif.

4.2.3 Protein Quantification

Gel-based methods are used, including differential staining of gels with fluorescent dyes (gel electrophoresis variation). Gel-free methods include several labelings or chemical modification methods, such as isotope-encoded affinity tags (ICATs), metal-coded affinity markers (MeCATs), and composite fractional radial chromatography (COFRADIC). Modern-day gel electrophoresis research often leverages software-based image analysis tools primarily to analyze biomarkers by measuring the individual, in addition to showing the separation of one or more protein "points" on a scanned image of a two-dimensional electrophoresis product. In addition, these tools match the stains between gels of similar samples to show, for example, proteomic differences between early and advanced stages of the disease.

4.2.4 Protein Sequence Analysis

This is more than a branch of bioinformatics, dedicated to searching databases for potential proteins or peptide matches, but also functional assignment of domains, prediction of function from the sequence, and evolutionary relationships of proteins.

4.2.5 Structural Proteomics

Related to determining the high-throughput of protein structures in the three-dimensional space. Common methods are X-ray crystallography and NMR (nuclear magnetic resonance) spectroscopy.

4.2.6 Interaction Proteomics

This relates to the investigation of protein interactions at the atomic, molecular, and cellular levels.

4.2.7 Protein Modification

Almost all proteins are modified from the sequence of pure amino acids translated, which is called post-translational modification. Specialized methods have been developed to study phosphoproteomics and glycoproteomics.

4.2.8 Cellular Proteomics

A new branch of proteomics that aims to determine the location of protein-protein interactions in whole cells during major cell events. Centers on the use of techniques such as X-ray tomography and optical fluorescence microscopy.

4.2.9 Experimental Bioinformatics

A branch of bioinformatics, as applied to proteomics, was formulated by Mathias Mann. It involves the mutual design of experimental approaches and bioinformatics to develop (extract) new kinds of information from experiments with proteomics.

4.3 THE MAIN TECHNOLOGIES USED IN PROTEOMICS

One- and two-dimensional gel electrophoresis is used to determine the relative mass of a protein and its isoelectric point. An X-ray and NMR crystallography study are used to characterize the three-dimensional structure of peptides and proteins. However, low-resolution techniques, such as circular dichroism, Fourier transform infrared spectroscopy, and small-angle X-ray scattering, can be used to study the secondary composition of proteins. Tandem mass spectrometry (MS/MS) is used in conjunction with reverse phase chromatography or two-dimensional electrophoresis to identify (by de novo peptide sequencing) and to determine all the levels of proteins present in cells. No-tandem MS, often MALDI-TOF, is used to identify proteins by mass imprinting of the peptide. Less common is this approach is used with high-resolution chromatography and/or mass spectrometry. This procedure is becoming less used, and the technical world no longer accepts absolute discovery of a protein based solely on peptide mass fingerprint data.

Affinity chromatography, two-hybrid yeast techniques, fluorescence resonance energy transfer (FRET), and surface plasmon resonance (SPR) are used to determine protein-protein and DNA-binding interactions. A CT scan uses X-rays to locate the proteins or protein complexes in a healthy cell, much related to the images of cells taken from light microscopes.

Software-based image analysis is used to automate the quantification and spot detection within and between gel samples. While this technology is widely used, intelligence has yet to be mastered. For example, industry-leading software tools tend to agree on analyzing well-separated, well-defined protein spots but present different results and tendencies with less point and less segregation – necessitating manual verification of results.

4.4 APPLICATIONS OF PROTEOMICS IN FOOD SAFETY

The goal of food safety is to prevent any consumer risk to consumers. It is a very complex approach that includes, particularly in the case of food of animal origin, animal management (including welfare) up to manufacturing industries. The main problem with food safety is food poisoning associated with foodborne bacteria, but it is also true that accidental contamination of non-biological materials, alternation of protein shape or contents during food processing, preservation, and cooking, including adulteration and allergy, involve food safety. This section provides some information about how proteomic technologies can help detect foodborne pathogens.

4.4.1 Bacteria

Bacteria are an essential component of food processing, maturation, and ripening. However, there are many instances where bacteria can pose a serious food safety burden, especially in light of increasing antibiotic resistance. This section provides some information about how proteomic technologies can help detect foodborne pathogens. Among the most common pathogens are *E. coli, S. aureus, Campylobacter* spp., and *L. monocytogenes*. Proteomics can provide significant support in understanding the mechanisms of infection, antibiotic resistance, and biofilm formation of food-borne pathogens. There is a lot of literature describing these developments discovered through proteomic techniques. The aim of this section is to focus on recent proteomic developments in the discovery of foodborne pathogens in order to avoid disease outbreaks or health risks. *Escherichia coli* is one of the most common food-borne pathogens responsible for health risks and disease outbreaks. A direct method for gastrointestinal bleeding, *Escherichia coli* O157:H7 has been described by Ochoa and Harrington (2005). This method uses an enrichment step by magnetic beads coated with antibodies specific to O157 antigens. After this enrichment step, the authors were able to detect 2×10^6 cells/mL by analyzing MALDI MS. More recently, Fagerquist and colleagues have successfully applied MALDI-TOF-TOF and MS/MS for the characterization, using a top-down approach, of different subspecies of *Escherichia coli* (STEC) producing Shiga toxins (Fagerquist et al. 2014). Remaining in the area of toxin producers and foodborne pathogens, another burden is represented by *Staphylococcus aureus* that can affect animals and humans. Milk and dairy products can be affected by the presence of mastitis, especially in dairy cows. Subclinical mastitis is one of the burdens most related to milk hygiene and quality worldwide (Coulona et al. 2002). The presence of this pathology negatively interferes with the quality and usability of the milk in its transformation processes. High numbers of somatic cells (somatic cell count) in milk represent an index of mastitis (Harmon 1994) that is also associated with a variable proteome and with different amounts of key important compounds such as fatty acids and lactose (Coulona et al. 2002). In this area, proteomics has provided many advances in the detection of subclinical mastitis in the serum and milk of infected cows. Recently, Turk et al. (2012) and Alonso-Fauste et al. (2012) discovered, both in serum and milk from cows with mastitis, several good candidates of putative biomarkers for subclinical mastitis. In both studies, the technique applied was two-dimensional electrophoresis and gun MS analysis. This information provides relevant insights into the transformation of processed foods. Its use is limited in food science because it is long and cost-consuming. There is still a lot of work to be done in order to improve process automation to reduce costs and time consumption.

4.4.2 Fungi

The big problem in the food chain is the contamination of food, especially grains, with mycotoxins. In special environmental conditions, when temperature and humidity are favorable, molds multiply and can produce mycotoxins. Mycotoxins are toxic secondary metabolites produced by several species of fungi, mainly belonging to the genera *Aspergillus, Penicillium,* and *Fusarium.* The main classes of mycotoxins are ochratoxins, aflatoxins, fumonisins, zearalenone, trichtothecenes, tremor toxins, and ergot alkaloids. In general, it enters the food chain through polluted crops to produce food and forage, especially grains. The presence of mycotoxins in food and feed can be harmful to human and animal health as it can cause adverse effects of various types, such as cancer and mutagenesis, gastrointestinal failure, and kidney failure. Several mycotoxins are also immunosuppressive and decrease resistance to infectious diseases. In this field, proteomics (Doyle 2011) and, to a greater extent, metabolomics (Capriotti et al. 2012) have been used to characterize fungi metabolites and secreted proteins in order to build the most comprehensive knowledge base of secreted proteins and other metabolites (Bhatnagar et al. 2008; Giacometti et al. 2013). Immunohistochemical techniques and chromatography are used routinely to detect mycotoxins. Currently, liquid chromatography coupled to tandem mass spectrometry (LC-MS) is the method of choice for multiple detections of mycotoxins and confirmation purposes (Capriotti et al. 2012; Berthiller et al. 2015). In the past ten years, proteomics has either been used to build a knowledge base (Pechanova et al. 2013) or investigates how different environmental or artificial conditions during fungal growth can modulate fungi stress response (Qin et al. 2007; Kniemeyer 2011; Stoll et al. 2014) or proteome changes during mycotoxin producing conditions (Taylor et al. 2008; Bruns et al. 2010; Crespo-Sempere et al. 2011; Choi 2012). Recently, few proteomic based studies have been conducted to investigate how mycotoxins modulate immunity in vitro (Nogueira da Costa et al. 2011), mitochondrial dynamics (Li et al. 2014) or induce selective toxicity (Mu et al. 2013; Shen et al. 2013; Pan et al. 2014; Zhang et al. 2014).

4.4.3 Other Pathogens

More than bacterial and fungal pathogens, there are also many protozoa and helminths that are responsible for food hazards. Among them are the *Toxoplasma gondii*, *Giardia intestinalis*, and *Taenia* spp. These organisms can be transmitted through water, soil, or contact with people or animals. However, it increases the incidence of its transmission with food, such as undercooked fish, crabs, mollusks, and meats and raw vegetables contaminated with human or animal feces. Cryptosporidiosis is a human gastrointestinal infection that can be a real burden for immunocompromised patients. There is, in fact, no current medicine to control its growth and prevent infection. In order to unravel the mechanisms underlying sporozoite transmission, Snelling and colleagues carried out an experiment of LC-MS/MS coupled with labeling on the N-end of stable isotopes of both oocysts in and out of sporozoites (Snelling et al. 2007).

4.5 DETECTION OF ALLERGENS

The real challenge is identifying the allergens. Oftentimes, hypoallergenic proteins or peptides become allergens when they are overused. Allergens are a matter of public health, mainly because of the dramatically increasing incidence in the last 20 years (Leung et al. 2014). Since there is no cure for allergy, the only way is to avoid anaphylaxis with correct dietary education, with responsible information that involves all the food chain, from farm to fork. Proteomics is the main tool for studying the presence, composition, and nature of food allergens. The risk is now evaluated only with IgE measurements to identify low, medium, or high allergens. It is also clinically important to highlight the difference between sensitization and elicitation proven by new methods. Proteomics can provide new methods for improved assays. There are two loops that can bind IgE: linear and harmonic. The linear elements are closely related to the basic protein structure and are thermoplastic and identifiable by antibodies even after the reduction process. The conformational ones are dependent on the secondary and tertiary protein structure and are thermolabile, and their binding with antibodies is not possible after protein reduction (Picariello et al. 2013). Proteomics can contribute in two ways to identify food allergens – a gel-free approach. It includes a gel-based approach to the two-dimensional electrophoresis workflow, two-dimensional immunohistochemistry, and an MS approach for identifying protein stains. The gel-free approach is characterized by the HPLC-MS/MS approach and the trypsin protein IgE correlation assay. Bioinformatic analysis to detect specific immune epitopes is essential at the end of experiments. Some examples of studies that have been recently performed using two-dimensional electrophoresis for the detection of allergens in several foods are related to beer (Picariello et al. 2015), beef (Apostolovic et al. 2014), milk (Hettinga et al. 2015; Odedra 2015), rice (Goliáš et al. 2013), and fish (Tomm et al. 2013). The absolute amount was assessed by MRM quantities of antigens in the range from 0.5 to 0.7 μg/mg. The progress of this study is represented by using BSA as an internal standard that allowed technical variance to be reduced up to 7% of the scale. Koeberl and colleagues developed a method for the quantification always using MRM (Koeberl et al. 2014). Authors reported an interesting comparison of pros and cons of both immunological and mass spectrometry methods and described the importance of a good selection of each antigen of signature peptides and related transitions.

4.6 FOOD-PROCESSING PROCEDURES

Large-scale food production and processing include the application of mechanical, chemical, and physical treatments to preserve foods by slowing or stopping the natural processes of rotting and increasing preservation time. Depending on the type of food, several processing procedures can be applied individually or in combination. Freezing, heating, drying, fermentation, salting, and the use of chemicals are some of the most popular classic procedures. Other processing treatments are less common (e.g., microwaves, hyper pressure, and pulsed electric fields) or very specific to many foods (e.g., irradiation). Depending on the type of processing techniques, these can improve or lose the nutritional value of food. Over the past ten years, proteomics has been successfully applied to study protein and protein modification in food before and after transformation to obtain valuable information about the molecular changes at the protein level associated with each type of treatment. Heat treatment is one of the most used and studied nutritional transformations. With this kind of treatment, we can obtain food that is microbiologically safe and extend the shelf life. Obviously, the nutritional value of each food is influenced by heat treatments. Milk and dairy products are subjected to different types of thermal treatments from pasteurization (72°C for 15 s) to sterilization by ultra-high-temperature treatment (UHT; 135–150°C for 2–6 s). These actions led to the Maillard reaction, which is the non-enzymatic hydrolysis of amino groups (mainly lysine residues in milk proteins) by reducing sugars (lactose is the main reducing sugar in milk) (Van Boekel 1998). The products of this complex reaction can vary depending on the duration of heating. In milk, lactulosyllysine (bound to many milk proteins) is the main product in the early stage of the heat treatment, and many other reaction products are formed during the advanced stage (longer heat treatment) of the Maillard reaction. In the late nineties, before the advent of proteomics, antibody-based methods was used to detect lactosylated caseins (Fogliano et al. 1997; Tauer et al. 1999) and lactosylated proteins in pasteurized and UHT milk (Pallini et al. 2001). However, these methods were not applicable to characterizing the lactose-binding site. For this reason, several strategies based on mass spectrometric methodologies for the structural analysis of milk proteins have been developed. In 1997, using the recently developed LC-ESI-MS technique in milk whey protein, Leonil and colleagues demonstrated that beta-lactoglobulin concentrate (WPC) was specifically modified by covalent binding of a lactose residue on Lys47 under mild heat treatments due to the early Maillard reaction (Leonil et al. 1997). Using roughly the same approach, Fogliano and colleagues analyzed purified samples subjected to three different thermal treatments: pasteurized (72–85°C for 15–30 s), UHT (142–145°C for 2–5 s), and sterilized (115–120°C for 10–30 min). Lys-100 was determined by mass spectroscopy and structural analysis as the preferential lactosylated site of β-Lg during industrial heat treatments (Fogliano et al. 1998). The 2-DE/MS proteomic approach, combined with multivariate statistics, was also applied to investigate storage time and freezing temperature in fish meat. The authors reported that frozen storage time has a significant effect on the protein profile compared to different freezing temperatures. In particular, the abundance of fragments of several glycolytic and cytoskeletal proteins was directly correlated to the storage time (Kjaersgard et al. 2006).

4.7 PRODUCT ADULTERATION

Food fraud is a worldwide problem today. All valuable ingredients in every food are subject to adulteration. In general, food is adulterated when a valuable ingredient is omitted or replaced in whole or in part with other, lower-quality ingredients, but the definition can be broader and more complex. The use of rapid analysis with high sensitivity and specificity is critical to verify food quality and safety and to ensure consumer health. An adulteration common in the food industry is characterized by congenital contamination in processed foods. Von Bargen et al. (2014) recently applied a targeted proteomic method to detect specific peptides of horse meat and pork in beef products. The authors were able to detect up to 0.24% horse or pork in the beef matrix using an MRM/MRM3 strategy combined with an improved rapid extraction strategy. For the quantitative detection of chicken meat in a mixed-meat food with high reproducibility and sensitivity, Santandreu et al. (2010) implemented a method based on a non-gel fractionation step combined with AQUA labeling MS and detection of selected mucin-3 peptides on the conventional LC-ion trap MS/MS. With this experimental procedure, they were able to detect as low as 0.5% w/v contaminating chicken in pork meat with high confidence (Sentandreu et al. 2010). The two-dimensional gel-based strategy was applied by Montowska and co-workers, and they analyzed differences in the amount of myosin light chain (MLC) in different meat products made from cows, pigs, chickens, turkeys, ducks, and geese

(Montowska and Pospiech 2012). Using this approach, it was possible to detect up to 10% of different meats that degrade at least three isoforms of MLC. In the same samples, the authors searched for other protein markers suitable for use in documenting meat products. Several blood plasma proteins, metabolic enzymes, and regulatory proteins were found as potential targets to build specific tests (Montowska and Pospiech 2013).

Meat adulteration not only involves the fraudulent use of a mixture of meat of various kinds. Oftentimes, soybean proteins are added to meat as emulsifiers to improve their functional properties. Moreover, the low cost of these proteins enhances their use in doses exceeding the permissible limit. In 2006, Leitner used the 2D-LC-MS/MS approach that confidently identified five major high-abundance variants of glycine and all three chains of alpha-conglycine as a marker of soybean proteins in processed meats. Meat adulteration not only involves the fraudulent use of a mixture of meat of various kinds. Oftentimes, soybean proteins are added to meat as emulsifiers to improve their functional properties. Fish-based foods are affected by similar problems, including the fraudulent substitution of high-quality fish with low-quality ones for higher gains. In 2008, Mazzeo and colleagues developed and successfully applied a MALDI-TOF-based method for validating fish. By analyzing protein samples from 25 different fish muscle tissues, it was able within a few minutes to determine a strict distinction between the analyzed species based on the characteristic features of parvalbumins in the MALDI linear spectrum after PMF (Mazzeo et al. 2008). Contrarily to several IEF- and SDS-PAGE-based approaches (Etienne et al. 2000; Rehbein et al. 2000), MALDI-TOF is faster and easily discriminates very close species based if coupled with bioinformatic analysis. Other investigations applied both 2-DE and MALDI-TOF to analyze *Parvalbumin isoforms* in closely related species of the Meluccidae family (Carrera et al. 2006) or different types of tuna fish. Recently Wulff presented an interesting approach for the authentication of fish products (Wulff et al. 2013). The evaluation of the quality of dairy products is mainly based on the traditional procedures genetic (Mayer and Fiechter 2013), chromatographic (Cserháti et al. 2005; Mayer and Fiechter 2013), electrophoretic (Cserháti et al. 2005; Mayer and Fiechter 2013), and immunoenzymatic (Hurley et al. 2004b) methods. In addition, several proteomic-based techniques have been implemented to assess the validity of dairy products and to quickly and accurately detect fraud. To highlight differences in the protein profile of milk from five different species (cow, goat, buffalo, horse, and camel), Hinz and co-workers applied a classical 2-DE/MS-based approach (Hinz et al. 2012). Other similar attempts have been made using gel-based (Yang et al. 2014) or gel-free approaches. An ITRAQ-based approach was applied by Yang et al. (2013) to obtain a quantitative differential and functional expression pattern of 211 proteins from the milk whey fraction of cow, yak, buffalo, goat, and camel. As suggested by the authors, the results form a knowledge base for assessing the adulteration of expensive dairy with cow's milk or low-quality milk. The MALDI-TOF MS approach proved to be a fast, simple, and accurate analytical method for assessing the presence of cow's milk in sheep's or water buffalo's milk or for the detection of powdered milk in fresh milk (Cozzolino et al. 2001), down to a 1% of adulteration level (Calvano et al. 2013).

4.8 CHEMICALS AND OTHER CONTAMINANTS

Not only is proteomics useful for the detection of biological hazards, but as described below, it can also provide a reliable indirect index of contamination with xenobiotics. One example is represented by the documented differential protein expression of oysters in relation to $HgCl_2$ contamination. Zhang and colleagues described the differential protein expression of 13 proteins, and four of them showed interesting features as possible biomarkers to be applied for the detection of Hg contamination in food (Zhang et al. 2013). Illicit corticosteroid therapy also represents a burden on food safety. Guglielmetti and colleagues reported bovine paroxonase/arylesterase 1 (PON1) as a specific and reliable biomarker for corticosteroid therapy (Guglielmetti et al. 2014). In both cases, the method used is two-dimensional electrophoresis combined with MS, and the proposed protein represents an indirect biomarker for detecting dangerous chemical contamination.

4.9 PROTEOMIC APPLICATION IN HEALTHCARE

4.9.1 The Application of Proteomics in Human Health

People are able to modify themselves in response to the atmosphere through mental, physical, psychological, and social changes (Huber et al. 2011). Human health could divide into physical and mental health. Physical health relates to maintaining the state of the human body in good health, dietary type, and environmental factors. Mental health is related to the psychological state of a person, while physical health is greatly affected by mental health and vice versa. Both genetic and environmental factors are associated with complex human traits. The genetic factor accounts for approximately 50% plus the environmental factor in human health traits. The human trait is affected not only by variation in DNA but also by modification of gene expression (Georgiades et al. 2017). The structure of the gut microbiome and the rapid metabolism of the resveratrol system determine the end product of the metabolites. Resveratrol affects cardiovascular risk factors, such as increased blood cholesterol or trimethylamine N-oxide levels (Bird et al. 2017). In human health, the average risk indicators for arsenic as an example of the environmental factor were below 1. This result demonstrated that there were no non-carcinogenic risks to arsenic. In addition, the cancer risk from arsenic was within the acceptable range (less than 1×10^{-4}), indicating a low to very low risk for the exposed population (Zhou et al. 2017). A complex and interconnected link between sleep apnea and cardiovascular disease occurs where sleep disturbances adversely affect the structure and function of the heart and blood vessels. Disruptive sleep apnea is associated with an increased incidence of heart failure, stroke, atrial fibrillation, and coronary heart disease. Thus, sustained stress restores obstructive sleep apnea. Moreover, various clinical observations of the treated patient are also recorded continuously, such as drowsiness, quality of life, and mood, and at the same time, cardiovascular endpoints, such as blood pressure, ejection fraction, vascular parameters, and arrhythmia, are also treated (Drager et al. 2017). Metabolic examination is performed to identify nutrient components such as lipoic acid, pectin, and polysaccharides. These components have a synergistic and complementary role with female and male hormones that play an important and significant role in the state of human health. These nutrients and hormones protect human health from colon cancer and preserve human health (Koriem 2017a). From the previous data, it is evident that the human diet, exercise, and sleep are the main factors that affect the status of human health.

4.9.2 The Application of Proteomics in Human Diet

A healthy complementary diet is very important and required to maintain human health. Healthy and complete food items should contain plant and animal products. This food is essential for supplying energy with energy, maintaining the human physiological process in hemostasis, building human muscles, and regulating blood pressure and body temperature. The relationship between diet and human health or disease is critically important in both biomarker discovery and clinical applications. In one study, a protein analysis was performed after ingesting sweetened dried cranberries in the urine and feces of a sample of ten healthy people. Protein analysis was based on the mass spectra of different urine proteins. The intake of sweetened dried cranberries caused many changes in 22 proteins in the urinary tract and multiple sequences of 16S fecal ribosome genes RNA genes that negatively impacted human health (Bekiares et al. 2017). In another study, a proteomic test showed that a low dose of freeze-dried oregano suppressed tumor frequency by 55.5%, tumor incidence by 44%, and tumor volume by 44.5% compared to control animals. Mouse tumor cells analysis showed that Ki67 and VEGFR-2 were decreased, while caspase-3 expression increased after low-dose freeze-fried oregano treatment (Kubatka et al. 2017). The tremendous and very rapid developments in proteomic research in the last decade have helped discover the relationship between human-related microbes and the role of the human immune system. This research can help prevent and treat chronic diseases, including allergies. Advances in proteomic studies are useful for understanding the environmental impact on human health and the human impact on all surrounding organisms, which are very important to human health. This concept can affect health and disease in all human life (Renz et al. 2017). Obesity is a major health crisis worldwide. The proteomic studies correlate with brain lipid toxicity that occurs in impaired brain function on a high-fat diet. There are significant differences in brain proteins that occurred in mass-spectrometry-based proteomic analysis. These proteins are mainly associated with oxidative stress, glycolysis, and calcium signaling (Smine et al. 2017). The proteomic approach helps maintain digestive function and health. Meta-proteomics and real-time PCR and DNA fingerprints are two of the primary methods implemented. The human diet with lower fat and higher fiber increased the activity of beneficial bacteria and excretion of fecal fatty acids, especially butyrate, while the human diet with high fat and less fiber stimulated another bacterium that has a negative impact on human health (Heinritz et al. 2016). In another research, the results obtained showed that the inflammatory proteins in the liver were greater after oral administration of saturated fatty acid compared to inflammatory proteins in the liver after oral administration of monounsaturated fatty acids in the high-fat diet. Dietary administration of monounsaturated fatty acids in a high percentage of lipids caused an important and important process of cholesterol transmission between different groups in the liver. From these results, it can be concluded that new biomarkers of a damaged liver were developed and reflected from the in vivo reverse cholesterol transporter estimated from protein levels on high-density lipoproteins (HDL) (O'Reilly et al. 2016). There is a big difference in both the progressive age and the professional environment. This can greatly increase the triggering of human resistance. These observations were recently reported using lung matrix proteomic analysis. There was stimulation of myofibroblasts and a growth diversion of the factor-beta signaling pathway in the case of additional matrix proteins deposition (Calhoun et al. 2016).

4.9.3 The Application of Proteomics in Human Exercise

Human training program exercise improves or maintains fitness, general health, and wellness. Exercise supports muscles, restores the cardiovascular system, and promotes hemostasis in the human body. Changes in food quality, habits, and exercise increase susceptibility to obesity. A lazy lifestyle causes an imbalance in blood flow that affects cardiovascular function in pregnant women. Nitric oxide composition and bioavailability are controlled by endothelial cell antioxidant activity. These observations disturb the health of the mother's blood vessels and the vascular functioning of the placenta and thus the healthy growth of the fetus and blood flow to the placenta. All of the above observations are controlled by neonatal proteomic and metabolism (Cid and González 2016). This proteomic assay focuses on an exercise-related proteomic that is characterized by the generation of adenosine triphosphate generation, oxygen delivery, antioxidant activity, and regulation of mitochondrial protein synthesis. A vigorous and intense training program controls the processes of oxidative phosphorylation and the carboxylic acid cycle within the human body. The metabolism of amino acids and the leakage of calcium ions into the cytosol are controlled by exercise. Proteomics are controlled by exercise style, strength, intensity, schedule, and muscle type. These analyses of molecular networks are controlled by a sports training program in health and disease, and these findings support the therapeutic effect of exercise (Padrão et al. 2016). A two-dimensional proteomic analysis was performed. One-sided lower limb suspension caused a reduction in the muscle-fibrous protein content, metabolism (glycolytic and oxidative stress), and antioxidant defense system protein content. Long-term, unilateral lower-limb suspension did not prevent the beneficial and beneficial effects of exercise on human muscle (Brocca et al. 2015). The proteomic analysis aims to evaluate intensive and long-term training exercises in healthy and sick populations. This exercise reduces lipids while increasing enzyme activity and harmful bases for vascular progression. There are differential changes in the DNA expression of methyl and microRNA (miRNA) in skeletal muscle in an intense and vigorous exercise program (Rowlands et al. 2014). Both maternal separation stress and exercise separation stress are performed by the proteomic technique through isobaric labeling and MS/MS using matrix/ionization with laser. Maternal separation stress controls hippocampal proteins that occur in energy metabolism, such as enolase, triosephosphate isomerase, and nucleoside diphosphate kinase B. Maternal separation stress alters the synaptic plasticity such as the neurocan core protein, tenascin-R, alpha-synuclein, Bal–667, and Prevacan. Exercise stops many changes by inhibiting the secretions of hippocampal proteins linked to energy metabolism, such as nucleoside diphosphate kinase B, enolase, and triosephosphate isomerase. The exercise also stops synaptic plasticity proteins, such as Bal–667, brevican, α-synuclein, tenascin-R, and the essential neurotransmitter proteins. Therefore, both exercise stress and maternal separation pressures have conflicting effects on hippocampus proteins in the brain (Dimatelis et al. 2013).

4.9.4 The Application of Proteomics in Human Sleep

Sleep is a vital factor in maintaining human health. Sleep is extremely important for growth and development in childhood. Persistent sleep disturbance is compatible with long-term health problems. Proteomic analysis reveals that humans with myopia show higher serum melatonin levels than those found in people without deficiency. This indicates the important and fundamental roles of human exposure to light and the rhythm of the circadian rhythm in the mechanism of development of myopia in humans (Kearney et al. 2017). The red blood cell proteomic technology revealed that obstructive sleep apnea (OSA) is associated with many and varied proteins. Red blood cell samples were taken and collected from patients with moderate and severe obstructive sleep apnea in the pre- and post-night period. The MS technology identified 31 proteins, including 21 unique and different proteins, as a result of the existence of post-translation modification regulations. Most of the proteins are associated with catalytic activity, oxidoreductase, peroxidase, hydrolase, adenosine tri-phosphatase, and antioxidant activity. In the morning, a greater number of differential proteins were observed, including response to chemical stimuli, oxidation reduction, regulation of catalytic activity, and stress response in OSA (Feliciano et al. 2017). The effect of sleep on the level of melatonin in the brain where proteomic and genomic studies related to melatonin receptor 1 and melatonin receptor 2 reveals 378 different proteins. Some of these proteins are presynaptic proteins that interact with melatonin receptor 1 but not with melatonin receptor 2, and these observations indicate a major role of melatonin receptor 1 in neurotransmission. The melatonin receptor 1 appears in the hypothalamus, striatum, and cortex, so melatonin receptor 1 is part of the presynaptic protein network (Benleulmi-Chaachoua et al. 2016). The general public health concerns that cause and maintain many adverse effects on cardiovascular health is sleep apnea. Advances and advanced proteomic research are essential to identifying new disease mediators as important diagnostic and treatment targets for many diseases, including OSA (Feliciano et al. 2015). OSA is linked to obesity and diabetes. These complications include metabolic irregularity and cardiovascular imbalance. The incidence of complication disorders in obesity and diabetes can be improved through new and advanced techniques, such as analyzing proteomics that improves health outcomes for the negative consequences of sleep apnea and thus reduces the risk of sleep disorders (Seetho and Wilding 2013). Modern technology is applied like proteomics in OSA. PCR is the most widely applied technique, especially in the field of sleep medicine, and provides good and bright insights into the conditions related to OSA, enabling the diagnosis and management of complex sleep disorders (Tan et al. 2014).

4.9.5 The Application of Proteomics in Human Disease

Human disease refers to an abnormal human condition that affects a specific part of the person or the entire human body. This includes disturbance of the human structure or function. There are external factors, such as pathogens, and internal factors, such as hypersensitivity (sensitivity and autoimmunity), that cause human disease. Any condition that causes human distress, social problems, pain, dysfunction, or death is called human disease. Human disease is usually accompanied by human disorders, syndromes, infections, injuries, disabilities, unusual behaviors, and abnormal personalities. A proteomic study using mass spectrometry (nLC-MS/MS) technology assists in mapping the proteomic landscape of diffuse UV-spread human melanoma cells. The data obtained led to a molecular network that explored the dual nature of UV rays of both anti-tumor and anti-neoplastic agents in cytological assays for metastatic melanoma. This proteomic technology helps develop new biomarkers and expand new treatments for disease (Konstantakou et al. 2017). The term "proteoform" has been used to describe all molecular variation formulas in which a protein molecule can occur from a single gene. There have been many, many efforts to develop techniques to characterize proteoform (Chen et al. 2017). In a new and recent clinical study, chemokine receptor proteomic investigations showed significant and significant differences created and recorded between cells obtained from both chronic lymphocytic leukemia and small lymphocytic lymphoma patients. As a result, higher expression of transporter receptor and lower expression of adhesion molecules was detected in chronic lymphocytic leukemia cells (CLCs) compared to small lymphoma cells, so small lymphocytic lymphoma cells were more advanced than chronic lymphocytic leukemia (CLL) (Tooze et al. 2017). In another study, there are four plasma proteins and these proteins: (1) sex-hormone-binding globulin (SHBG), (2) apolipoprotein C-1, (3) gelsolin, and (4) complement component C4-A expressed in stomach cancer patients. The SHBG protein is frequently expressed in GC patients, and GC patients have SHBG levels above the control level. Sex, age, and disease stage affect patient group level. These results demonstrated that LC associated with mass spectra is more suitable for detecting plasma biomarkers, and SHBG is a sensitive and accurate plasma biomarker for GC control (Cheng et al. 2018). Protein structure and function are affected in developmental and metabolic disturbances that occurred after exposure to low levels of di-n-butyl phthalate in the application of proteomic assays. Both BPA and di-n-butyl phthalate control the expression levels of several proteins, which provide us with good information for actions of BPA and di-n-butyl phthalate on the evolutionary systems (Dong et al. 2018). Proteomic study has been applied previously in Parkinson's disease, where resveratrol therapy affected specific unregulated biological processes, such as redox homeostasis, cellular reduction, and protein homeostasis. Resveratrol was also effective in restoring heat shock protein network and protein degradation systems. Administration of resveratrol caused an increase in glutathione level with reduced oxidized glutathione/decreased glutathione and reduced free thiol content in the patient's cells compared to normal fibroblasts. Thus, resveratrol maintains cellular homeostasis in parkin metastatic fibroblasts (Vergara et al. 2017). In general, there are four basic types of human diseases: (1) infectious diseases, (2) deficiency diseases, (3) genetic diseases, and (4) physiological diseases.

4.9.6 The Application of Proteomics in Human Infectious Disease

There are many external microbial agents that cause infectious diseases in humans. These agents include viruses, bacteria, fungi, and parasites. The viral envelope contains the main factor for the effect of the virus, which is called spike (S) glycoprotein. The S protein contains 29 glycosylation sites. These aids in protein folding and protein function S. The proteomic technique used for infectious bronchitis virus protein S reveals eight sites. These sites are important for the functions of infectious bronchitis S protein (Zheng et al. 2018). About 101 proteins were expressed in the bile sample of primary sclerosing cholangitis patients compared to the control group. The majority were intracellular and associated with ribosomal and protozoal pathways. Another 91 proteins were identified in the control's bile sample; most of them were from the extracellular space and were associated with cellular adhesion, the coagulation cascade, and the complementary system (Rupp et al. 2018). Lipids communicate with proteomic to play a vital role in infectious diseases. The role of lipids in biological processes includes many processes, such as biological components, host lipids, and proteins. There are many molecules of phosphatases, kinases, and lipases included in lipid technology (Koriem 2017b). Twelve proteins were isolated and identified from falciparum malaria. These proteins replicated the inherent parasite epitopes by applying the fluorescence technique (Nikolaeva et al. 2020). Proteomic methods, such as liquid chromatographic mass spectra and the matrix-assisted laser absorption/ionization with flight time/flight time, revealed the presence of a genin that contains trypsin-like activities that aid in the digestion of trypsin factor family peptides (Chaiyarit et al. 2017). The quantitative proteomic method identified protein virulence and drug resistance in three clinical samples of *Escherichia coli* strains. Therefore, protein assays should be applied in microbiological diagnostic laboratories to determine drug resistance in *Escherichia coli* infection (Kalule et al. 2018).

4.9.7 The Application of Proteomics in Human Deficiency Disease

Lack of essential and vital nutrients, such as vitamins and minerals, is the main cause of human deficiency disease. Proteomic tests and histological assays were applied to verify the aggressive behavior reported in cutaneous squamous cell carcinoma (cSCC) patients. The cSCC patients showed signs of UVB injury, high mutational rates, tissue damage, and inflammation. Histological analysis confirmed these results. The cSCC patients are of high risk associated with enhanced bacterial challenge. Histological analysis revealed the association of bacterial colonization with worst prognosis. Protein identification could serve as potential diagnostic markers and therapeutic targets in high-risk cSCC patients (Föll et al. 2018). There is an effective termination between the Baf60a and Baf60c subunits of SWI/SNF chromatin remodeling complex as regulators of metabolic gene programs in maintaining oxidative and glycolytic metabolism in skeletal muscle fibers and endurance, which is responsible for impaired skeletal muscle energy metabolism linking to the pathogenesis of insulin resistance/glucose intolerance in T2D. The transcriptional assay identifies the thermogenic program of muscle and myokine secretion as a major stimulus involved in the metabolism of muscle fibers by demonstrating a complete energy balance between them. The Baf60 skeletal muscle deficit explains the disconnect between exercise toughness and adequate metabolic balance (Meng et al. 2018). There are 315 proteins occurring in soil-borne parasitic worms (*Ancylostoma caninum*, ESPs [AcES]) using a new advanced proteomic technology compared to only 105 previously identified. The largest group of proteins are SCP/TAPs (110 of the 315 proteins), while the richest constituents of AcES are tissue inhibitors of the metalloprotease family. There are also new groups of candidates vaccines and immunomodulatory proteins (Morante et al. 2017). Proteomic tests were also performed to study the effect of riboflavin deficiency on protein expression in HepG2 hepatocytes. The liquid chromatography method linked to mass spectra (LC-MS/MS) was used to determine riboflavin deficiency. The obtained cell viability and apoptosis results confirmed that riboflavin was essential in maintaining the cellular activity of hepatocyte HepG2 cells. The proteomic test identified 37 proteins after riboflavin deficiency. Observations after riboflavin deficiency showed an escalating regulation of the following biochemical cycles: (1) steroid catabolism, (2) apoptosis, (3) endoplasmic reticulum stress, and (4) the pathway of Parkinson's disease, while riboflavin insufficiency caused decreased regulation of many biochemical processes, such as (1) fatty acid metabolism, (2) the tricarboxylate citrate cycle, (3) oxidative phosphorylation, (4) iron metabolism (Xin et al. 2017). There are four proteins associated with emphysema, and these proteins can be summarized as follows: (1) C-reactive protein, (2) adipocyte-binding protein, (3) leptin, and (4) tissue plasminogen activator. Leptin is associated with the progression of emphysema and depends on age and gender. All four proteins mentioned above were associated with BMI after further modification (Beiko et al. 2017). The proteomic tests have been used to identify aortic valve disease. The proteomic-specific functions, pathways, and interactions depended on valve stiffening associated with age and genotype. Protein differences were dependent on Emilin1 deficiency, such as pathways, functions, and biomechanical abnormalities (Angel et al. 2017). The proteomic shows that biosynthetic actions in each mutation, such as (1) cell wall, (2) cell membrane phospholipids, and (3) ergosterol, were rejected at both transcriptomic and translational levels. In mitochondrial activities, such as function, glycolysis/gluconeogenesis, and ROS scavengers, the genetic differences contrasted with proteinaceous data in mutations. Thus, the loss of energy production in mutations is compensated for by increased protein levels in glycolysis, glycogenesis, and anti-ROS in mutagenic survival (She et al. 2018).

4.9.8 The Application of Proteomics in Human Genetic Disease

This type of disease begins through genetic disorders that occur in the human genetic map. The majority of genetic disorders are rare and affect a single person in a community or communities. Genetic disease has two main types: (1) hereditary disease, which is passed from the genes of parents to the fetus, and (2) mutational disease, which results from new mutations in the DNA. Proteomic and metabolic tests are connected together, especially in inherited metabolic disorders. MS techniques are successes in this case. MS is the method most used in both proteomic and metabolomic tests due to its ability to analyze a wide range of molecules, their optimal dynamic range, their great sensitivity, and the rapid identification of many metabolite molecules in many body fluids and small samples used, such as dried blood spots.

These techniques maintain the timely diagnosis of inherited metabolic disorders and facilitate early treatment application (Costanzo et al. 2017). In another study, the proteomic test recorded an upward upregulation of seven proteins, and these proteins are as follows: (1) C-reactive protein, (2) heat shock protein 27, (3) keratin KB40, (4) T-complex protein-10, (5) chaperonin containing T-complex protein-1, (6) albumin, and (7) keratin. There is a downregulation of three other proteins, and these proteins are as follows: (1) apolipoprotein A1, (2) precursor phospholipase A2, and (3) phospholipase C-α. There are a higher upregulation of 118 genes and a lower downregulation of 28 genes out of 146 total genes. These genes are associated with inflammation and mucin production (Lee et al. 2018). The proteomic approaches showed molecular fingerprints for the I complex, which had a significant specialty in synaptic mitochondria. There are at least 30% of mitochondrial enzyme activity changes that correlate with protein richness. Molecular differences between mitochondrial subgroups could have an effect on synaptic morphology in vivo (Graham et al. 2017). Differently expressed proteins have been associated with the inflammatory immune response. The protein-protein interactions test revealed a new relationship between the vitamin-binding protein D and the methylenetetrahydrofolate reductase genotype C677T, and this relationship was established through a molecular genotype (Zhang et al. 2017). The proteomic assay related to physiological analysis showed that H_2O_2 stress caused stressful phenotypes, such as increased H_2O_2 content in vivo, decreased photosynthesis rate, higher osmolarity, accumulation of antioxidants, and increased activities of several reactive oxygen species that cleanse enzymes (Yu et al. 2017). Alzheimer's disease damages protein synthesis at an early stage. Exposure to oxygen improved mental function and reduced mitochondrial damage in Alzheimer's disease. Increased exposure to oxygen halted the damage in protein synthesis, and thus, the synthesis of many different proteins involved in mRNA binding, transcription regulation, and translation has been reported. The methionine oxidation and all body oxidation levels were similar in the oxygen exposure group and the control group. These observations indicated that the oxygen exposure did not cause any increase in the levels of peptide oxidation. Exposure to oxygen increased the regulation of many different proteins involved in antioxidant defense (Wang et al. 2017).

4.9.9 The Application of Proteomics in Human Physiological Disease

A physiological disease occurs when the normal function of the human body is affected by a defect in the functions of human organs. In other words, a physiological disease is an abnormal human condition that modifies normal body functions, leading to pain and weakness, and is associated with certain symptoms and signs. Protein, metabolism, and transcription techniques have been used to visualize human organs with physiological application in non-alcoholic fatty liver disease in a simple screen. All of these technologies aid in the detection of the vital signs of disease, knowledge of disease, and evaluation of new drug development (Cole et al. 2017). IgM M phosphorylcholine induced increased regulatory T cells in healthy donors, systemic lupus erythematosus (SLE) patients, and atherosclerotic cells, while control antibodies did not. T cells in SLE of patients caused levels of regulatory T cells while causing increased levels of Th17 cells compared to control. In this study, a decrease in the secretion of IL-17 and TNFα was observed in SLE patients and atherosclerotic cells in immunoglobulin M (IgM) antibodies. The de novo protein sequencing method was used and revealed that IgM peptide was expressed in anti-PC compared to control antibody (Sun et al. 2017). Kruppel-like factor 15 (KLF15) is vital in controlling the lipid cycle in adipocytes. As a result, the mice with a deficiency of KLF15 in adipose tissue showed a reduction in obesity and a protection against obesity. This result relates to KLF15, which controls many genes in triglyceride formation, and the lipolysis action reduces the process. Therefore, an increase in fat storage is observed. In conclusion, KLF15 is a necessary lipid regulator of adipocyte lipid metabolism and energy balance (Matoba et al. 2017). There is an increase in photosynthetic-related proteins like rubisco, ATP synthase delta chain, plastocyanin, eIF4 metabolism-related proteins, and protease subunits. There is also an increase in proteins associated with the cytoskeleton, such as the protein transporting phosphatidylinositol and porphylline in the tea variety Dongchall at low temperature and light. The histone H4, the histone H2A.1, congeners, the putative protein, and the linear protein 28 control the development of winter buds and their adaptation to adverse conditions (Liu et al. 2017). The proteolytic method showed that a secreted exosome was found in the human sweat as 1,062 proteins were detected in the outer body of the sweat, and these proteins included 997 different proteins and 896 unique proteins compared to urine, saliva, and exogenous plasma. Several antimicrobial and immunomodulatory peptides are found in the outer sweat. Therefore, the outer particle of sweat plays an important and major role in skin immunity. The sweat proteomic assay helps in determining the physiological importance of exosomes in immune homeostasis (Wu and Liu 2018). There are 245 and 379 IDs that were identified through the proteomic tests ProteinPilot and the Mascot software, respectively. There are 133 protein identifiers identified by the shaker peptide assay. Also, there is a well-established relationship between 127 proteins pathways and 349 different genes. These data are critically important in characterizing sheep circulating in cell protein using liquid chromatography associated with mass spectra. This peptide spectroscopy data contributes to the protein library, which aids in identifying the bulk and diverse proteins in sheep serum (Chemonges et al. 2017). There was a main and significant decline in tyrosine nitrate in the YYCFQGNQFLR peptide. This nitrate occurs in the site of hemopexin binding to human hemopexin. These nitrates are similar to the hemopexin nitrate in rabbits and rats. Tyrosine nitrate was detected in both in vivo and in vitro models by immune fermentation and selective reaction control (Hahl et al. 2017).

4.9.10 The Protective Role of Proteomics in Human Health and Disease

Cathelicidins are peptides to be taken by mouth. These peptides are originated from defense. Cathelicidins play a vital and important role within the human body as antimicrobial, immunomodulatory, wound-healing, angiogenic and cancer-fighting agents (Khurshid et al. 2017). New technologies such as proteomics, metabolomics, genomics, and transcription allow the discovery and classification of large and diverse microorganisms in many media of the ecosystem, such as the digestive system, the skin, the airway, and the genitourinary system and to identify all genomes in these ecosystems also as their genetic products. These aforementioned tests revealed that everyone has their own ecosystem that plays a vital role in human health and disease. These techniques aid in understanding the pathogenesis of human diseases. Technologies aid in diagnostic, curative, and preventive studies in medicine (Blum 2017). Many different pathogens bind to natural killer (NK) cells by stimulating immunity. Respiratory virus (human metapneumovirus [HMPV]) is responsible for acute respiratory infection in children worldwide. In 70% of children (below 5 years old), HMPV infection may be fatal. The NK p46 is a normal cytotoxic receptor in humans for HMPV-infected cells. The NK cells that are most active are NK lung cells and NK blood cells, regardless of HMPV infection (Diab et al. 2017). Nitric oxide and S-nitrosylation-dependent superoxide of the cysteine protein affect both terminated and disease proteins. Proteomic tests revealed 93 proteins and 111 nitroxyl-modified proteins in human heart failure patients. There was an increase in macrophage cell leakage, free radical secretion, and cell death, while a decrease in fatty acid metabolism was recorded in human heart failure patients. The most obvious proteins detected by proteomic analysis are (1) ATP-synthase, (2) thrombospondin-1, and (3) vinculin, as these proteins can be used as biomarkers to detect heart failure (Koo et al. 2016). Several inflammatory diseases, such as (1) obesity, (2) poor wound healing from diabetes syndromes, and (3) atherosclerosis are closely related to dysfunction of monocytes and macrophages. The identification of specific S-glutathionylated proteins and the mechanisms that control protein alteration in monocytes and macrophages can aid both preventive and treatment research focusing on atherosclerosis and metabolic disease (Short et al. 2016). *SORBS1* is a human gene that plays an important and major role in the transmission of insulin signaling, and this gene contains an open homology domain and three SH3 domains in the C peripheral region. An association has been observed between genetic changes of *SORBS1*, blood pressure, hypertension, and age when the hypertension occurs (Chang et al. 2016). There was a significant difference in glutathione types and metabolic status of patients with terminal liver disease in transplantation surgery compared with healthy controls. The following acids play a significant and vital role in HCC patients with the use of proteomic tests: citric acid, succinic acid, myristic acid, L-methionine, D-threitol, fumaric acid, pipecolic acid, isoleucine, glycolic, hydroxy-butyrate, steraric acid, and hexanoic acid. Therefore, the types of glutathione and metabolic patterns determined the severity of liver disease and the degree of hepatocellular carcinoma in patients (Sanabria et al. 2016). Sepsis infection, meningitis, and pneumonia are caused in pigs and humans by *Streptococcus suis* type 2. Streptococcus toxic shock syndrome exerts its influence through the *virD4* gene in both pigs and humans. Streptococcus toxic shock syndrome infection, meningitis, and pneumonia decreased by 65%. The percentage of bacteria decreases in the liver and brain. And the lower expression of inflammatory cytokines was found by detection of the *virD4* gene. Therefore, the *virD4* gene plays an important role in the pathogenesis of streptococcus toxic shock syndrome through its anti-phagocytic activity and higher regulation of its expression (Jiang et al. 2016). Expression of sodium/potassium transporting ATPase interacting with two genes (*NKAIN2*) in prostate cancer cell progression by inhibiting apoptosis, increasing cell movement and attack. Knockdown of *NKAIN2* increases prostate cancer cell progression by inhibiting apoptosis and increasing cell movement and attack. The *NKAIN2* gene is similar to a new tumor suppressor gene that has decreased activity in prostate cancer. It stops the disease progression by inducing apoptosis and suppressing the growth, movement, and attack of cancer cells (Mao et al. 2016). There is a specific and important region that plays a vital and essential role in cases of T2D. This region is Cg19693031, which lies within the 3'-untranslated region of the protein interacting with thioredoxin. Therefore, the thioredoxin-interacting protein is expressed in diabetic animals and humans, and the 3'-untranslated regions of this protein play as major promoters in gene expression (Florath et al. 2016).

4.9.11 Treating the Role of Proteomics in Human Health and Disease

The proteomic test is used to screen the Cisd2 protein, a key regulator of mice age and the gene for Wolfram syndrome in humans, within the calf muscle after midlife in mice. The results showed that there was a 70% deficiency of Cisd2 protein in an aging animal model of the leg. There is also a defect in the regulation of calcium signaling, Sercal activity is significantly impaired. Therefore, Cisd2 protein is essential for calf muscle and is a therapeutic protein for muscle aging (Huang et al. 2018). Cdc42BPA protein and Cdc42 signaling cycle are important for the occurrence of colon cancer. Turning off Cdc42BPA and Cdc42 signaling reduces the incidence of colon cancer cells. Cdc42BPA protein expression is increased in colon cancer tissues and is upregulated in metastases in lymph nodes. The metastases and death of colon cancer patients depend on the expression of the Cdc42BPA protein. Thus, the incidence of colon cancer depends on Cdc42BPA and Cdc42 signals, and the Cdc42BPA protein is used to diagnose and treat colon cancer (Hu et al. 2018). Hair examination is a key factor in controlling many biological disorder processes, such as (1) long term compliance with drugs, (2) chronic alcohol abuse, and (3) forensic toxicology. The proteomic method is applied to understand the morphology of human hair and is used as a diagnostic tool in medicine where human hair is made mostly of proteins (Adeola et al. 2018). Genome regulation controls both normal and diseased conditions. The genome base is controlled by chromatin remodeling complexes. These chromatin-remodeling complexes are studied by the proteolytic method. The proteomic assay includes (1) determination of the content, (2) determining of regulation, and (3) investigation of the dynamics of complexes under different cellular states (Eubanks et al. 2017). Proteinology provides important informational data on the role of various proteins in health and diseases, such as inflammatory bowel disease. These studies help to understand the effects of different proteins in different periods of disease and the different pathways that increase or decrease in different periods of an inflammatory process. Proteomics explains the expressions of proteins in different biochemical processes, such as (1) inflammation, (2) cellular structure, (3) stress of the endoplasmic reticulum, and (4) energy reduction in both inflammation and therapy. The role of mesenteric lymphocytes, exosomes, and the muco-intestinal barrier, and the beneficial effects of some therapeutic drugs and food ingredients on enteritis can also be achieved by controlling protein expression (Mourad et al. 2017).

Forty-eight proteins were expressed in apical periodontitis compared with healthy periodontitis by the application of the protease method. Thirty of the 48 proteins were expressed in all four lesions. Expression of heat shock protein 27 and sorbin family B's member 1 was double-expressed in epithelial periodontitis. An increase in expression of heat shock protein 27 was recorded in epithelial cells, while expression of member 1 of the sorbin family B was detected in neutrophils and epithelial cells (Cavalla et al. 2017). The human respiratory system is greatly susceptible to diseases and complications. There are many different lung diseases, such as lung cancer, tuberculosis, and chronic obstructive pulmonary disease, and these diseases are the most common causes of death worldwide.

Cystic fibrosis is the most common genetic disease in Caucasians. It has many and varied effects on the lungs. Respiratory proteomic plays an important role in explaining disease mechanism and lung pathology, as well as biomarkers and treatment strategies. A protease test has the ability to isolate proteins from a specific cell mass. The higher the protein isolate is, the more protein discovery (Tan et al. 2018). Cystic fibrosis transmembrane conductance regulator (CFTR) is a dynamic process controlled by multiple protein processes. Proteomic testing is a better method for the human respiratory system, cystic fibrosis epithelial cell lines, and specific molecular mechanisms that have occurred in cystic fibrosis. There are several molecular mechanisms that regulate CFTR-associated pathways, such as (1) thermal shock response, (2) cytoskeleton crosstalk and signal transduction, (3) chronic inflammation, and (4) CFTR alteration. These data are important in understanding cystic fibrosis and pharmacological treatments for cystic fibrosis in order to alleviate the instability of the 508CFTR membrane and thus extend the life of patients with cystic fibrosis (Puglia et al. 2018). The expression of cystathionine β-synthase (CBS) in renal tubular epithelial cells in human and rat renal tissue was inversely proportional with the progression of the fibrous disease. In CBS, the worsening extracellular matrix decreased the induced tumor growth factor 1, exacerbating extracellular matrix deposition in vitro. Inflammatory factors were increased in CBS hexokinase-2 reductase cells stimulated by IL-1. CBS is a new inhibitor in renal fibrosis and a novel therapeutic agent in patients with chronic kidney disease (Yuan et al. 2017). Both the epithelium of the human stomach and the mucous layers are affected by *Helicobacter pylori* (gram-negative bacteria). *Helicobacter pylori* is the main cause of chronic gastritis, peptic ulceration, and stomach cancer. Proteins have an impact on many branches of medicine, such as (1) understanding the molecular basis of infection, (2) identifying a specific drug, and (3) discovering disease biomarkers. The role of bacteria and their most virulent factor in the development of gastric cell transformation and cancer have been investigated by proteomic tests (Bernardini et al. 2017).

4.9.12 The Application of Proteomics in Epidemic Diseases

Epidemics (pandemics) wreak havoc on human life and are not just problems from the ancient world. A series of recent viral outbreaks, including HIV, Ebola, influenza, Zika, and SARS-CoV-2, have risen to the rank of epidemics. The recent and ongoing coronavirus disease (COVID-19) caused by SARS-CoV-2 has caused more than one million deaths and infected more than thirty-seven million people worldwide, according to a WHO report. Prevention, early diagnosis, and early treatment are the keys to managing the epidemic. Proteomics can play an important role in understanding host-pathogen interactions, diagnosing infections, developing vaccines, and creating treatments for pandemic pathogens, such as SARS-CoV-2. It is worth noting that COVID-19 appeared in Wuhan, China, and was first reported as pneumonia of an unknown cause to the WHO office in China on December 31, 2019. Furthermore, it was elevated to a pandemic by WHO on March 11, 2020. COVID-19 is a serious threat for patients with comorbidities, such as compromised immune systems, respiratory diseases, cardiovascular diseases, hypertension, diabetes, and other diseases. This disease has destabilized the healthcare systems and economies worldwide. COVID-19 can infect any age, gender, or ethnicity and can infect healthy people. Body fluids, including nasal aerosol and saliva, are major modes of transmission for spreading COVID-19. There are several emergency drugs for COVID-19, including remdesivir, dexamethasone, and favipiravir. Early treatment with favipiravir and remdesivir may be beneficial during the ongoing COVID-19 pandemic. Both favipiravir and remdesivir are prodrugs that inhibit the RNA-dependent RNA polymerase (RdRp) enzyme and prevent virus replication. RdRp is one of the favorite targets for antiviral drug discovery. In the *Proteomics in Pandemic Disease* special issue, Zhao and Bourne (2020) suggest four classes of binding modes for RdRp-binding pockets that can help the in silico screening of RdRp inhibitors. Nucleotide analogs, such as triphosphates of sofosbuvir, alovudine, AZT, abacavir, lamivudine, and emtricitabine, can inhibit the RdRp of SARS-CoV-2, as studied by Chien et al. (2020).

Furthermore, Zeng et al. (2020) proposed 41 drugs for repurposing, including dexamethasone for COVID-19, using the deep learning framework and AI methodology. Moreover, by a computational approach including homology modeling, molecular docking, molecular dynamic simulations, and binding affinity calculations, Martin and Cheng (2020) found potential targets for toremifene in SARS-CoV-2, such as heptad repeat 1 (HR1) and methyltransferase nonstructural protein (NSP) 14. Using in silico studies, Barros et al. (2020) found that the antimalarial drug metaquine and anti-HIV antiretroviral saquinavir interact with four SARS-CoV-2 receptors, including Nsp9 replicase, main protease (Mpro), NSP15 endoribonuclease, and spike protein (S protein), interacting with human ACE2; therefore, they may be repurposed for COVID-19 treatment. The bioinformatic analysis of BCG antigens by Glisic et al. (2020) suggested that four bacterial proteins, Rv0934, Rv3763, Rv3875, and Rv2997, have similar properties as the S1 protein of SARS-CoV-2; therefore, they might be effective against SARS-CoV-2. A molecular docking and dynamics simulation analysis suggested that noscapine binds with the main protease of SARS-CoV-2 and produces conformational changes (Kumar et al. 2020). Furthermore, Maffucci and Contini (2020) used an in silico approach to finding drug candidates against the main proteinase and spike protein of SARS-CoV-2. This led to the finding that indinavir, polymyxin B, daptomycin, terlipressin, and thymopentin can be repurposed against the SARS-CoV-2 infection. Interestingly, the studies by Stamatakis et al. (2020)

suggested that the antigenic peptides generated from the S1 spike glycoprotein of SARS-CoV-2 using aminopeptidases ERAP1, ERAP2, and IRAP might be helpful in selecting better epitopes for immunogenic studies and the design of a vaccine for COVID-19.

Several topics have been encouraged that connect proteomics and pandemic diseases, including proteomic technologies, biomarker discovery, pathogenesis, mechanistic details of proteins, protein-protein interactions, signaling pathways, post-translational modifications, computational proteomics, prevention and vaccination, drug repurposing, and therapeutic agents and their mode of action. It will be thrilling to find the bridge between proteomics and pandemic diseases, especially for COVID-19.

4.10 FOOD SAFETY: NEW PROTEOMIC TECHNOLOGIES AND FUTURE PERSPECTIVES

For the foreseeable future, the individuation of qualitative and quantitative protein biomarkers might become pivotal also in food testing to determine food safety and authenticity (D'Alessandro and Zolla 2012). Since both concepts are somewhat closely intertwined, proteomics may provide valuable information for identifying, for example, the milk that was used to produce a specific cheese, thus determining the origin of food production of approved and guaranteed "controlled origin". In practice, methods based on LC-MS have been developed, for example, to assess the addition of pig or beef gelling agents to pork, beef, lamb, or chicken, which is of obvious commercial interest, particularly in light of religious issues regarding some meat consumption (Grundy et al. 2007). Likewise, MS-based methods of screening bovine serum to look for the effects of performance-enhancing agents have been proposed, which are used in cattle (particularly in lean veal) and other meat-producing types to increase food conversion and lean meat production (Della Donna et al. 2009). On the other hand, not only is food safety a matter of determining the origin of a product, but it also evaluates its edibility through biochemical assessment of product purity, both from a chemical and microbiological standpoint. As for the latter, the recent epidemic of *Escherichia coli* mutant, which included northern Germany and nearly paralyzed the vegetable trade within Europe at the beginning of June 2011, could be a warning sign. Nonetheless, big strides in the field of the application of MS to microbiology are still defining an ongoing revolution that might spread its benefits to the food safety endeavor, in addition to the introduction of BrukerDaltonics' MALDI-Biotyper (Seng et al. 2009). This technology allows for rapid and >99% accurate identification of bacteria and microorganisms (and region-specific substrains) cultured from routine clinical samples through the identification of species-specific proteomic profiles. Its application to the field of food safety might result in something more than a suggestive perspective, contributing to diminishing the likelihood of untoward risks rising from the assumption of unsafe food.

4.11 CLINICAL PROTEOMICS: AN OUTLOOK FOR THE NEAR FUTURE

Clinical proteomic plays a vital and important role in human health and disease, especially in both preventive and curative studies. In the future, the physician and pathologist will use these different proteomic analyses at many disease management points. A paradigm shift will directly affect clinical practice by influencing all of the following critical elements of patient care and management: early detection of disease using proteomic patterns of body-fluid samples, diagnosis based on proteomic signatures as a complement to histopathology, individually selecting therapeutic formulations that better target the protein network, disease-specific and real-time evaluation of therapeutic efficacy and toxicity, and rational reorientation of therapy based on changes in the diseased protein network associated with drug resistance.

REFERENCES

Adeola, H. A., Van Wyk, J. C., Arowolo, A., Ngwanya, R. M., Mkentane, K., and Khumalo, N. P. 2018. Emerging diagnostic and therapeutic potentials of human hair proteomics. *Proteomics Clinical Applications* 12(2):1700048.

Alonso-Fauste, I., Andrés, M., Iturralde, M., Lampreave, F., Gallart, J., and Álava, M. A. 2012. Proteomic characterization by 2-DE in bovine serum and whey from healthy and mastitis affected farm animals. *Journal of Proteomics* 75(10):3015–30.

Angel, P. M., Narmoneva, D. A., Sewell-Loftin, M. K., et al. 2017. Proteomic alterations associated with biomechanical dysfunction are early processes in the emilin1 deficient mouse model of aortic valve disease. *Annals of Biomedical Engineering* 45(11):2548–62.

Apostolovic, D., Tran, T. A. T., Hamsten, C., Starkhammar, M., CirkovicVelickovic, T., and Van Hage, M. 2014. Immunoproteomics of processed beef proteins reveal novel galactose-α-1,3-galactose-containing allergens. *European Journal of Allergy and Clinical Immunology* 69(10):1308–15.

Barros, R. O., Junior, F. L. C. C., Pereira, W. S., Oliveira, N. M. N., and Ramos, R. M. 2020. Interaction of drug candidates with various SARS-CoV-2 receptors: An in silico study to combat COVID-19. *Journal of Proteome Research* 19(11):4567–75.

Beiko, T., Janech, M. G., Alekseyenko, A. V., et al. 2017. Serum proteins associated with emphysema progression in severe alpha-1 antitrypsin deficiency. *Chronic Obstructive Pulmonary Disease* 4(3):204–16.

Bekiares, N., Krueger, C. G., Meudt, J. J., Shanmuganayagam, D., and Reed, J. D. 2017. Effect of sweetened dried cranberry consumption on urinary proteome and fecal microbiome in healthy human subjects. *OMICS* 22(2):145–53.

Benleulmi-Chaachoua, A., Chen, L., Sokolina, K., et al. 2016. Protein interactome mining defines melatonin MT1 receptors as integral component of presynaptic protein complexes of neurons. *Journal of Pineal Research* 60(1):95–108.

Bernardini, G., Figura, N., Ponzetto, A., Marzocchi, B., and Santucci, A. 2017. Application of proteomics to the study of *Helicobacter pylori* and implications for the clinic. *Expert Review of Proteomics* 14(6):477–90.

Berthiller, F., Breda, C., Crews, C., et al. 2015. Developments in mycotoxin analysis: An update for 2013–2014. *World Mycotoxin Journal* 8(1):5–35.

Bhatnagar, D., Rajasekaran, K., Payne, G., Brown, R., Yu, J., and Cleveland, T. 2008. The "omics" tools: Genomics, proteomics, metabolomics and their potential for solving the aflatoxin contamination problem. *World Mycotoxin Journal* 1(1):3–12.

Bird, J. K., Raederstorff, D., Weber, P., and Steinert, R. E. 2017. Cardiovascular and anti-obesity effects of resveratrol mediated through the gut microbiota. *Advances in Nutrition* 8(6):839–49.

Blum, H. E. 2017. The human microbiome. *Advances in Medical Sciences* 62(2):414–20.

Brocca, L., Longa, E., Cannavino, J., et al. 2015. Human skeletal muscle fibre contractile properties and proteomic profile: Adaptations to 3 weeks of unilateral lower limb suspension and active recovery. *Journal of Physiology* 593(24):5361–85.

Bruns, S., Bruns, S., Seidler, M., et al. 2010. Functional genomic profiling of *Aspergillus fumigatus* biofilm reveals enhanced production of the mycotoxin gliotoxin. *Proteomics* 10(17):3097–107.

Calhoun, C., Shivshankar, P., Saker, M., et al. 2016. Senescent cells contribute to the physiological remodeling of aged lungs. *Journals of Gerontology Series A Biological Sciences and Medical Sciences* 71(2):153–60.

Calvano, C. D., De Ceglie, C., Aresta, A., Facchini, L. A., and Zambonin, C. G. 2013. MALDI-TOF mass spectrometric determination of intact phospholipids as markers of illegal bovine milk adulteration of high-quality milk. *Analytical and Bioanalytical Chemistry* 405(5):1641–9.

Capriotti, A. L., Caruso, G., Cavaliere, C., Foglia, P., Samperi, R., and Laganà, A. 2012. Multiclass mycotoxin analysis in food, environmental and biological matrices with chromatography/mass spectrometry. *Mass Spectrometry Reviews* 31(4):466–503.

Carrera, M., Cañas, B., Piñeiro, C., Vázquez, J., and Gallardo, J. M. 2006. Identification of commercial hake and grenadier species by proteomic analysis of the parvalbumin fraction. *Proteomics* 6(19):5278–87.

Cavalla, F., Biguetti, C., Jain, S., et al. 2017. Proteomic profiling and differential messenger RNA expression correlate HSP27 and serpin family B member 1 to apical periodontitis outcomes. *Journal of Endodontics* 43(9):1486–93.

Chaiyarit, P., Jaresitthikunchai, J., Phaonakrop, N., Roytrakul, S., Potempa, B., and Potempa, J. 2018. Proteolytic effects of gingipains on trefoil factor family peptides. *Clinical Oral Investigations* 22(2):1009–18.

Chang, T. J., Wang, W. C., Hsiung, C. A., et al. 2016. Genetic variation in the human SORBS1 gene is associated with blood pressure regulation and age at onset of hypertension: A SAPPHIRe cohort study. *Medicine (Baltimore)* 95(10):e2970.

Chemonges, S., Gupta, R., Mills, P. C., Kopp, S. R., and Sadowski, P. 2017. Characterisation of the circulating acellular proteome of healthy sheep using LC-MS/MS-based proteomics analysis of serum. *Proteome Science* 15:11.

Chen, B., Brown, K. A., Lin, Z., and Ge, Y. 2017. Top-down proteomics: Ready for prime time? *Analytical Chemistry* 90(1):110–27.

Cheng, C. W., Chang, C. C., Patria, Y. N., et al. 2018. Sex hormone-binding globulin (SHBG) is a potential early diagnostic biomarker for gastric cancer. *Cancer Medicine* 7(1):64–74.

Chien, M., Anderson, T. K., Jockusch, S., et al. 2020. Nucleotide analogues as inhibitors of SARS-CoV-2 polymerase, a key drug target for COVID-19. *Journal of Proteome Research* 19(11):4690–7.

Choi, Y. E. 2012. Proteomic comparison of *Gibberella moniliformis* in limited-nitrogen (fumonisin-inducing) and excess-nitrogen (fumonisin-repressing) conditions. *Journal of Microbiology and Biotechnology* 22(6):780–7.

Cid, M., and González, M. 2016. Potential benefits of physical activity during pregnancy for the reduction of gestational diabetes prevalence and oxidative stress. *Early Human Development* 94:57–62.

Cole, B. K., Feaver, R. E., Wamhoff, B. R., and Dash, A. 2017. Non-alcoholic fatty liver disease (NAFLD) models in drug discovery. *Expert Opinion on Drug Discovery* 13(2):193–205.

Costanzo, M., Zacchia, M., Bruno, G., Crisci, D., Caterino, M., and Ruoppolo, M. 2017. Integration of proteomics and metabolomics in exploring genetic and rare metabolic diseases. *Kidney Diseases (Basel)* 3(2):66–77.

Coulona, J. B., Gasquib, P., Barnouin, J., Ollier, A., Pradel, P., and Pomiès, D. 2002. Effect of mastitis and related-germ on milk yield and composition during naturally-occurring udder infections in dairy cows. *Animal Research* 51(5):383–93.

Cozzolino, R., et al. 2001. Identification of adulteration in milk by matrix-assisted laser desorption/ionization time-of-flight mass spectrometry. *Journal of Mass Spectrometry* 36(9):1031–7.

Crespo-Sempere, A., Gil, J. V., and Martinez-Culebras, P. V. 2011. Proteome analysis of the fungus *Aspergillus carbonarius* under ochratoxin A producing conditions. *International Journal of Food Microbiology* 147(3):162–9.

Cserháti, T., Forgács, E., Deyl, Z., and Miksik, I. 2005. Chromatography in authenticity and traceability tests of vegetable oils and dairy products: A review. *Biomedical Chromatography* 19(3):183–90.

D'Alessandro, A., and Zolla, L. 2012. We are what we eat: Food safety and proteomics. *Journal of Proteome Research* 11(1):26–36.

Della Donna, L., Ronci, M., Sacchetta, P., et al. 2009. A food safety control low mass-range proteomics platform for the detection of illicit treatments in veal calves by MALDI-TOF-MS serum profiling. *Biotechnology Journal* 4(11):1596–609.

Diab, M., Glasner, A., Isaacson, B., et al. 2017. NK-cell receptors NKp46 and NCR1 control human metapneumovirus infection. *European Journal of Immunology* 47(4): 692–703.

Dimatelis, J. J., Hendricks, S., Hsieh, J., et al. 2013. Exercise partly reverses the effect of maternal separation on hippocampal proteins in 6-hydroxydopamine-lesioned rat brain. *Experimental Physiology* 98(1):233–44.

Dong, X, Qiu, X., Meng, S., Xu, H., Wu, X., and Yang, M. 2018. Proteomic profile and toxicity pathway analysis in zebrafish embryos exposed to bisphenol A and di-n-butyl phthalate at environmentally relevant levels. *Chemosphere* 193:313–20.

Doyle, S. 2011. Fungal proteomics: From identification to function. *FEMS Microbiology Letter* 321(1):1–9.

Drager, L. F., McEvoy, R. D., Barbe, F., Lorenzi-Filho, G., and Redline, S. 2017. Sleep apnea and cardiovascular disease: Lessons from recent trials and need for team science. *Circulation* 136(19):1840–50.

Etienne, M., Jérôme, M., Fleurence, J., et. al. 2000. Identification of fish species after cooking by SDS-PAGE and urea IEF: A collaborative study. *Journal of Agricultural and Food Chemistry* 48(7):2653–8.

Eubanks, C. G., Dayebgadoh, G., Liu, X., and Washburn, M. P. 2017. Unravelling the biology of chromatin in health and cancer using proteomic approaches. *Expert Review of Proteomics* 14(10):905–15.

Fagerquist, C. K., Zaragoza, W. J., and Carter, M. Q. 2014. Top-down proteomic identification of Shiga toxin 2 subtypes from Shiga toxin-producing *Escherichia coli* by matrix-assisted laser desorption ionization – tandem time of flight mass spectrometry. *Applied and Environmental Microbiology* 80(9):2928–40.

Feliciano, A., Torres, V. M., Vaz, F., et al. 2015. Overview of proteomics studies in obstructive sleep apnea. *Sleep Medicine* 16(4):437–45.

Feliciano, A., Vaz, F., Valentim-Coelho, C., et al. 2017. Evening and morning alterations in obstructive sleep apnea red blood cell proteome. *Data Brief* 11:103–10.

Fields, Stanley. 2001. Proteomics in genomeland. *Science* 291(5507):1221–4.

Florath, I., Butterbach, K., Heiss, J., et al. 2016. Type 2 diabetes and leucocyte DNA methylation: An epigenome-wide association study in over 1,500 older adults. *Diabetologia* 59(1):130–8.

Fogliano, V., Monti, S. M., Ritieni, A., Marchisano, C., Peluso, G., and Randazzo, G. 1997. An immunological approach to monitor protein lactosylation of heated food model systems. *Food Chemistry* 58(1):53–8.

Fogliano, V., Monti, S. M., Visconti, A., et al. 1998. Identification of a beta-lactoglobulin lactosylation site. *Biochimica et Biophysica Acta* 1388(2):295–304.

Föll, M. C., Fahrner, M., Gretzmeier, C., et al. 2018. Identification of tissue damage, extracellular matrix remodeling and bacterial challenge as common mechanisms associated with high-risk cutaneous squamous cell carcinomas. *Matrix Biology* 66:1–21.

Georgiades, E., Klissouras, V., Baulch, J., Wang, G., and Pitsiladis, Y. 2017. Why nature prevails over nurture in the making of the elite athlete. *BMC Genomics* 18(8):835.

Giacometti, J., Tomljanović, A. B., and Josić, D. 2013. Application of proteomics and metabolomics for investigation of food toxins. *Food Research International* 54(1):1042–51.

Glisic, S., Perovic, V. R., Sencanski, M., Paessler, S., and Veljkovic, V. 2020. Biological rationale for the repurposing of BCG vaccine against SARS-CoV-2. *Journal of Proteome Research* 19(11):4649–54.

Goliáš, J., Humlová, Z., Halada, P., Hábová, V., Janatková, I., and Tučková, L. 2013. Identification of rice proteins recognized by the IgE antibodies of patients with food allergies. *Journal of Agricultural and Food Chemistry* 61(37):8851–60.

Graham, L. C., Eaton, S. L., Brunton, P. J., et al. 2017. Proteomic profiling of neuronal mitochondria reveals modulators of synaptic architecture. *Molecular Neurodegeneration* 12(1):77.

Grundy, H. H., Reece, P., Sykes, M. D., Clough, J. A., Audsley, N., and Stones, R. 2007. Screening method for the addition of bovine blood-based binding agents to food using liquid chromatography triple quadrupole mass spectrometry. *Rapid Communications in Mass Spectrometry* 21(18):2919–25.

Guglielmetti, C., Mazza, M., Pagano, M., et al. 2014. Identification by a proteomic approach of a plasma protein as a possible biomarker of illicit dexamethasone treatment in veal calves. *Food Additives & Contaminants: Part A* 31(5):833–8.

Hahl, P., Hunt, R., Bjes, E. S., Skaff, A., Keightley, A., and Smith, A. 2017. Identification of oxidative modifications of hemopexin and their predicted physiological relevance. *Journal of Biological Chemistry* 292(33):13658–71.

Harmon, R. 1994. Physiology of mastitis and factors affecting somatic cell counts. *Journal of Dairy Science* 77(7):2103–12.

Heinritz, S. N., Weiss, E., Eklund, M., et al. 2016. Intestinal microbiota and microbial metabolites are changed in a pig model fed a high-fat/low-fiber or a low-fat/high-fiber diet. *PLoS One* 11(4):e0154329.

Herrero, Miguel, et al. 2012. Foodomics: MS-based strategies in modern food science and nutrition. *Mass Spectrometry Reviews* 31(1):49–69.

Hettinga, K. A., Reina, F. M., Boeren, S., et al. 2015. Difference in the breast milk proteome between allergic and nonallergic mothers. *PLoS One* 10(3):e0122234.

Hinz, K., O'Connor, P. M., Huppertz, T., Ross, R. P., and Kelly, A. L. 2012. Comparison of the principal proteins in bovine, caprine, buffalo, equine and camel milk. *Journal of Dairy Research* 79(2):185–91.

Hu, H. F., Xu, W. W., Wang, Y., et al. 2018. Comparative proteomics analysis identifies Cdc42-Cdc42BPA signaling as prognostic biomarker and therapeutic target for colon cancer invasion. *Journal of Proteome Research* 17(1):265–75.

Huang, Y. L., Shen, Z. Q., Wu, C. Y., et al. 2018. Comparative proteomic profiling reveals a role for Cisd2 in skeletal muscle aging. *Aging Cell* 17(1):e12705.

Huber, M., Knottnerus, J. A., Green, L., et al. 2011. How should we define health? *BMJ* 343:d4163.

Hurley, I. P., Coleman, R. C., Ireland, H. E., and Williams, J. H. H. 2004a. Measurement of bovine IgG by indirect competitive ELISA as a means of detecting milk adulteration. *Journal of Dairy Science* 87:215–21.

Hurley, I. P., Ireland, H. E., Coleman, R. C., and Williams, J. H. H. 2004b. Application of immunological methods for the detection of species adulteration in dairy products. *International Journal of Food Science and Technology* 39(8):873–8.

Inda, L. A., Razquin, P., Lampreave, F., Alava, M. A., and Calvo, M. 1998. Rapid, sensitive, enzyme-immunodotting assay for detecting cow milk adulteration in sheep milk – a modern laboratory project. *Journal of Chemical Education* 75:1618–21.

Jiang, X., Yang, Y., Zhou, J., et al. 2016. Roles of the putative type IV-like secretion system key component VirD4 and PrsA in pathogenesis of *Streptococcus suis* type 2. *Frontier in Cellular and Infection Microbiology* 6:172.

Kalule, J. B., Fortuin, S., Calder, B., et al. 2018. Proteomic comparison of three clinical diarrhoeagenic drug-resistant *Escherichia coli* isolates grown on CHROMagar™STEC media. *Journal of Proteomics* 30(180):25–35.

Kearney, S., O'Donoghue, L., Pourshahidi, L. K., Cobice, D., and Saunders, K. J. 2017. Myopes have significantly higher serum melatonin concentrations than non-myopes. *Ophthalmic Physiological Optics* 37(5):557–67.

Khurshid, Z., Naseem, M., Yahya, I., et al. 2017. Significance and diagnostic role of antimicrobial cathelicidins (LL-37) peptides in oral health. *Biomolecules* 7(4):80.

Kjaersgard, I. V., Norrelykke, M. R., and Jessen, F. 2006. Changes in cod muscle proteins during frozen storage revealed by proteome analysis and multivariate data analysis. *Proteomics* 6(5):1606–18.

Kniemeyer, O. 2011. Proteomics of eukaryotic microorganisms: The medically and biotechnologically important fungal genus *Aspergillus. Proteomics* 11(15):3232–43.

Koeberl, M., Clarke, D., and Lopata, A. L. 2014. Next generation of food allergen quantification using mass spectrometric systems. *Journal of Proteome Research* 13(8):3499–509.

Konstantakou, E. G., Velentzas, A. D., Anagnostopoulos, A. K., et al. 2017. Deep-proteome mapping of WM-266-4 human metastatic melanoma cells: From oncogenic addiction to druggable targets. *PLoS One* 12(2): e0171512.

Koo, S. J., Spratt, H. M., Soman, K. V., et al. 2016. S-nitrosylation proteome profile of peripheral blood mononuclear cells in human heart failure. *International Journal of Proteomics* 2016:1384523.

Koriem, K. M. M. 2017a. A lipidomic concept in infectious diseases. *Asian Pacific Journal of Tropical Biomedicine* 7(3):265–74.

Koriem, K. M. M. 2017b. Protective effect of natural products and hormones in colon cancer using metabolome: A physiological overview. *Journal of Tropical Biomedicine* 7(10):957–66.

Kubatka, P., Kello, M., Kajo, K., et al. 2017. Oregano demonstrates distinct tumour-suppressive effects in the breast carcinoma model. *European Journal of Nutrition* 56(3):1303–16.

Kumar, N., Sood, D., van der Spek, P. J., Sharma, H. S., and Chandra, R. 2020. Molecular binding mechanism and pharmacology comparative analysis of noscapine for repurposing against SARS-CoV-2 protease. *Journal of Proteome Research* 19(11):4678–89.

Lee, Y., Hwang, Y. H., Kim, K. J., et al. 2018. Proteomic and transcriptomic analysis of lung tissue in OVA-challenged mice. *Arch Pharm Res* 41(1):87–100.

Leonil, J., Molle, D., Fauquant, J., Maubois, J. L., Pearce, R. J., and Bouhallab, S. 1997. Characterization by ionization mass spectrometry of lactosyl beta-lactoglobulin conjugates formed during heat treatment of milk and whey and identification of one lactose-binding site. *Journal of Dairy Science* 80(10):2270–81.

Leung, P. S., Shu, S. A., and Chang, C. 2014. The changing geoepidemiology of food allergies. *Clinical Reviews in Allergy and Immunology* 46(3):169–79.

Li, Y., Zhang, B., Huang, K., et al. 2014. Mitochondrial proteomic analysis reveals the molecular mechanisms underlying reproductive toxicity of zearalenone in MLTC-1 cells. *Toxicology* 324:55–67.

Liu, S., Gao, J., Chen, Z., et al. 2017. Comparative proteomics reveals the physiological differences between winter tender shoots and spring tender shoots of a novel tea (*Camellia sinensis* L.) cultivar ever growing in winter. *BMC Plant Biology* 17(1):206.

Maffucci, I., and Contini, A. 2020. In silico drug repurposing for SARS-CoV-2 main proteinase and spike proteins. *Journal of Proteome Research* 19(11):4637–48.

Mao, X., Luo, F., Boyd, L. K., et al. 2016. NKAIN2 functions as a novel tumor suppressor in prostate cancer. *Oncotarget* 7(39):63793–803.

Martin, W. R., and Cheng, F. 2020. Repurposing of FDA-approved toremifene to treat COVID-19 by blocking the spike glycoprotein and NSP14 of SARS-CoV-2. *Journal of Proteome Research* 19(11):4670–7.

Matoba, K., Lu, Y., Zhang, R., et al. 2017. Adipose KLF15 controls lipid handling to adapt to nutrient availability. *Cell Reports* 21(11):3129–40.

Mayer, H. K. 2005. Milk species identification in cheese varieties using electrophoretic, chromatographic and PCR techniques. *International Dairy Journal* 15(6–9):595–604.

Mayer, Helmut K., and Gregor Fiechter. 2013. Electrophoretic techniques. *Comprehensive Analytical Chemistry* 60:251–78.

Mazzeo, M. F., Giulio, B. D., Guerriero, G., et al. 2008. Fish authentication by MALDI-TOF mass spectrometry. *Journal of Agricultural and Food Chemistry* 56(23):11071–6.

Meng, Z. X., Tao, W., Sun, J., Wang, Q., Mi, L., and Lin, J. D. 2018. Uncoupling exercise bioenergetics from systemic metabolic homeostasis by conditional inactivation of Baf60 in skeletal muscle. *Diabetes* 67(1):85–97.

Montowska, M., and Pospiech, E. 2012. Myosin light chain isoforms retain their species-specific electrophoretic mobility after processing, which enables differentiation between six species: 2DE analysis of minced meat and meat products made from beef, pork and poultry. *Proteomics* 12(18):2879–89.

Montowska, M., and Pospiech, E. 2013. Species-specific expression of various proteins in meat tissue: Proteomic analysis of raw and cooked meat and meat products made from beef, pork and selected poultry species. *Food Chemistry* 136(3–4):1461–9.

Morante, T., Shepherd, C., Constantinoiu, C., Loukas, A., and Sotillo, J. 2017. Revisiting the ancylostoma caninum secretome provides new information on hookworm-host interactions. *Proteomics* 17:23–4.

Mourad, F. H., Yau, Y., Wasinger, V. C., and Leong, R. W. 2017. Proteomics in inflammatory bowel disease: Approach using animal models. *Digestive Diseases and Sciences* 62(9):2266–76.

Mu, P., Xu, M., Zhang, L., et al. 2013. Proteomic changes in chicken primary hepatocytes exposed to T-2 toxin are associated with oxidative stress and mitochondrial enhancement. *Proteomics* 13(21):3175–88.

Nikolaeva, D., Illingworth, J. J., Miura, K., et al. 2020. Functional characterization and comparison of *Plasmodium falciparum* proteins as targets of transmission-blocking antibodies. *Molecular and Cellular Proteomics* 19(1):155–66.

Nogueira da Costa, A., Mijal, R. S., Keen, J. N., Findlay, J. B. C., and Wild, C. P. 2011. Proteomic analysis of the effects of the immunomodulatory mycotoxin deoxynivalenol. *Proteomics* 11(10):1903–14.

Ochoa, M. L., and Harrington, P. B. 2005. Immunomagnetic isolation of enterohemorrhagic *Escherichia coli* O157: H7 from ground beef and identification by matrix-assisted laser desorption/ionization time-of-flight mass spectrometry and database searches. *Analytical Chemistry* 77(16):5258–67.

Odedra, K. M. 2015. Milk allergy in adults and children. *Nursing Standard* 29(44):43–8.

O'Reilly, M., Dillon, E., Guo, W., et al. 2016. High-density lipoprotein proteomic composition, and not efflux capacity, reflects differential modulation of reverse cholesterol transport by saturated and monounsaturated fat diets. *Circulation* 133(19):1838–50.

Padrão, A. I., Ferreira, R., Amado, F., Vitorino, R., and Duarte, J. A. 2016. Uncovering the exercise-related proteome signature in skeletal muscle. *Proteomics* 16(5):816–30.

Pallini, M., Compagnone, D., Di Stefano, S., Marini, S., Coletta, M., and Palleschi, G. 2001. Immunodetection of lactosylated proteins as a useful tool to determine heat treatment in milk samples. *Analyst* 126(1):66–70.

Pan, X., Whitten, D. A., Wilkerson, C. G., and Pestka, J. J. 2014. Dynamic changes in ribosome-associated proteome and phosphoproteome during deoxynivalenol-induced translation inhibition and ribotoxic stress. *Toxicological Sciences* 138(1):217–33.

Pandey, Akhilesh, and Mann, Matthias. 2000. Proteomics to study genes and genomes. *Nature* 405(6788):837–46.

Pechanova, O., Pechan, T., Rodriguez, J. M., Williams, W. P., and Brown, A. E. 2013. A two-dimensional proteome map of the aflatoxigenic fungus *Aspergillus Flavus. Proteomics* 13(9):1513–8.

Picariello, G., Mamone, G., Addeo, F., Nitride, C., and Ferranti, P. 2013. Proteomic-based techniques for the characterization of food allergens. *Foodomics: Advanced Mass Spectrometry in Modern Food Science and Nutrition*:69–99.

Picariello, G., Mamone, G., Cutignano, A., et al. 2015. Proteomics, peptidomics, and immunogenic potential of wheat beer (Weissbier). *Journal of Agricultural and Food Chemistry* 63(13):3579–86.

Puglia, M., Landi, C., Gagliardi, A., et al. 2018. The proteome speciation of an immortalized cystic fibrosis cell line: New perspectives on the pathophysiology of the disease. *Journal of Proteomics* 170:28–42.

Qin, G., Tian, S., Chan, Z., and Li, B. 2007. Crucial role of antioxidant proteins and hydrolytic enzymes in pathogenicity of *Penicillium expansum*: Analysis based on proteomics approach. *Molecular and Cellular Proteomics* 6(3):425–38.

Rehbein, H., Kündiger, R., Pineiro, C., and Perez-Martin, R. I. 2000. Fish muscle parvalbumins as marker proteins for native and urea isoelectric focusing. *Electrophoresis* 21(8):1458–63.

Renz, H., Holt, P. G., Inouye, M., Logan, A. C., Prescott, S. L., and Sly, P. D. 2017. An exposome perspective: Early-life events and immune development in a changing world. *Journal of Allergy and Clinical Immunology* 140(1):24–40.

Rowlands, D. S., Page, R. A., Sukala, W. R., et al. 2014. Multi-omic integrated networks connect DNA methylation and miRNA with skeletal muscle plasticity to chronic exercise in type 2 diabetic obesity. *Physiological Genomics* 46(20):747–65.

Rupp, C., Bode, K. A., Leopold, Y., Sauer, P., and Gotthardt, D. N. 2018. Pathological features of primary sclerosing cholangitis identified by bile proteomic analysis. *Biochimica et Biophysica Acta* 1864(4 Pt B):1380–9.

Sanabria, J. R., Kombu, R. S., Zhang, G. F., et al. 2016. Glutathione species and metabolomic prints in subjects with liver disease as biological markers for the detection of hepatocellular carcinoma. *HPB (Oxford)* 18(12):979–90.

Seetho, I. W., and Wilding, J. P. 2013. Screening for obstructive sleep apnoea in obesity and diabetes – potential for future approaches. *European Journal of Clinical Investigation* 43(6):640–55.

Seng, P., Drancourt, M., Gouriet, F., et al. 2009. Ongoing revolution in bacteriology: Routine identification of bacteria by matrix-assisted laser desorption ionization time-of-flight mass spectrometry. *Clinical Infectious Diseases* 49(4):543–51.

Sentandreu, M. A., Fraser, P. D., Halket, J., Patel, R., and Bramley, P. M. 2010. A proteomic-based approach for detection of chicken in meat mixes. *Journal of Proteome Research* 9(7):3374–83.

She, X., Zhang, P., Gao, Y., et al. 2018. A mitochondrial proteomics view of complex I deficiency in *Candida Albicans. Mitochondrion* 38:48–57.

Shen, X. L., Zhang, Y., Xu, W., et al. 2013. An iTRAQ-based mitoproteomics approach for profiling the nephrotoxicity mechanisms of ochratoxin A in HEK 293 cells. *Journal of Proteomics* 78:398–415.

Short, J. D., Downs, K., Tavakoli, S., and Asmis, R. 2016. Protein thiol redox signaling in monocytes and macrophages. *Antioxid Redox Signal* 25(15):816–35.

Smine, S., Obry, A., Kadri, S., et al. 2017. Brain proteomic modifications associated to protective effect of grape extract in a murine model of obesity. *Biochimica et Biophysica Acta* 1865(5):578–88.

Snelling, W. J., Lin, Q., Moore, J. E., and Millar, B. C. 2007. Proteomics analysis and protein expression during sporozoite excystation of *Cryptosporidium parvum* (Coccidia, Apicomplexa). *Molecular and Cellular Proteomics* 6(2):346–55.

Stamatakis, G., Samiotaki, M., Mpakali, A., Panayotou, G., and Stratikos, E. 2020. Generation of SARS-CoV-2 S1 Spike glycoprotein putative antigenic epitopes in vitro by intracellular aminopeptidases. *Journal of Proteome Research* 19(11):4398–406.

Stoll, D. A., Link, S., Kulling, S., Geisen, R., and Schmidt-Heydt, M. 2014. Comparative proteome analysis of *Penicillium verrucosum* grown under light of short wavelength shows an induction of stress-related proteins associated with modified mycotoxin biosynthesis. *International Journal of Food Microbiology* 175:20–9.

Sun, J., Lundström, S. L., Zhang, B., et al. 2017. IgM antibodies against phosphorylcholine promote polarization of T regulatory cells from patients with atherosclerotic plaques, systemic lupus erythematosus and healthy donors. *Atherosclerosis* 268:36–48.

Tan, H. L., Kheirandish-Gozal, L., and Gozal, D. 2014. The promise of translational and personalised approaches for pediatric obstructive sleep apnoea: An "Omics" perspective. *Thorax* 69(5):474–80.

Tan, H. W., Xu, Y. M., Wu, D. D., and Lau, A. T. Y. 2018. Recent insights into human bronchial proteomics – how are we progressing and what is next? *Expert Review of Proteomics* 15(1):113–30.

Tauer, A., Hasenkopf, K., Kislinger, T., Frey, I., and Pischetsrieder, M. 1999. Determination of Nε-carboxymethyllysine in heated milk products by immunochemical methods, *European Food Research and Technology* 209:72–6.

Taylor, R. D., Saparno, A., Blackwell, B., et al. 2008. Proteomic analyses of *Fusarium graminearum* grown under mycotoxin inducing conditions. *Proteomics* 8(11):2256–65.

Tomm, J. M., van Do, T., Jende, C., et al. 2013. Identification of new potential allergens from Nile perch (*Latesniloticus*) and cod (*Gadusmorhua*). *Journal of Investigational Allergology and Clinical Immunology* 23(3):159–67.

Tooze, J. A., Hamzic, E., Willis, F., and Pettengell, R. 2017. Differences between chronic lymphocytic leukaemia and small lymphocytic lymphoma cells by proteomic profiling and SNP microarray analysis. *Cancer Genetics* 218–219:20–38.

Turk, R., Piras, C., Kovacic, M., et al. 2012. Proteomics of inflammatory and oxidative stress response in cows with subclinical and clinical mastitis. *Journal of Proteomics* 75(14):4412–28.

Van Boekel, M. 1998. Effect of heating on Maillard reactions in milk. *Food Chemistry* 62(4):403–14.

Vergara, D., Gaballo, A., Signorile, A., et al. 2017. Resveratrol modulation of protein expression in parkin-mutant human skin fibroblasts: A proteomic approach. *Oxidative Medicine and Cellular Longevity* 2017:2198243.

Von Bargen, C., Brockmeyer, J., and Humpf, H. U. 2014. Meat authentication: A new HPLC-MS/MS based method for the fast and sensitive detection of horse and pork in highly processed food. *Journal of Agricultural and Food Chemistry* 62(39): 9428–35.

Wang, H., Hong, X., Li, S., and Wang, Y. 2017. Oxygen supplementation improves protein milieu supportive of protein synthesis and antioxidant function in the cortex of Alzheimer's disease model mice – a quantitative proteomic study. *Journal of Molecular Neuroscience* 63(2):243–53.

Wilkins, Marc R., et al. 1996. From proteins to proteomes: large scale protein identification by two-dimensional electrophoresis and arnino acid analysis. *Bio/technology* 14(1):61–5.

Wu, C. X., and Liu, Z. F. 2018. Proteomic profiling of sweat exosome suggests its involvement in skin immunity. *Journal of Investigative Dermatology* 138(1):89–97.

Wulff, T., Nielsen, M. E., Deelder, A. M., Jessen, F., and Palmblad, M. 2013. Authentication of Fish products by large-scale comparison of tandem mass spectra. *Journal of Proteome Research* 12(11):5253–9.

Xin, Z., Pu, L., Gao, W., et al. 2017. Riboflavin deficiency induces a significant change in proteomic profiles in HepG2 cells. *Scientific Reports* 7:45861.

Yang, Y. X., Bu, D., Zhao, X., Sun, P., Wang, J., and Zhou, L. 2013. Proteomic analysis of cow, yak, buffalo, goat and camel milk whey proteins: Quantitative differential expression patterns. *Journal of Proteome Research* 12(4):1660–7.

Yang, Y. X., Zheng, N., Yang, J. H., et al. 2014. Animal species milk identification by comparison of two-dimensional gel map profile and mass spectrometry approach. *International Dairy Journal* 35:15–20.

Yu, J., Jin, X., Sun, X., et al. 2017. Hydrogen peroxide response in leaves of poplar (*Populus simonii* × *Populus nigra*) revealed from physiological and proteomic analyses. *International Journal of Molecular Sciences* 18(10):e2085.

Yuan, X., Zhang, J., Xie, F., et al. 2017. Loss of the protein cystathionine β-synthase during kidney injury promotes renal tubulointerstitial fibrosis. *Kidney and Blood Pressure Research* 42(3):428–43.

Zeng, X., Song, X., Ma, T., et al. 2020. Repurpose open data to discover therapeutics for COVID-19 using deep learning. *Journal of Proteome Research* 19(11):4624–36.

Zhang, B., Shen, X. L., Liang, R., et al. 2014. Protective role of the mitochondrial Lon protease 1 in ochratoxin A-induced cytotoxicity in HEK293 cells. *Journal of Proteomics* 101:154–68.

Zhang, Q. H., Huang, L., Zhang, Y., Ke, C. H., and Huang, H. Q. 2013. Proteomic approach for identifying gonad differential proteins in the oyster (*Crassostrea angulata*) following food-chain contamination with HgCl2. *Journal of Proteomics* 94:37–53.

Zhang, Z., Yan, Q., Guo, J., et al. 2017. A plasma proteomics method reveals links between ischemic stroke and MTHFR C677T genotype. *Science Report* 7(1):13390.

Zhao, Z., and Bourne, P. E. 2020. Structural insights into the binding modes of viral RNA-dependent RNA polymerases using a function-site interaction fingerprint method for RNA virus drug discovery. *Journal of Proteome Research* 19(11):4698–705.

Zheng, J., Yamada, Y., Fung, T. S., Huang, M., Chia, R., and Liu, D. X. 2018. Identification of N-linked glycosylation sites in the spike protein and their functional impact on the replication and infectivity of coronavirus infectious bronchitis virus in cell culture. *Virology* 513:65–74.

Zhou, Y., Niu, L., Liu, K., Yin, S., and Liu, W. 2017. Arsenic in agricultural soils across China: Distribution pattern, accumulation trend, influencing factors, and risk assessment. *Science of the Total Environment* 616–617:156–63.

5 Metabolomics and Potential Nutrition-Specific Markers for Nutritional Safety, Quality, and Health Status

Ramachandran Chelliah, Inamul Hasan Madar, Syeda Mahvish Zahra, Khanita Suman Chinnanai, Mahamuda Begum, Ghazala Sultan, Umar Farooq Alahmad, Iftikhar Aslam Tayubi, and Deog-Hwan Oh*

CONTENTS

* Corresponding author email: ramachandran865@gmail.com

DOI: 10.1201/9781003142195-5

5.1 INTRODUCTION

There are many lifestyle habits, nutrition, and extrinsic influences that contribute to the occurrence and progression of diseases, such as overweightness and several cardiovascular disorders leading to impaired health (García-Cañas et al. 2012; Ibáñez et al. 2012). Besides that, trace elements included in food ingredients may help avoid or postpone diseases (Capozzi and Bordoni 2013). Today, the difficulty is to tailor dietary guidance for various demographics, and optimal diet modification for particular populations is critical (Brennan 2015). It is even more challenging to foresee when the trajectory of the patient's health state would shift in a certain direction and the emergence of impending ailments before the actual presence of any symptoms (German et al. 2005; Gibney et al. 2005).

To reiterate the above discussion, public health is nevertheless dependent on the expression of genes but on the multiplicity of mechanisms (lifestyle, microbial composition). Environmental factors, especially constituents of food eaten, may affect the expression of genetic information after it has been acquired; post-translational modifications and metabolism can impact proteins and formulations of metabolites. The metabolic evolution to proceed, as shown in Figure 5.1, types can be maintained under conditions of homeostasis. Implemented therapy is an outstanding example of the ability to recognize and intervene on biomarkers, illustrating the principle of homeostasis following nutrition intervention (line in black) where anomaly got corrected as soon as identified, and the impact of pathogenesis predicted deviation from homeostasis in case of an unidentified pathology issue until identified and corrected as depicted in Figure 5.2. The technological advancements in analytical methods didn't only influence how these biological

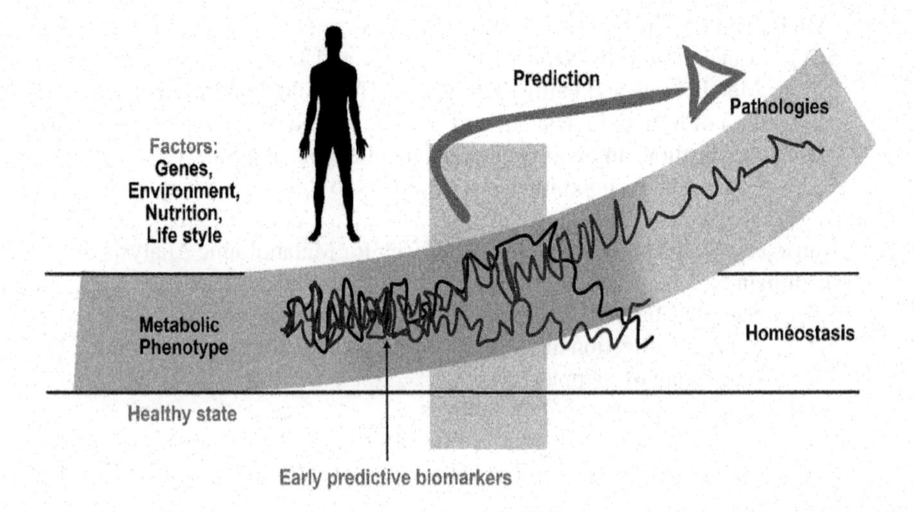

FIGURE 5.1 The role of early predictive biomarkers in the identification of disease pathogenesis.

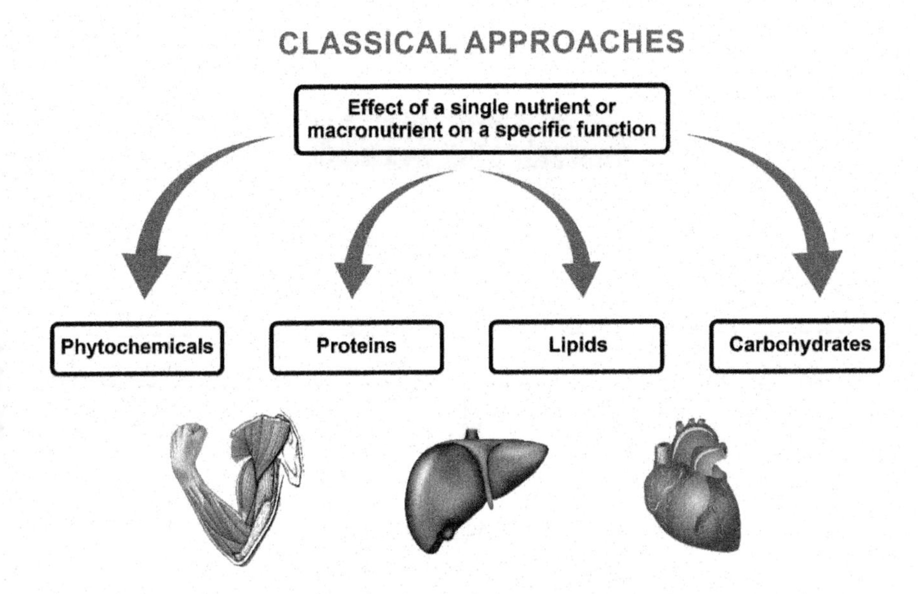

FIGURE 5.2 Schematic diagram of the classical approaches to find the effect of specific nutrients and macronutrients on a specific function.

fields of science and nutrition science disciplines evolved but also contributed to the emergence of bioinformatics, data-mining techniques, and fractionation methods. A contrasting difference between conventional and integrated neo-techniques has been well established in Figure 5.3. Conventional ways didn't emphasize nutritional components interaction while studying certain specific outcomes on organ systems, while neo-techniques, like utilization of omics – that is, at the level of genomics, transcription, proteomes, and eventually metabolites – led to huge data gathering at the complex edge and pooling information of interactional complexity of associations of dietary or other factors, which further maintain progress in the field of metabolomics.

5.2 METABOLOMIC APPROACHES

5.2.1 Metabolomic Workflow, Technologies, and Tools

The analysis of small molecules contained in biological materials is referred to as metabolomics. In recent times, the use of metabolomics in nutritional science has grown, with new research promoting various applications. Different concepts have appeared in the literature as the field has progressed, especially in metabolites quantification methods. Metabolomics, metabonomics, and nutri-metabolomics, for example, have all been used interchangeably. Similarly, untargeted and tailored

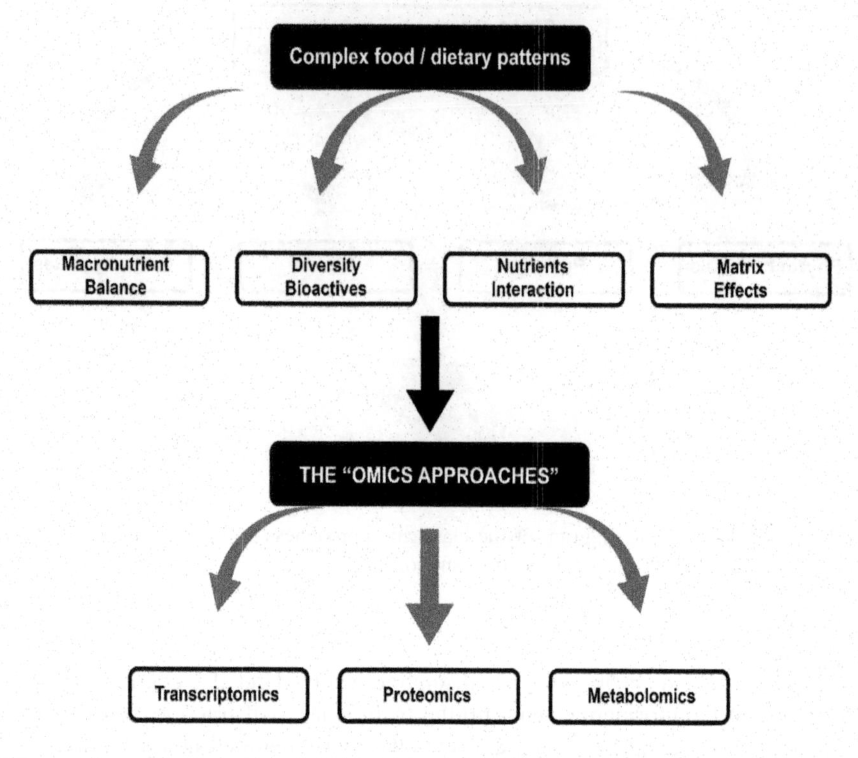

FIGURE 5.3 Integrative approaches used to study the complex dietary compounds at the genome, proteome, and metabolome level.

methods have been referred to as nutritional phenotyping, metabolic profiling, and metabolomic fingerprinting. In short, the metabolomics could be studied by involving two broader schemes, as depicted in Figure 5.4:

1. Untargeted approaches for concurrent analysis of hundreds/thousands of descriptive multivariate measurements, which are exclusive and well-defined to nutritional health status.
2. Targeted approaches for the identification and quantification of pre-allocated metabolites sets (Cajka and Fiehn 2016).

Most important to note is that these approaches can incorporate several factors and varying stimuli, such as dietary substances, into the structure of the tissues and biofluids. However, in more latest days, there has been a tendency to use these two tactics in tandem, with impressive success. Although targeted/focused approaches reveal new metabolites and set theories on new hypotheses, such approaches allow for well-established theories and reliable quantification. In each method, the analysis of data and processing steps varies and can differ from platform to platform, creating

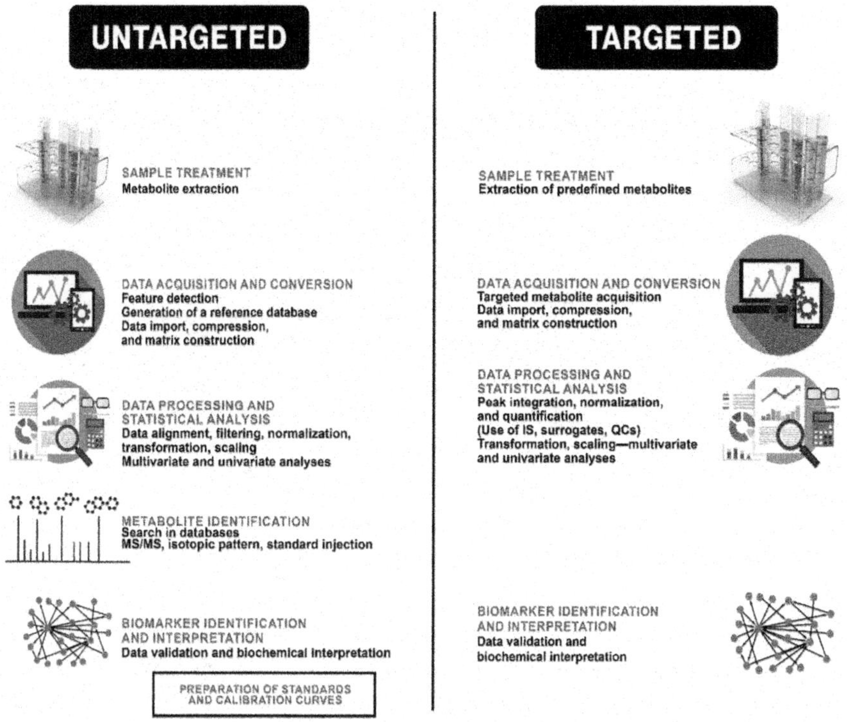

FIGURE 5.4 The targeted and untargeted approaches used for studying metabolomic data of dietary compounds for biological and clinical interpretation.

many options (Fiehn 2016; Gorrochategui et al. 2016; Misra et al. 2017; Pontes et al. 2017). Substantial improvements have been made in statistical techniques through computations, metabolic data analysis, and database maintenance. (Barupal et al. 2018; Tsugawa 2018). The use of metabolic agents in nutrition research continues to flourish and positively influences the research carried out. The standard metabolomic pathway, as represented in Figure 5.5, follows these main phases: it begins with the planning of the experiment and sample creation, following by LC-MS, NMR, and CE-MS (capillary electrophoresis mass spectrometry) (Smith et al. 2015) or by using a multidirectional strategy to achieve efficiency benefits of the metabolite sets.

5.2.2 Metabolome and Pathway Analysis: The Biological Interpretation

Metabolomics has become more and more widely used as part of nutritional analyses over the last decade. Overall, nutrition research provides knowledge on the interdependence of health and nutrition. Intervention with diet involves using whole grains or specific extracts of substances, like phytonutrients, minerals, and vitamins. Evaluation of nutritional interventions is complex because their long-term consequences are obscure and difficult to detect. At the same time, the application of metabolomics can offer insight into the significance of dietary interventions.

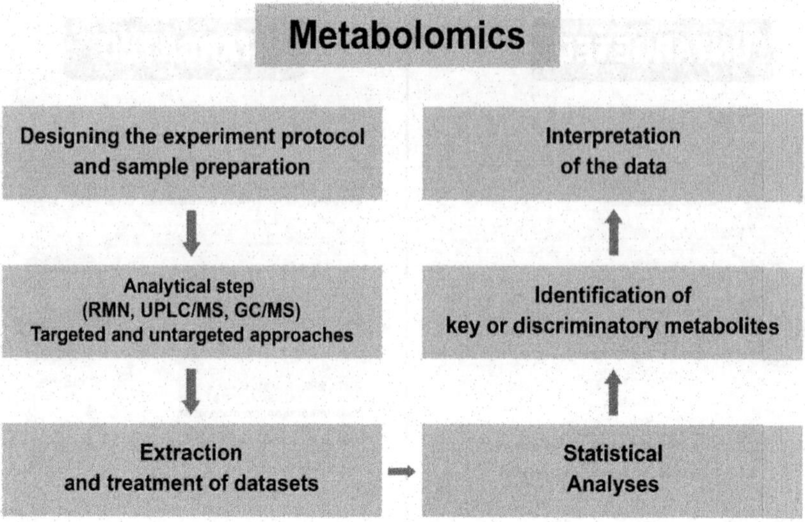

Metabolomics

Designing the experiment protocol and sample preparation

Analytical step (RMN, UPLC/MS, GC/MS) Targeted and untargeted approaches

Extraction and treatment of datasets

Statistical Analyses

Identification of key or discriminatory metabolites

Interpretation of the data

FIGURE 5.5 The major steps involved in a metabolomic study of body fluids.

For inspection and generation of metabolomic data in nutrition, NMR and MS combined with chromatography are the most widely used analytical approaches. NMR-based metabolomics is a stable and dependable method with comparatively little sample formulation (Nagana Gowda and Raftery 2017; Markley et al. 2017). In nutritional metabolomics, one-dimensional 1 H NMR is the most commonly used NMR technique. Two dimensional NMR approaches ^{1}H J-resolved (J-RES) and $^{1}H^{13}C$ heteronuclear single quantum correlation (HSQC) may be helpful for metabolite detection (Brennan 2014; van Duynhoven and Jacobs 2016). MS, on the other hand, is dependent on the mass-charge ratio (m/z). All the present molecules show a unique pattern in the form of peaks that represent their strength. Direct infusion mass spectrometry (DIMS) in direct MS-based platforms allows high-throughput and fast metabolite screening due to the requirement of minimal sample preparation, which eliminates the need for prior chromatographic or electrophoretic separation, allowing for shorter analysis times (González-Domìnguez et al. 2017; Khamis et al. 2017). However, the majority of the MS-based methods necessitate the use of a separation technique before the study. Although DIMS analysis provides sufficient metabolomic coverage, chemical isomers, and small variations in monoisotopic weights can only be detected employing ultra-high-resolution instruments, including Orbitrap-MS.

MS is often used in conjunction with gas chromatography, liquid chromatography, and capillary electrophoresis. The methods help reduce the biological samples with higher complexity and enhance the MS study of various groups of molecules by allowing them to enter the detectors at a specific interval of time. On these platforms, there are a wide variety of ionization and mass selection methodologies, but the most common nutritional analysis methods are ESI (electronic impact) and APCI (atmospheric pressure chemical ionization). Using ESI sources is a worry for both DIMS and hyphenation techniques. Molecular approaches have proven themselves to be quite valuable in the nutrition field. An NMR analysis analyzed a population sample and classified them according to their dietary patterns (Garcia-Perez et al. 2017). NMR spectroscopy has been effectively used for food biomarkers identification and estimation of food intake. Tartaric acid was used as a dose-responsive urinary biomarker to measure grape intake in a dietary intervention trial (Garcia-Perez et al. 2016); also in the cross-sectional study, the quantification of proline betaine allowed the evaluation of citrus consumption (Garcia-Perez et al. 2016).

The discovery of four biomarkers linked to milk intake in a twin cohort and their confirmation in separate populations demonstrates the importance of MS approaches. (Pallister et al. 2017). Using metabolomics of urine and fecal samples, the implications of breastfeeding, formula feeding, and bifidobacteria supplements on infants were successfully examined (Dessì et al. 2016; Bazanella et al. 2017). Therefore, the appropriate platform choice solely depends on the research objectives and the considered metabolites. Every analytical platform, on the other hand, has its own set of pros and cons. For instance, NMR-based metabolomics offers high replicability and confirms structural and metabolic pattern details that can be effectively utilized to identify undiscovered metabolites. Nevertheless, MS-based approaches have higher throughput sensitivity (Emwas 2015). Besides, to ensure the optimum metabolic coverage, the wide range of metabolites and their variations (from pico- to millimolar) necessitates the utility of several metabolic platforms. Many new research papers have emerged in the literature that has studied metabolites in recent years to examine childhood nutrition.

5.3 APPLICATION OF METABOLOMICS IN FOOD SCIENCE AND NUTRITION

Some examples of metabolomic applications include identifying and using diet-based and biochemical biomarkers, customized eating plans, and comprehensive interventional research in epidemiology for health. If metabolomics is successfully established for nutrient intake-based research, it can help deliver personalized nutrition after assessment, improving concept clearance about health concerning diet.

5.3.1 Applications in Food Quality, Authentication, and Safety

Food production and distribution have grown, making it necessary for food scientists worldwide to find residues, toxins, and pollutants in edible commodities. Of the various methods, implications of the metabolite studies through MS have found uses in the study of food quality protection and assurance of access to safe food components (Antignac et al. 2011). The use of nutrient metabolomics to detect adulteration in baby formula is an example of evidence-based science. (Inoue et al. 2015). The system changes must be made for systemic effects that conflict with recognition, and matrix effects must also be included in the food metabolite testing and characterization (Hird et al. 2014). Identifying bacterial contamination and toxic compounds further helps in assuring the public that the food is safe for consumption.

A potential challenge in freshly developed and consumed products involves pathogenic prokaryotic organisms, such as *Salmonella, Campylobacter, Escherichia coli*, and a few strains of *Bacillus*. Meanwhile, *Listeria monocytogenes* can be found in products involving processing. Among eukaryotes, *Alternaria, Aspergillus, Penicillium*, and *Fusarium* are concern oriented, which can cause harmful metabolites (Giacometti et al. 2012). GC-MS metabolomics and other omics tools, like DNA microarray, lipid-omics, and LC-MS/MS proteomics, have been more accurate in determining food spoiling pathogens and associated toxins compared to biochemical methods, even ELISA (Giacometti et al. 2012). There is an increased worry over food authentication as it is a key to fighting food theft, but it is also a method of determining the quality of food consumed for human health. Omics techniques, especially metabolomics with bioinformatic approaches, are a better solution for food quality assurance.

GC-MS, LC-MS, and NMR involving metabolomics have been utilized to investigate food composition concerning practices of agriculture (Johanningsmeier et al. 2016), also in dairy products (Boudonck et al. 2009). Such omics techniques have also been implicated to convert raw ingredients to final products (Johanningsmeier et al. 2016) and ensures the safety of the subsequent foodstuffs. A food item is typically produced through a combined application of physical and chemical treatments (heat treatment, extrusion, gel formation, cooking, etc.) that cause shape and compositional changes in the food product. Proteomics of packaged foods has always been a complex task (Picariello et al. 2012), owing to the increased complexity of proteins (protein-protein interaction, proteomics of processed foods, etc.).

5.3.2 Evaluation of Food Intake: Biomarkers to Reveal Exposure to Nutrients

Nutritional epidemiology is a critical method for assessing the diet-health relationship and, as a result, deciding human health policy and providing advice to particular populations. Dietary habits and assessment of dietary consumption of food nutrients and bioactive compounds have usually been performed using food frequency questionnaires, 24-hour recalls, or dietary records, whether in nutritional epidemiology or intervention trials (Tucker et al. 2013). However, due to the wide variety of foods eaten, such data are exceedingly difficult to obtain, even though the process of data collection has been modernized (Hedrick et al. 2012). Furthermore, people have trouble measuring the amount of food eaten. It is also worth noting that nutrient composition is affected by both the processing area and agricultural practices.

Polyphenols (a family of around 500 unique compounds) have been suggested to have possible beneficial effects on a variety of diseases, including heart attack and stroke, neurodegenerative diseases, and cancer, according to several reports, including cohort studies (Vauzour et al. 2010). This is the scenario with the correlation between flavonoid consumption and certain cardiovascular risk factors (Wang et al. 2014) since not all flavonoids' subclasses have the same protective impact. As a result, pinpointing particular compounds that have been ingested is critical in this form of research.

5.4 NUTRIMETABOLOMICS: AN INTEGRATED APPROACH FOR METABOLOMIC ANALYSIS IN HUMAN NUTRITIONAL STUDIES THROUGH SERUM/PLASMA

5.4.1 Sample Characteristics and Pre-Analytical Processing

The serum and plasma derived from blood are the widely used samples in human metabolomic experiments because they are comparatively easy to access due to the blood metabolome representing significant variations in metabolism. The serum is obtained post-clotting process, whereas plasma is obtained without clotting, as displayed in Figure 5.6. In whole blood, centrifugation extracts serum and plasma from macroparticles, such as coagulated material and cells. In whole blood, centrifugation separates serum and plasma from macroparticles, such as flocculated components and cells. Since it appears to lack fibrinogen, prothrombin, and other

SERUM	PLASMA
Clot for 30 min at room temperature; centrifuge 10 min at 4°C and 2,500 × g.	**Mix with anticoagulant; centrifuge 10 min at 4°C and 2,500 × g.**
Serum samples can show features of polymeric materials, peptides, and xanthines (the latter ones probably from the clot).	Anticoagulants may interfere with NMR signals and MS analysis.
There is higher content of peptides and protein fragments.	The presence of anticoagulant cations can cause problems in metabolomic and lipidomic analysis by binding to negatively charged phospholipids and causing ion enhancement.
Incubation affects the analyte peak area less in serum than in plasma what may result in reduced peak areas of plasma amino acids and carbohydrates with GC-MS detection.	Lithium ions from heparin can exacerbate matrix effects by increasing the signals of plastic polymers from Vacutainer containers.
Metabolite concentrations were found generally higher in serum yet still highly correlated with plasma.	EDTA was poorly suited for the analysis of polar metabolites. Sodium citrate can cause problems in determining citric acid and its derivatives.
	Sodium and potassium formate ion clusters from K-EDTA and sodium citrate creates adducts in MS spectra.
	The presence of anticoagulant residues may affect further extraction processes, including derivatization efficiency in case of GC-MS analysis.
	Isolation of plasma yields a greater sample volume per volume of whole blood drawn.
	There is an absence of platelet microparticles and post-coagulation protein fragments.

FIGURE 5.6 Difference between the collection, storage, and analytical techniques of serum and plasma.

clotting proteins, it has a higher viscosity than plasma. Ex vivo protein degradation, on the other hand, is more vulnerable to serum, which results in a vast amount of small peptides that can make extracting valuable information difficult (Wedge et al. 2011).

About the fact that metabolite concentrations in serum are typically higher, the two matrices are highly correlated. Furthermore, as phenotypes are compared, serum uncovers more possible biomarkers when compared to the plasma of blood (Denery et al. 2011; Yu et al. 2011; Barri and Dragsted 2013).

5.4.2 Sample Collection and Pre-Storage

The pre-analytical era, which includes sample selection, post-collection processing, and preservation, is a major source of heterogeneity in metabolomic study (Godzien et al. 2015; Yin et al. 2015). Standard operating procedures (SOPs) must be used in the metabolomic pipeline to achieve a significant level of reproducibility and repeatability. As a result, the sample storage container and metabolic quenching process must be carefully chosen. Until beginning, an investigation inspects sample tubes/containers and ensure that no pollutants are present or that no contaminants spill into the tests from the tubes since this may affect the results. A satiating metabolic protocol must be used, followed by the processing of the sample to inactivate enzymatic reactions to produce a precise representation of the metabolome during sampling. Since the blood from arteries and veins have different biochemical components, it is important to use the same blood collection site in the study, regardless of the sample type (serum/plasma).

The two techniques for extracting blood are vacuum (e.g., Vacutainer tubes) and aspiration (e.g., Monovettes). Various metabolomic experiments use Vacutainer tubes because they are a simple and standardized means of collecting blood. The constant volume of blood collected is ensured by the vacuum in the tubes. To avoid red cell lysis and reduce protease generation, plasma tubes should be positioned horizontally *on* ice (not *in* ice). In contrast, serum tubes should be incubated at room temperature for 30 minutes for clot formation (Rist et al. 2013). Plasma test samples should be treated immediately after blood is drawn, but serum needs a pre-clotting period at room temperature, which can introduce many metabolic variances (Denery et al. 2011; Yu et al. 2011; Barri and Dragsted 2013). As a result, SOPs are specifically essential while obtaining serum samples to ensure that all samples in the study have the same clotting period. The amount of time between blood collection and centrifugation and the temperature at which the samples are stored all affect metabolomic profiles (Boyanton and Blick 2002).

5.4.3 Aliquoting of Samples

Both samples for metabolomic analysis must be aliquoted in the same batch tubes to eliminate analytical variations. For each test, at least three aliquots are highly recommended and can be proceeded through targeted or untargeted analysis, as illustrated in Figure 5.7 (Ulaszewska et al. 2019).

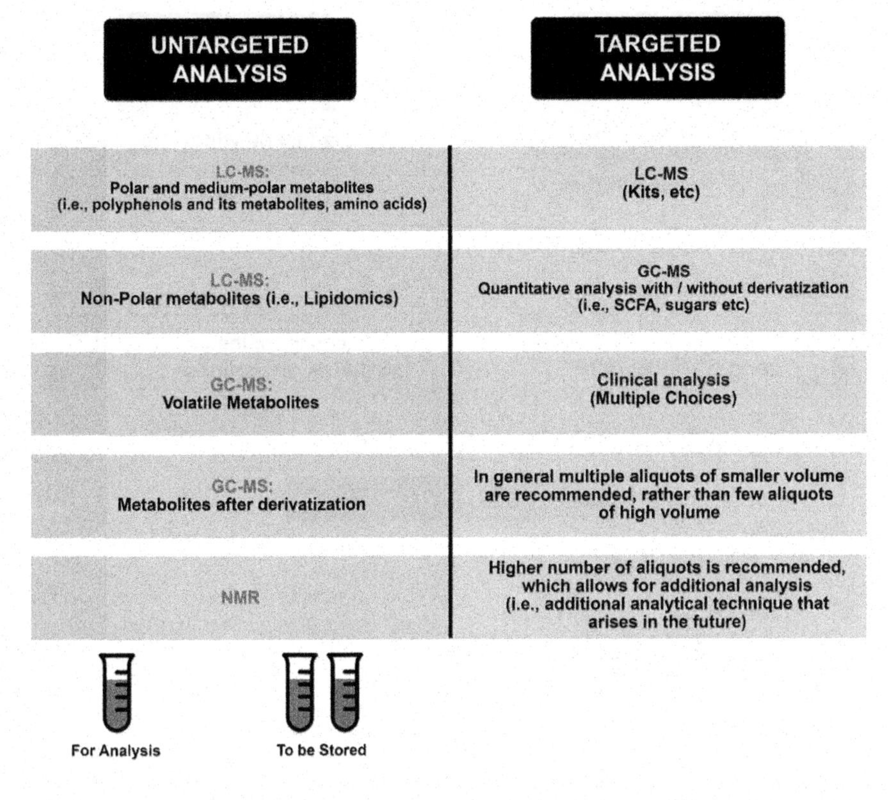

FIGURE 5.7 The different types of possible analytical techniques of biospecimens.

5.4.4 Storage and Thawing of Samples

Both plasma/serum samples must be put in cryovials as soon as possible after sampling and stored at −80°C in an ultra-cold freezer or liquid nitrogen containers before the examination, with temperatures and storage data being monitored continuously, as illustrated in Figure 5.8.

Because of the high abundance of enzymes in plasma and serum, there is general agreement that the metabolome is dysfunctional in nonfrozen samples. As the blood was retained at room temperature for several days, Clark and his colleagues found the increased concentration of fat-soluble vitamins and numerous plasma analytes (albumin, apolipoproteins A1 and B, cholesterol, HDL, total protein content, triglycerols, alanine transaminase, creatine kinase, creatinine, and glutamyl transferase) (Clarke et al. 2000). A recent metabolomic analysis based on the NMR also found that the plasma samples held at room temperature above 2.5 hours had significant impacts on lipoproteins and choline compounds (Pinto et al. 2014), while a 4°C sample cooling only maintains metabolite profiles for up to 24 hours (Yang et al. 2013; Kamlage et al. 2014). Anton et al. examined the effect on the levels of

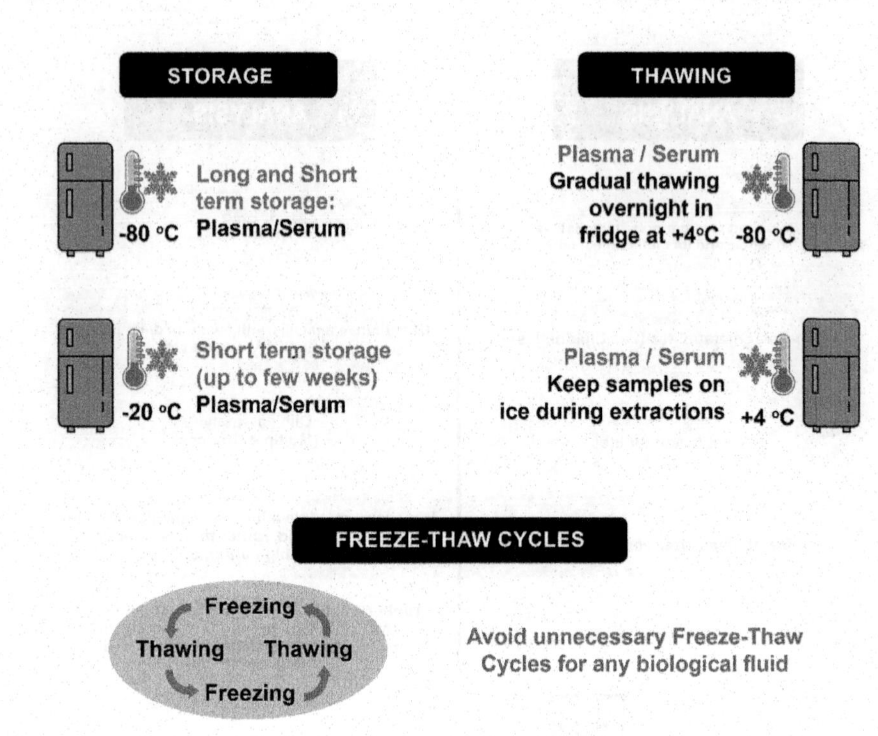

FIGURE 5.8 Various storage and thawing conditions ideal for biospecimens.

127 serum metabolites of the various storage conditions (room temperature, dry ice, wet ice, and for 12, 24, and 36 hours) (Anton et al. 2015). They also discovered a distinct characteristic of deterioration in the samples stored at room temperature (lysophosphatidylcholines, phosphatidylcholines, decadienylcarnitine, arginine, glycine, ornithine, phenylalanine, serine, leucine, isoleucine, ornithine, phenylalanine, and serine), while storing in ice resulted in fewer. Deep freezing at −80°C is the most frequent way of preserving blood-derived specimens and urine over a long period (Yang et al. 2013; Pinto et al. 2014; Moriya et al. 2016), although some authors claim that samples stored at −20°C may remain stable over short periods as well (i.e., a few weeks or months) (Zivkovic et al. 2009; Cuhadar et al. 2013; Pinto et al. 2014). Several researchers have examined the stability of plasma stored at −80°C for several years (5 to 17 years), indicating that certain metabolites, especially amino acids, acylcarnitines, glycerophospholipids, sphingomyelins, vitamins and, hexoses, deteriorate from prolonged storage, with concentration changes ranging from 13.7 to 14.5% (Haid et al. 2018; Lee and Kim 2017). The analysis of plasma samples after 14 to 17 years using untargeted UPLC-TOF (ultra-performance liquid chromatography–time-of-flight) method showed no significant differences (Hebels et al. 2013). Before being analyzed, samples must be thawed, as illustrated in Figure 5.8. Often scientists thaw plasma or serum samples at 4°C overnight. As a consequence of this mechanism, heat shock proteins are often grouped. While thawing blood samples at

room temperature removes lumps and thrombosis, it also raises the risk of enzymatic reactions and other sample modifications. Not all metabolites are influenced in the same manner by pre-analytical handling environments. As a result, sample integrity must be maintained during thawing.

5.4.5 Quality Control Samples for GC-MS and LC-MS Analyses

In GC-MS and LC-MS metabolomic trials, dealing with methodological instability is a big obstacle. Metabolomic workflows have also been monitored using test mixtures, intrinsic criteria, and pooled quality control (QC) samples. In the background of metabolomics, previous studies have established QC samples. The repetitive study of QC samples serves many purposes if numerous QC sample aliquots are primed autonomously: (1) in general, control of the analytical system's performance, such as retention time (tR) and signal strength reliability, mass calibration, and so on, and (2) determining the ultimate accuracy of a procedure (including sample preparation, intra-day, and inter-day). The QC samples indicate the qualitative and quantitative makeup of the samples to be assessed (Ulaszewska et al. 2019).

5.5 EVALUATION OF HEALTH STATUS: FROM HOMEOSTASIS TO A DISEASE STATE

Transition in nutrition means changing dietary intake and modifying physical activity levels. Inadequate dietary intake and habits, along with sedentary lifestyles, are root causes of increased prevalence of obesity because calorie intake is inversely proportional to calorie expenditure (Popkin 2011); obesity is a menace faced by all populations due to metabolic factors (e.g., oxidative strain to cells, glucose and lipid anabolic or catabolic issues, calorie excess or deficit) (Kaess et al. 2012) that set multifaceted challenges for understanding integrative metabolomic strategies and pathways involved in the progression of chronic diseases.

5.6 CONCLUSION

Advancement has been achieved on the development of test markers when high standards have been used in laboratory design, eliminating false-positive results, finding the most important metabolites, and increasing the efficacy of databases. Now, multi-omics advanced analytics is being developed to fully recreate the system-level interconnection and help elucidate the positioning of the microflora in metabolomic processes. Food safety and quality assurance have always been intensions to implicate the use of omics techniques, especially metabolomics. Nutritional biomarkers (models) are also used in efforts to investigate possible nutritional action, as well as to determine the risks and tendencies associated with functional changes and relatedness to the condition of dysfunctional metabolism, to learn the underlying causes and ramifications, and to identify new indicators that might forecast danger (obesity in relation to pathologic interfaces and metabolic syndrome). Investigations of the markers' ability are still required to validate nutrient sensitivity and to ascertain the full impact on the effectiveness of the metabolomic analysis for progress in individualized nutrition.

ACKNOWLEDGMENTS

The authors gratefully acknowledge Inamul Hasan Madar, Ghazala Sultan, and Deog-Hwan Oh for their expert technical support to fulfill the omics technologies in nutrition research of this research and helpful discussions. This work was funded by the National Research Foundation of Korea (NRF), grant number 2018007551, and Brain Korea (BK) 21 Plus Project, grant number 4299990913942.

REFERENCES

Antignac, J. P., Courant, F., Pinel, G., Bichon, E., Monteau, F., Elliott, C., and Bizec, B. 2011. Mass spectrometry-based metabolomics applied to the chemical safety of food. *Trends in Analytical Chemistry* 30:292–301.

Anton, G., Wilson, R., Yu, Z. H., et al. 2015. Pre-analytical sample quality: Metabolite ratios as an intrinsic marker for prolonged room temperature exposure of serum samples. *PLoS One 10*(3):e0121495.

Barri, T., and Dragsted, L. O. 2013. UPLC-ESI-QTOF/MS and multivariate data analysis for blood plasma and serum metabolomics: Effect of experimental artefacts and anticoagulant. *Analytica Chimica Acta* 768:118–28.

Barupal, D. K., Fan, S., and Fiehn, O. 2018. Integrating bioinformatics approaches for a comprehensive interpretation of metabolomics datasets. *Current Opinion in Biotechnology* 5:41–9.

Bazanella, M., Maier, T. V., Clavel, T., et al. 2017. Randomized controlled trial on the impact of early-life intervention with bifidobacteria on the healthy infant fecal microbiota and metabolome. *American Journal of Clinical Nutrition* 106(5):1274–86.

Boudonck, K. J., Mitchell, M. W., Német, L., et al. 2009. Discovery of metabolomics biomarkers for early detection of nephrotoxicity. *Toxicologic Pathology* 37(3):280–92.

Boyanton Jr, B. L., and Blick, K. E. 2002. Stability studies of twenty-four analytes in human plasma and serum. *Clinical Chemistry* 48(12):2242–7.

Brennan, L. 2014. NMR-based metabolomics: From sample preparation to applications in nutrition research. *Progress in Nuclear Magnetic Resonance Spectroscopy* 83:42–9.

Brennan, L. 2015. Metabotyping: Moving towards personalised nutrition. In *Metabolomics as a Tool in Nutrition Research* 137–44. Woodhead Publishing, London.

Cajka, T., and Fiehn, O. 2016. Toward merging untargeted and targeted methods in mass spectrometry-based metabolomics and lipidomics. *Analytical Chemistry* 88(1):524–45.

Capozzi, F., and Bordoni, A. 2013. Foodomics: A new comprehensive approach to food and nutrition. *Genes and Nutrition* 8(1):1–4.

Clarke, V. A., Lovegrove, H., Williams, A., and Machperson, M. 2000. Unrealistic optimism and the Health Belief Model. *Journal of Behavioral Medicine* 23(4):367–76.

Cuhadar, S., Koseoglu, M., Atay, A., and Dirican, A. 2013. The effect of storage time and freeze-thaw cycles on the stability of serum samples. *Biochemia Medica* 23(1):70–7.

Denery, J. R., Nunes, A. A., and Dickerson, T. J. 2011. Characterization of differences between blood sample matrices in untargeted metabolomics. *Analytical Chemistry* 83(3):1040–7.

Dessì, A., Murgia, A., Agostino, R., et al. 2016. Exploring the role of different neonatal nutrition regimens during the first week of life by urinary GC-MS metabolomics. *International Journal of Molecular Sciences* 17(2):265.

E Smith, R., Tran, K., and M Richards, K. 2015. Recent advances in metabolomics. *Current Metabolomics* 3(1):54–64.

Emwas, A. H. M. 2015. The strengths and weaknesses of NMR spectroscopy and mass spectrometry with particular focus on metabolomics research. In *Metabonomics* 161–93. Humana Press, New York, NY.

Fiehn, O. 2016. Metabolomics by gas chromatography – mass spectrometry: Combined targeted and untargeted profiling. *Current Protocols in Molecular Biology* 114(1):30–4.

García-Cañas, V., Simó, C., Herrero, M., Ibáñez, E., and Cifuentes, A. 2012. Present and future challenges in food analysis: Foodomics. *Analytical Chemistry* 84(23):10150–9.

Garcia-Perez, I., Posma, J. M., Chambers, E. S., et al. 2016. An analytical pipeline for quantitative characterization of dietary intake: Application to assess grape intake. *Journal of Agricultural and Food Chemistry* 64(11):2423–31.

Garcia-Perez, I., Posma, J. M., Gibson, R., et al. 2017. Objective assessment of dietary patterns by use of metabolic phenotyping: A randomised, controlled, crossover trial. *The Lancet Diabetes and Endocrinology* 5(3):184–95.

German, J. B., Watkins, S. M., and Fay, L. B. 2005. Metabolomics in practice: Emerging knowledge to guide future dietetic advice toward individualized health. *Journal of the American Dietetic Association* 105(9):1425–32.

Giacometti, J., Tomljanovic, A. B., and Josic, D. 2012. Application of proteomics and metabolomics for investigation of food toxins. *Food Res.* 54:1042–51.

Gibney, M. J., Walsh, M., Brennan, L., Roche, H. M., German, B., and van Ommen, B. 2005. Metabolomics in human nutrition: Opportunities and challenges. *American Journal of Clinical Nutrition* 82(3):497–503.

Godzien, J., Alonso-Herranz, V., Barbas, C., and Armitage, E. G. 2015. Controlling the quality of metabolomics data: New strategies to get the best out of the QC sample. *Metabolomics* 11(3):518–28.

González-Domínguez, R., Sayago, A., and Fernández-Recamales, Á. 2017. Direct infusion mass spectrometry for metabolomic phenotyping of diseases. *Bioanalysis* 9(1):131–48.

Gorrochategui, E., Jaumot, J., Lacorte, S., and Tauler, R. 2016. Data analysis strategies for targeted and untargeted LC-MS metabolomic studies: Overview and workflow. *TrAC Trends in Analytical Chemistry* 82:425–42.

Haid, M., Muschet, C., Wahl, S., Römisch-Margl, W., Prehn, C., Möller, G., and Adamski, J. 2018. Long-term stability of human plasma metabolites during storage at −80°C. *Journal of Proteome Research* 17(1):203–11.

Hebels, D. G., Georgiadis, P., Keun, H. C., et al. 2013. Performance in omics analyses of blood samples in long-term storage: Opportunities for the exploitation of existing biobanks in environmental health research. *Environmental Health Perspectives* 121(4):480–7.

Hedrick, V. E., Dietrich, A. M., Estabrooks, P. A., Savla, J., Serrano, E., and Davy, B. M. 2012. Dietary biomarkers: Advances, limitations and future directions. *Nutrition Journal* 11(1):1–14.

Hird, S. J., Lau, B. P. Y., Schuhmacher, R., and Krska, R. 2014. Liquid chromatography-mass spectrometry for the determination of chemical contaminants in food. *TrAC Trends in Analytical Chemistry* 59:59–72.

Ibáñez, C., Valdés, A., García-Cañas, V., et al. 2012. Global Foodomics strategy to investigate the health benefits of dietary constituents. *Journal of Chromatography A* 1248:139–53.

Inoue, K., Tanada, C., Sakamoto, T., Tsutsui, H., Akiba, T., Min, J. Z., Todoroki, K., Yamano, Y., and Toyo'oka, T. 2015. Metabolomics approach of infant formula for the evaluation of contamination and degradation using hydrophilic interaction liquid chromatography coupled with mass spectrometry. *Food Chemistry* 181:318–24.

Johanningsmeier, S. D., Harris, G. K., and Klevorn, C. M. 2016. Metabolomic technologies for improving the quality of food: Practice and promise. *Annual Review of Food Science and Technology* 7:413–38.

Kaess, B. M., Pedley, A., Massaro, J. M., Murabito, J., Hoffmann, U., and Fox, C. S. 2012. The ratio of visceral to subcutaneous fat, a metric of body fat distribution, is a unique correlate of cardiometabolic risk. *Diabetologia* 55(10):2622–30.

Kamlage, B., Maldonado, S. G., Bethan, B., et al. 2014. Quality markers addressing pre-analytical variations of blood and plasma processing identified by broad and targeted metabolite profiling. *Clinical Chemistry* 60(2):399–412.

Khamis, M. M., Adamko, D. J., and El-Aneed, A. 2017. Mass spectrometric based approaches in urine metabolomics and biomarker discovery. *Mass Spectrometry Reviews* 36(2):115–34.

Lee, J. E., and Kim, Y. Y. 2017. Impact of preanalytical variations in blood-derived biospecimens on omics studies: Toward precision biobanking? *Omics: A Journal of Integrative Biology* 21(9):499–508.

Markley, J. L., Brüschweiler, R., Edison, A. S., Eghbalnia, H. R., Powers, R., Raftery, D., and Wishart, D. S. 2017. The future of NMR-based metabolomics. *Current Opinion in Biotechnology* 43:34–40.

Misra, B. B., Fahrmann, J. F., and Grapov, D. 2017. Review of emerging metabolomic tools and resources: 2015–2016. *Electrophoresis* 38(18):2257–74.

Moriya, T., Satomi, Y., and Kobayashi, H. 2016. Intensive determination of storage condition effects on human plasma metabolomics. *Metabolomics* 12:179.

Nagana Gowda, G. A., and Raftery, D. 2017. Recent advances in NMR-based metabolomics. *Analytical Chemistry* 89(1):490–510.

Pallister, T., Haller, T., Thorand, B., et al. 2017. Metabolites of milk intake: A metabolomic approach in UK twins with findings replicated in two European cohorts. *European Journal of Nutrition* 56(7):2379–91.

Picariello, G., Mamone, G., Addeo, F., and Ferranti, P. 2012. Novel mass spectrometry-based applications of the "omic" sciences in food technology and biotechnology. *Food Technology and Biotechnology* 50(3):286–305.

Pinto, J., Domingues, M. R. M., Galhano, E., et al. 2014. Human plasma stability during handling and storage: Impact on NMR metabolomics. *Analyst* 139(5):1168–77.

Pontes, J. G. M., Brasil, A. J. M., Cruz, G. C., de Souza, R. N., and Tasic, L. 2017. NMR-based metabolomics strategies: Plants, animals and humans. *Analytical Methods* 9(7):1078–96.

Popkin, B. M. 2011. Is the obesity epidemic a national security issue around the globe? *Current Opinion in Endocrinology, Diabetes and Obesity* 18(5):328–31.

Rist, M. J., Muhle-Goll, C., Görling, B., Bub, A., Heissler, S., Watzl, B., and Luy, B. 2013. Influence of freezing and storage procedure on human urine samples in NMR-based metabolomics. *Metabolites* 3(2):243–58.

Tsugawa, H. 2018. Advances in computational metabolomics and databases deepen the understanding of metabolisms. *Current Opinion in Biotechnology* 54:10–17.

Tucker, K. L., Smith, C. E., Lai, C. Q., and Ordovas, J. M. 2013. Quantifying diet for nutrigenomic studies. *Annual Review of Nutrition* 33:349–71.

Ulaszewska, M. M., Weinert, C. H., Trimigno, A., et al. 2019. Nutrimetabolomics: An integrative action for metabolomic analyses in human nutritional studies. *Molecular Nutrition and Food Research* 63(1):e1800384.

Van Duynhoven, J. P., and Jacobs, D. M. 2016. Assessment of dietary exposure and effect in humans: The role of NMR. *Progress in Nuclear Magnetic Resonance Spectroscopy* 96:58–72.

Vauzour, D., Rodriguez-Mateos, A., Corona, G., Oruna-Concha, M. J., and Spencer, J. P. 2010. Polyphenols and human health: Prevention of disease and mechanisms of action. *Nutrients* 2(11):1106–31.

Wang, X., Ouyang, Y. Y., Liu, J., and Zhao, G. 2014. Flavonoid intake and risk of CVD: A systematic review and meta-analysis of prospective cohort studies. *The British Journal of Nutrition* 111(1):1–11.

Wedge, D. C., Allwood, J. W., Dunn, W., et al. 2011. Is serum or plasma more appropriate for intersubject comparisons in metabolomic studies? An assessment in patients with small-cell lung cancer. *Analytical Chemistry* 83(17):6689–97.

Yang, W., Chen, Y., Xi, C., et al. 2013. Liquid chromatography-tandem mass spectrometry-based plasma metabonomics delineate the effect of metabolites' stability on reliability of potential biomarkers. *Analytical Chemistry* 85(5):2606–10.

Yin, P., Lehmann, R., and Xu, G. 2015. Effects of pre-analytical processes on blood samples used in metabolomics studies. *Analytical and Bioanalytical Chemistry* 407(17):4879–92.

Yu, Z., Kastenmüller, G., He, Y., et al. 2011. Differences between human plasma and serum metabolite profiles. *PLoS One* 6(7):e21230.

Zivkovic, A. M., Wiest, M. M., Nguyen, U. T., Davis, R., Watkins, S. M., and German, J. B. 2009. Effects of sample handling and storage on quantitative lipid analysis in human serum. *Metabolomics* 5(4):507–16.

6 Nutriomic Approaches in Diabetic Practices

Srinivasan Kameswaran, Bellemkonda Ramesh, M. Subhosh Chandra, Ch. Venkatrayulu, M. Srinivasulu, Prathap Reddy Kallamadi, and G. Sudhakara*

CONTENTS

6.1 THE BACKGROUND

Diabetes mellitus (DM) is a metabolic issue described by delayed times of hyperglycemia (Priyadarsini et al. 2015), which incorporates regular urination, thirst, and hunger (Colvin 1997). The three main types of DM are as follows (Haw et al. 2017): Type 1 diabetes (T1D), also known as insulin-dependent diabetes or juvenile

* Corresponding author email: rammygp@gmail.com

DOI: 10.1201/9781003142195-6

diabetes, is caused by the pancreas being unable to produce enough insulin due to the loss of beta cells. T2D, otherwise called non-insulin-dependent diabetes or adult-type diabetes, starts with insulin resistance, and its progression may include insulin insufficiency. Gestational diabetes mellitus (GDM) refers to high blood sugar in pregnant women with no previous history of DM. Inability to treat any of these kinds in time causes numerous complexities (Yazdanpanah et al. 2017). Acute complications include diabetic ketoacidosis, hyperglycemia, and even death. Chronic complications include cardiovascular disease, stroke, chronic kidney disease, foot ulcers, and eye damage. According to the International Diabetes Federation (IDF), there were 425 million diabetic patients worldwide in 2017, and it is estimated that this number will increase to 629 million by 2045 (Cho et al. 2018). In 2017, DM patients in China ranked first worldwide, which is a value of 114,294.8 (www.idf.org). However, since DM is highly heterogeneous, individual treatments are required (Moucheraud et al. 2019). Comprehensive knowledge of the pathogens of DM becomes urgently necessary. Most of the studies combined clinical cases and summarized and suggested factors that might enhance the occurrence of DM. Due to the application of multi-data nutritional data analysis methods in DM research, obtaining potential molecular markers of pathogenicity is very simple and provides an acronym for further research, clinical diagnosis, and treatment. Human nutrients typically include the genes of protein-based human nutrition, human-component-based metabolism, the biology of microbial-based human diets, system-based diet, and systems biology. This chapter analyzes nutriomics over the years, describes the research progress and molecular mechanisms, and provides a reference for subsequent DM research (VanBuren et al. 2018).

6.2 NUTRITION AND DIABETES

A variety of dietary factors have been linked to the development of T1D and type 1 autoimmunity. For example, one study found that eating vegetables every day during pregnancy decreased the risk of a child developing type 1 autoimmunity (Brekke and Ludvigsson 2009). Another study found that consuming more iron in the first four months of life (via infant formula or supplements) was linked to a higher risk of developing T1D (Ashraf et al. 2010). Other researches, on the other hand, have found no connection between diet and the development of T1D. For example, Virtanen et al. (2011) discovered only a weak protective effect of a few foods consumed during pregnancy on the offspring's development of type 1 autoimmunity (the foods in question were butter, low-fat margarine, berries, and coffee; the majority of foods had no link).

6.2.1 Omega-3 Fatty Acids

Norris et al. (2007) discovered that omega-3 fatty acids, which can be found in fish, flax seeds, walnuts, soy, canola, and greens, prevent children at genetic risk of T1D from developing T1D-related autoantibodies. Omega-3 fatty acids may help to reduce inflammation, and a lack of omega-3s in Western diets can make people more prone to it. However, the same authors later discovered that omega-3 levels were not linked to T1D development in these children (Miller et al. 2011). As a result, omega-3s can be protective against the formation of type 1 autoantibodies but less so later in the disease phase.

The mother's dietary consumption of omega-3 fatty acids during pregnancy had no impact on the risk of autoimmunity in children, according to a previous study of the same children (Fronczak et al. 2003). Cod liver oil, on the other hand, has been linked to a lower risk of T1D in offspring when taken during pregnancy. This oil contains both omega-3 fatty acids and vitamin D, and one or both can play a role (Stene et al. 2000). The fatty acids present in milk and ruminant meat fat intakes were linked to an increased risk of type 1 autoimmunity, according to (Virtanen et al. 2010). Linoleic acid, on the other hand, was linked to lower levels of autoimmunity in children who were genetically predisposed to T1D. For six months, a group of people with metabolic syndrome (a set of disorders common in people with T1D or T2D) were given either omega-3 fatty acid supplements or a placebo. When compared to people who did not take the supplements, those who did had lower markers of autoimmunity and inflammation, as well as more weight loss (Ebrahimi et al. 2009). Adequate omega-3 intake during pregnancy can reduce the risk of obesity in children. Higher levels of omega-6s in umbilical cord blood compared to omega-3s have been linked to obesity in children under the age of three (Donahue et al. 2011).

6.2.2 Chemicals and Omega-3s

The effects of nutritional factors can also be influenced by the presence of environmental contaminants in food. Some pollutants may cause foods to lose their beneficial effects. For example, researchers concluded in a study linking insulin resistance to persistent organic pollutants that the beneficial aspects of omega-3 fatty acids in salmon oil do not mitigate the detrimental effects of persistent organic pollutants in that oil (Ruzzin et al. 2010). While fish is a good source of omega-3 fatty acids, an editorial in the *American Journal of Clinical Nutrition* suggests that plant-based sources are preferable (Feskens 2011). Studies on fish consumption and T2D are mixed: some show a connection between higher dietary omega-3 intake and a lower risk of T2D, while others show no link and even show that higher fish consumption raises the risk of T2D (Djoussé et al. 2011; Villegas et al. 2011). It's possible that the chemicals found in fish are to blame for these discrepancies. A research found that plant-based omega-3s had different effects on T2D than marine-based omega-3s (Brostow et al. 2011), and it was speculated that this might be due to toxins found in fish.

T2D and insulin resistance have been related to a high-fat diet, especially one high in saturated fats. Saturated fatty acids (but not unsaturated fats) tend to stimulate immune cells, causing them to develop an inflammatory protein, which causes cells to become insulin resistant (Wen et al. 2011). Excess body fat was found to be more common in mothers who ate more trans fats, as well as in their breastfed infants (Anderson et al. 2010).

Is it possible for the consequences of a high-fat diet to be passed on to future generations? A high-fat diet that induces obesity in mothers has been shown in animal studies to influence the metabolism and weight of their offspring. But what about fathers who eat a high-fat diet? Female offspring of heavier father rats (fed a high-fat diet) had defects in their insulin and glucose levels, similar to their fathers, according to one report. They were not heavier than the controls, unlike their fathers (Ng et al. 2010). Other researchers fed mice a high-fat diet with a fat composition close to that of a typical Western diet, then bred and fed them the same diet for generations. Despite not consuming more calories, the offspring grew increasingly heavier and produced higher insulin levels over four generations. Dietary changes were linked to changes in gene expression (Massiera et al. 2010).

6.2.3 Sweeteners and Glycemic Index

The glycemic index is a metric that determines how quickly a food increases blood glucose levels after consumption. Foods with a high glycemic index cause blood glucose levels to rise faster, triggering insulin output (in those that do produce insulin) and then lowering blood glucose levels. A higher glycemic index diet is linked to a quicker progression to T1D, according to one prospective study. However, the community on this diet did not have higher levels of autoantibodies, indicating that the diet may influence disease progression but not disease initiation. Oxidative stress, which is triggered by elevated blood glucose levels during meals or insulin resistance, could be involved. A high glycemic index diet, whatever the mechanism, can put additional stress on beta cells that are already under autoimmune attack (Lamb et al. 2008). Evidence supporting the active reduction of blood fats continues to accumulate, and many major diabetes societies now recommend that people with DM should reduce their fat intake and increase their carbohydrate intake to approximately 50% of total calories (Kayode et al. 2009). High-fiber foods are advocated (Jenkins et al. 1984). It has been emphasized that, although prior to providing detailed advice, comparative data may be required on the physiological effects of foods containing carbohydrates. Consumption of sugar-sweetened beverages has been linked with T2D, obesity, and metabolic syndrome. A meta-analysis of 11 prospective studies (of 300,000 people) discovered that those who consumed one to two sweetened beverages per day had a 26% higher chance of developing T2D than those who drink not more than one serving per month. The danger of growing metabolic syndrome was 20% higher. Sugar-sweetened drinks include carbonated drinks, fruit juices, iced tea, and energy drinks such as Vitaminwater (Malik et al. 2010). High-fructose corn syrup is another sweetener linked to obesity. The rats that received high-fructose corn syrup gained more weight than those that received sucrose, despite eating the same number of calories (Bocarsly et al. 2010).

6.2.4 Zinc

A few researchers have discovered that high levels of zinc in drinking water may be protective against T1D. For example, Zhao et al. (2001) reported that in southwest England, higher levels of zinc and magnesium were linked to lower rates of T1D. In Norway, an experiment found that higher levels of zinc in water were linked with a lower chance of developing T1D, but the consortium was not statistically significant

(Stene et al. 2002). Low zinc levels in drinking water were linked to a higher incidence of T1D in a study conducted in Finland (Ulf et al. 2011).

6.2.5 Nicotinamide and Other Antioxidants

Nicotinamide is a component of vitamin B3 that has been shown to prevent DM in animals and prevent beta-cell damage (Gale et al. 2004). Even better, one study found that it prevents the development of T1D in children with type 1 autoantibodies (Elliott et al. 1996). On the basis of these and other studies, a large double-blind, placebo-controlled trial was conducted in Europe, the United States, and Canada, called the European Diabetes Intervention Trial of Nicotinamide (ENDIT). This trial gave nicotinamide to first-degree relatives of T1D patients who had already developed type 1 autoantibodies. Unfortunately, they found no difference in DM progression between the two groups during the five-year follow-up period. The study gave high doses of the vitamin, up to three grams per day (30–50 times higher than the RDA) (Gale et al. 2004).

Another double-blind, placebo-controlled study in Sweden gave high doses of antioxidants (including nicotinamide, vitamin C, vitamin E, beta-carotene, and selenium) to people after they had already been diagnosed with T1D and also found that they had no effect in protecting beta cells from free-radical damage (Ludvigsson et al. 2001). There is no evidence linking levels of alpha- or beta-carotene antioxidants with the development of related type 1 autoimmunity in another study as well (Prassad et al. 2011). According to Uusitalo et al. (2008), taking antioxidants and trace minerals (such as retinol, beta-carotene, vitamin C, vitamin E, selenium, zinc, and manganese) during pregnancy had no impact on the risk of children developing type 1 autoimmunity. Antioxidant supplements were not found to be protective against metabolic syndrome, a group of conditions common in people with T1D or T2D (Czernichow et al. 2009). However, they discovered that people with the highest levels of antioxidants (beta-carotene, vitamin C, and vitamin E) at the start of the research had a lower risk of developing metabolic syndrome, likely due to a diet rich in plant foods. Although these studies found no positive results regarding antioxidant supplements, they also found no evidence that they were harmful. In T1D, free radicals can play a role in the inflammatory process that destroys beta cells (Ludvigsson et al. 2001). As a result, antioxidants are thought to protect the body from oxidative stress caused by free radical production. However, some animal evidence suggests that antioxidant supplements may increase insulin resistance, implying that the relationship is not as straightforward as it appears. Researchers found that giving mice an antioxidant made them more likely to develop insulin resistance (Loh et al. 2009). This finding can explain why antioxidant supplements haven't been found to protect people with T1D.

6.3 PRODUCTION OF FOOD: AGEs

Heat-processed foods contain advanced glycation end products (AGEs), which have been related to T1D and T2D in animal studies. They tend to predispose people to oxidative stress and inflammation, and they can damage the fetus if consumed by the mother while pregnant. A study has found that the levels of AGEs that a mother eats are correlated with insulin levels in the baby. It was discovered that if mothers' AGE levels are elevated and infant food is high in AGEs, the offspring's risk of DM is increased (Mericq et al. 2010).

6.3.1 Protein

Researchers fed mother rats a low-protein diet and discovered that their offspring had a higher incidence of DM. They also discovered that one of the offspring's genes had been "silenced" – a gene linked to the development of T2D. As a result, nutrition can have an effect on gene expression, which has been related to the development of T2D (Sandovici et al. 2011).

6.4 HUMAN NUTRIGENOMICS AND DIABETES

Human nutrigenomics, a new field in the study of nutrition proposed in the year 2000 (Jimenez-Sanchez et al. 2008), is the study of molecular biological processes and the effects of nutrients and food chemicals on humans (Roberts et al. 2001). The study of transcription, translation, and expression of human genes and metabolic mechanisms enables the development of nutritional recommendations of high predictive value to prevent disease, reduce the risk of unforeseen consequences, and control chronic diseases (Müller and Kersten 2003). Protein-based human dietary genomics has three research directions (Trujillo et al. 2006): food genomics, transcription, and proteomics.

6.4.1 Nutritional Genomic Advances in Diabetes Research

Genomics was first proposed by Roderick and colleagues in 1986, using DNA techniques of mapping, sequencing, and bioinformatics to analyze the structure and function of all genomes in living organisms (Jain et al. 2018). The food genomic research methods are consistent with functional genomic research (Reddy et al. 2018), mainly including DNA chip technology, biomarkers, and protein technologies. Genome-wide association studies (GWASs) are commonly used in nutritional genomics to investigate the pathogeneses of diseases like DM. GWAS includes the identification of existing sequence variants, which include single-nucleotide polymorphisms (SNPs) in human genome-wide applications, from which disease-associated SNPs are screened (Pearson and Manolio 2008). Studies have shown that the use of binary logistic regression analysis for diabetes analysis can effectively identify DNA different sequence differences (Zhang et al. 2011; Barroso and McCarthy 2019). GWASs have undergone several updates and upgrades. The latest T2D GWAS showed that common variations explain approximately 20% of the overall T2D risk, which is equivalent to at least half of the overall heritability (Defesche et al. 2017; Mahajan et al. 2018). Analysis of SNPs common in T2D patients and matched controls identified three T2D-binding sites in non-coding regions near CDKN2A and CDKN2B, and IGF2BP2 and CDKAL1 introns, as well as transcription correlations near HHEX and SLC30A8. T2D-related sites were also identified and confirmed in non-coding regions by analyzing the common polymorphisms in T2D patients and matched controls (Richa et al. 2007). Jeong et al. (2019) used DNA microarray to analyze cases of diabetic nephropathy (DN) and control cases and found that rs3765156 in PIK3C2B was significantly associated with DN. Using epigenome analysis of primary TH1 and TREG cells isolated from healthy subjects and T1D, (Gao et al. 2019) identified four SNPs (rs1077211, rs1077212, rs3176792, and rs883868) that could alter optimizer activities (H3K4me1 and H3K27ac). After a candidate gene associated with DM has been found by GWAS, experimental verification (i.e., cellular and animal experiments) is necessary.

6.4.2 Transcriptomic Advances in Diabetes Research

Transcriptomics refers to the sum of all the genetic copies of an organism or cell under certain conditions, which contain encoding the RNA protein required by the cell for a specific time and environment and a set of RNA molecules derived from the gene that regulates expression (Yu et al. 2010). Transcription is based on the development of sequencing technology, which includes the marker expression sequence (EST) technique, gene expression serial analysis (SAGE), massive parallel signature sequencing (MPSS), and RNA-seq. Several updated databases can be used for searching, such as GEO, DDBJ, SRA, MIRBase, NONCODE, ERA, and DRA.

The creation of the transcription database facilitated research related to the DM program. Wieczorek et al. (2019) examined transcriptional data from the salivary gland tissues of T1D patients and found inhibitory lymphoid structures outside the uterus and Sjögren's syndrome by blocking the CD40-CD154 pathway interaction. Using DM-based microarray and normal glucose tolerance, transcriptional profiles of subcutaneous adipose tissue were generated by studies from Asia and India. Differentially expressed genes can be analyzed using weighted gene co-expression network analysis to clinically diagnose (Saxena et al. 2019). The researchers used a complete and small proportional analysis RNA to optimize clinical tissue samples from DM patients with cardiovascular disease and successfully completed the complete copy of human left ventricular tissue (Ford et al. 2019). Fang et al. (2019) developed RePACT, a sensitive single-cell analysis algorithm, to discover the previously unrecognized role of cohesin loading complex and NuA4/Tip60 histone acetyltransferase in regulating insulin transcription and release. Hong et al. (2019) identified a number of angiogenes in the transcriptional features of glomerular endothelial cells, including leucine-rich α-2-glycoprotein 1 (LRG1), which was upregulated in DM mouse models. Caberlotto et al. (2019) analyzed transcriptional data from the brains of post-mortem T3D (type 3 diabetes) and T2D patients to determine the major role of autophagy in the molecular basis of T3D and T2D. Dusaulcy et al. (2019) analyzed islet cell transcript data from controlled mice and DM-induced mice, revealed 11–39 genes expressed differently in the pancreatic alpha cell transcript of hyperglycemic mice compared to controls, and identified three new target genes (Adcyl, Upk3a, and Dpp6) after further analysis. In summary, transcription database generation and analysis provide a reliable basis for researching DM mechanisms and determining gene functions.

6.4.3 Proteomic Advances in Diabetes Research

Wilkins and Williams proposed the concept of proteomics for the first time at the first international workshop for proteomics in Italy in 1994 (Jorrin-Novo et al. 2018). Proteomics refers to the science of understanding the laws of life activities from the entire protein level, with the protein being the object of research. Proteomics is a mature technology in the pharmaceutical industry, primarily for the detection of biomarkers and drug targets (Kussmann et al. 2005). Proteomics is divided into expression proteins, structural proteomics, and functional proteomics, mainly through two-dimensional gel electrophoresis, mass spectrometry, and other methods to study protein function and disease mechanisms. Relevant nutritious proteins can be controlled from a nutritional perspective to achieve early prevention and early treatment using proteomic methods to study nutritional diseases. Determination of apolipoprotein M (apoM) by proportional and proteomic analysis of conditioned media from isolated adipocytes and stromal cells in human adipose tissue (AT), where the expression level is lower in subjects with metabolic syndrome and T2D and may be associated with insulin sensitivity (Sramkova et al. 2019). Abdulwahab et al. (2019) collected sera from healthy subjects and T2D patients to measure protein mass spectrometry and found that 62 proteins were differentially expressed in T2D, which were functionally grouped into 16 proteins, including heparin cofactor 2, and the Ig α-1 chain C, and zinc-α-2-glycoprotein, the largest of which was an immunostimulant protein. Muralidharan et al. (2019) used borate-affinity chromatography to isolate red blood cell glycoproteins without hemoglobin from controls and DM samples, and proteomic analysis, using the nanoLC/ESI-MS proteins platform, to determine the site-specific glycemic index of the red blood cell protein using indicators different for the glycemic level in the blood of DM patients. Ricci et al. (2019) evaluated peptide biomarkers using capillary electrophoresis and mass spectrometry (CE-MS) and showed that the urinary protein in renal cysts in pediatric and diabetic syndrome (RCAD) differs from the predominant polycystic kidney disease (PKD1, PKD2), congenital nephrotic syndrome (NPHS1, NPHS2, NPHS4, and NPHS9), and chronic kidney conditions, indicating that there are differences between the pathophysiology of these disorders. The sequential window acquisition (SWATH) was used for all theoretical MS fragmentation spectrometers to study the biological determinants associated with the response to diet and weight-loss programs in impaired glucose regulation groups (Malipatil et al. 2019). These authors have successfully distinguished individuals who may lose weight from those who may have increased insulin sensitivity. For instance, as insulin sensitivity improves, hemoglobin *A1c* (HbA1C) levels lower with weight reduction (Malipatil et al. 2019). A differential gel electrophoresis method for comparing protein groups in DM and normal human urine (Rao et al. 2007). Seven select proteins (α1B-glycoprotein, zinc-α2-glycoprotein, α2-HS-glycoprotein, VDBP, calgranulin B, A1AT, and hemopexin) and four regulator proteins (prealbumin, α1-microglobulin, and bikunin) may be used as additional tests to diagnose DM. The role of proteins in studying complications of DM is important. Sims and Evans-Molina 2014 used proteomics to display proteins particularly expressed inside the urine of patients with DM retinopathy and nephropathy to discover biomarkers for early prognosis. Chiang et al. (2012) used 2-DE and MALDI-TPF-MS to analyze protein expression in diabetic retinopathy patients and identified 11 differentially expressed proteins associated with nutrient transport, microscopic realignment, angiogenesis, antioxidants, and neuroprotection. Zoccali et al. (2019), on biomarkers of diabetic kidney disease (DKD), found that the DKD 273 classifier was a promising biomarker for early identification of non-proteinogenic patients at high risk of developing progressive DKD. Empagliflozin and SGLT2 inhibitors may positively affect DKD progression of non-albuminous diabetic patients. Mirza et al. (2014) summarized the proteinaceous relationship between T3D and T2D and identified a single group or group of potential blood-based protein biomarkers with high sensitivity and specificity for early diagnosis of AD and T2D.

6.5 NUTRITIONAL METABOLOMICS AND DIABETES IN HUMANS

Metabolism is a method of studying issues related to nutrition through metabolism principles and methods (Baenas and Wagner 2019). Metabolism focuses on the metabolic pathways of intrinsic small-molecule metabolites in organisms, organs, and tissues and their changes, which can reflect the endpoint of the physiological regulation process in real time. The information obtained is closest to the phenotype of the organism or the general state and is the final expression of the biological phenomenon. The trophic metabolites can be divided into metabolites, lipids, and minerals (Figure 6.1).

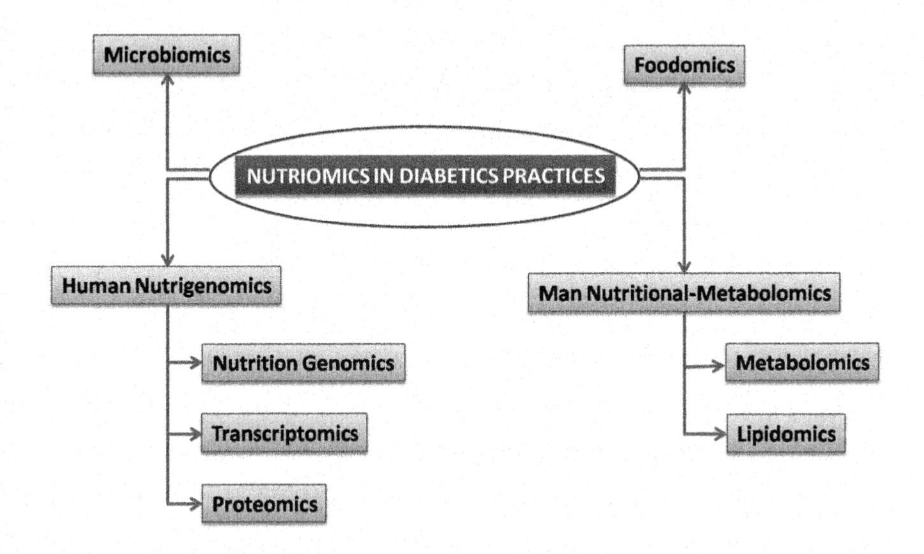

FIGURE 6.1 Human nutrition advance study in DM.

6.5.1 Metabolomic Advances in Diabetes Research

Nicholson et al. (1999) from Imperial College of Science and Technology in the United Kingdom proposed NMR-based metabonomics based on long-term graduated body fluids (Nicholson et al. 1999). Fiehn (2002) utilize GC to study the plant metabolism network and proposed metabolism at the same time. As the research progresses, the metabolic and metabolic processes are mixed together and now represent metabolomics (Ross and Babgi 2017). Metabolomics mainly analyzes the association of endogenous small molecular metabolites with physiological and pathological changes under the influence of internal and external factors (such as genetic variation, drug intervention, disease invasion, and environmental changes) through group indicators and is mainly divided into levels of metabolic target analysis, metabolic fingerprinting, metabolic profiling, metabolism analysis, and metabolic phenotypic analysis. Compared to food genomics, transcription, and proteomics, metabolism has the advantages of clear changes, fewer types and quantities, specific ingredients, common methods, and lower costs. Vangipurapu et al. (2019) studied metabolomic data on 20 amino acids from 4,851 patients with transverse metabolic syndrome and found that expressions of five amino acids (alanine, tyrosine, aspartic acid, isoleucine, and glutamic acid) were importantly associated with an increased risk of infection to T2D development. LC-MS for the non-targeted metabolism analysis of elevated glucose-induced changes in human proximal tubular H2 cell cultures to study proximal renal tubules in DM mechanisms in kidney disease progression (Bernardo-Bermejo et al. 2019). Using integrated proportional metabolism methods, Osataphan et al. (2019) showed that canagliflozin (CANA) regulates key nutrient-sensing pathways, activates AMPK 5-activated protein kinase (AMPK), and inhibits mTOR independently of insulin or glucagon sensitivity or signaling. The use of metabolites for the analysis of dietary nutrients contributes to the prevention and treatment of metabolic diseases through nutritional intervention.

6.5.2 Lipidomic Advances in Diabetes Research

Lipidomics is the study of lipid extracts to obtain lipid group information that reflects overall changes in lipids under specific physiological conditions (Murphy 2018). Nowadays, the many branches of lipids include adipocytes, computational lipidology, and neurolipidology.

Commonly used techniques related to lipids are thin-layer chromatography (TLC), electrostatic spray ionization mass spectrometry (ESI-MS), gas chromatography–mass spectrometry (GC-MC), high-performance liquid chromatography combined with the discovery of time-of-flight mass spectrometry (HPLC-TOF), high-performance liquid chromatography combined with quadrupole mass spectrometry (UPLC-TOF/MS), matrix-assisted flight time mass spectrometry (MALDI-TOF-MS), and shotgun lipidomics. Fat lipid research has shown that metabolic diseases, such as obesity and DM, are closely related to disorders of lipid metabolism (Gross and Han 2007). Lipidomics has enabled significant progress in discovering metabolic diseases, identifying lipid biomarkers and targeted drugs, and developing new drugs. He et al. (2019) established a lipid mass spectrum of 29 women with

GDM and 33 pregnant women without GDM and found that elevated GPR120 levels were associated with GDM. Lamichhane et al. (2019) compared cord blood lipids in T1D patients with that of healthy children and found that phospholipids, especially sphingomyelin, were lower in T1D progression. Wang et al. (2019) automatically screened obese rhesus monkeys and performed plasma lipid analysis on both normal and obese monkeys using GC-MS and UPLC-MS. These authors found that the lipids FFA C16:0 and 16:0-LPA may be a potential candidate for the diagnosis and study of obesity-related diseases. Zhang W et al. (2019) built a Paternò-Büchi reaction combined with LC-MS, using the C=C lipid derivative analysis platform online, and found that the C=C isomer could be used to discover lipid biomarkers, which could be used for screening, DM subsequent predictive. Pape et al. (2018) explored the role of hepatic triglycerides induced by a high-fat diet in the high-fat diet DM via MS-based fats and found associations between Per-Arnt-Sim kinase (PASK). Lamichhane et al. (2018) reported a longitudinal plasma lipid dataset of 40 children who progressed to T1D, 40 children with single-islet autoantibodies without T1D, and 40 matched controls. Their data could assist other researchers in studying the age-dependent development of autoimmunity to islet and T1D and the age-dependent nature of the general lipid spectrum. Six hundred ninety-two participants were randomized (639 non-cases and 53 T2D cases), and 207 plasma lipid metabolites were repeatedly measured (Razquin et al. 2018). They used principal component analysis to generate a global factor for lipid types and to assess the relationship between these lipid factors and the incidence of T2D. Lipid analysis and found that *Cyclocarya paliurus* may improve diabetic lipidosis by reducing the accumulation of hepatic lipid droplets and regulation of lipids in circulation in diabetic mice via PI3K signaling and MAPK signaling pathways (Zhai et al. 2018). Yang et al. (2018) analyzed large datasets generated by metabolites and lipids and revealed the role of metabolites, like lipids, amino acids, and bile acids, in the regulation of insulin sensitivity.

6.5.3 Metallomic Advances in Diabetes Research

Mineralogy is the comprehensive study of the distribution, existence, content, structural properties, and physiological functions of metallic and metallic elements in biological systems (Zhang Y et al. 2019). Mineral science covers morphological analysis of elements in biological structure, as well as distribution and analysis of elements in muscles, tissues, body fluids, and cells in living organisms; metallurgy structural analysis; metal group reactions mechanism; metalloprotein action and metalloenzyme recognition; multi-component analysis for biomolecules and metals; multi-component analysis for biomolecules and metals; and metabolic analysis of biomolecules and metals and design of inorganic drugs in chemotherapy, medicine, environmental sciences, food sciences, agriculture, toxicology, and biogeology. Other minerals in chemistry help in the functional biological sciences. Commonly used techniques include atomic absorption spectrometry, inductively coupled plasma mass spectrometry (ICP-MS), infrared spectroscopy, quantitative isotope analysis, X-ray absorption spectroscopy, and nuclear magnetic resonance (Biagioni et al. 2017). In recent years, increasing reports on mineralogy and metabolic diseases have guided the importance of healthy diets. Lindeque et al. (2015) evaluated the protective effects of metallothioneins (MTs) on obesity and effects induced by a high-fat diet, such as insulin resistance in male and female mice's MT-1-, MT-2-, and MT-3-knockout. Steinbrenner et al. (2011) summarized the current evidence of interference with selenium compounds and molecular pathways regulated by insulin and validated that excessive selenium intake in nutrition and high levels of selenium in plasma were potential risk factors for T2D. Roverso et al. (2019) recruited 76 pregnant women from the University Hospital of Padua (Italy); half of them had DM. Placenta samples were collected from whole maternal blood and umbilical cord blood, and mineral groups were determined by ICP-MS analysis. The results showed that the concentrations of calcium, copper, sodium, and zinc in the cord blood of GDM patients were higher than those of the controls, while potassium, iron, phosphorus, manganese, sulfur, rubidium, and silicon exhibited opposing patterns. Roverso et al. (2015) used a mineral database to analyze GDM and other DM types and found that selenium concentrations were higher in GDM than in the other groups. A combined metabolic method and metallurgy using a hypercholesterolemia rat model, including NMR spectroscopy, plasma MS, and mineral fingerprinting law (Liu et al. 2012). The consequences revealed that vanadium, manganese, sodium, and potassium will be biomarkers of hypercholesterolemia. The omics-driven study by Lopes et al. is based on the time-resolved H-NMR metabolism to study the outcomes of Roux-en-Y gastric bypass surgery (Lopes et al. 2016). The role of selenoprotein S (SelS) gene differentiation in subclinical risk and mortality in T2D patients was investigated (Cox et al. 2013).

6.6 DIABETES AND MICROBIOMICS

Microbial-based human nutritional metabolomics is gut microbiology (Sonnenburg and Sonnenburg 2019). In a healthy adult, the total number of gut microbes is enormous, and this microbial layer is referred to as the "human second genome". In December 2007, the National Institutes of Health introduced the Human Microbiome Program, which is a microbial genome study of the digestive system, mouth, vagina, skin, and nasal passages (US National Institutes of Health 2019). Human intestinal bacteria begin to colonize from the birth of the host and gradually mature as the host grows, reaching a relatively stable state. Microbial functions in the gut include nutritional and metabolic functions, mucosal barrier function, and immune function. Common research techniques used in gut microbiology include biochips, DGGE, and RT-PCR. The use of the gut microbiome to analyze changes in the structure and function of the human microbial community under health and disease conditions could improve the prevention and treatment of metabolic diseases.

Díaz-Rizzolo et al. (2020) divided 182 diabetic patients over 65 years of age into obese and non-obese groups, analyzed the outcome and biochemical parameters of the gut microbiome (FINDRISC), and found the significance of the gut microbiome. Larsen et al. (2010) reported that human T2D was associated with changes in the composition of the gut microbiota and that the gut microbiota could be altered to control metabolic diseases. For instance, the proportions of Firmicutes and Clostridia were altogether diminished in the DM group compared to the control group. Likewise, the Betaproteobacteria class was highly enriched in-group compared to the control group and positively linked to plasma glucose. In addition, Aydin et al. (2018) conducted a study of the gut microbiota's function in human obesity and T2D. Qiao et al. (2018) reported that the intestinal microbiotas of patients with T2D differed significantly in bacterial composition and diversity from the intestinal microbiotas of healthy subjects. A metabolic and standardized anthropometric evaluation of 30 clinically stable T2D patients and concluded that DM leads to intestinal bacterial overgrowth, increased intestinal permeability, and low-grade systemic inflammation (Pasini et al. 2019). Chronic exercise can also reduce excessive intestinal floral development, intestinal leakage, and systemic inflammation, according to the researchers. Ohtsu et al. (2019) found that oral administering of *Porphyromonas gingivalis* can alter the gut microbiota and exacerbate glycemic control in streptozotocin-induced DM mice. Chen et al. (2019) examined and compared the effects of green tea polyphenols (polyphenon E) and black tea polyphenols (theaflavins) on the gut microbiota and DM development in db/db mice. A review by Whang et al. (2018) presented evidence explaining the presumed interaction between antidiabetic agents and the gut microbiome and discussed the potential of microbiome modifiers in drug processing, microbial interactions, and drug metabolism.

6.7 DIABETES AND FOODOMICS

The word "foodomics" was first used in 2007 in network and academic conferences (Herrero et al. 2010) and refers to the use of omics analysis methods to study the components of complex diets, like proteins, peptides, carbohydrates, amino acids, fats, vitamins, and trace elements. Commonly used methods include genomics, transcription, proteomics, metabolism, and bioinformatics. Foodomic analysis contributes to explaining single genomes responses to specific food formulations; explaining the biochemical, molecular, and cellular mechanisms by which some of the active ingredients in food constitute health benefits and adverse effects; determining the role of bioactive food components in key molecular pathways; identifying genes and possible molecular biomarkers from pre-onset to onset; determining the general role and function of the gut microbiome; conducting studies of unintended effects of genetically modified crops; studying the application of food microbes as delivery systems; studying adaptations of food pathogen stress to response; ensuring food hygiene, handling, and storage; comprehensively assessing food safety, quality, and traceability; and investigating the molecular basis of biological processes including crop-pathogen interactions and physical and chemical changes during fruit ripening. The holistic method of environmental interactions explains the phenomena and defines the biological network (Cifuentes 2009).

The foodomic study involves studying food metabolites to provide a basis for a healthy diet. Mounting evidence indicates that healthy diets rich in vegetables, fruits, nuts, extra-virgin olive oil, and fish are beneficial for preventing and controlling different human diseases and metabolic disorders. This is the Mediterranean diet, and it is one of the healthiest diets in existence. Proteomic and metabolomic analyses revealed that Mediterranean diets had clinical implications for metabolic and microvascular activities, cholesterol and fasting blood glucose, and anti-inflammatory and antioxidative effects (Alkhatib et al. 2017). Therefore, a dietary study is useful in preventing and treating diseases (Santangelo et al. 2016). Olivas-Aguirre et al. (2016) studied the metabolites of cyanidin-3-o-glucoside (Cy3G) and found that they protect against *Helicobacter pylori* infection, age-related disease, T2D, cardiovascular disease, and metabolic syndrome. The mouse models of Janšáková et al. (2019) were used to verify advanced glycation end products (AGEs) in hot processed foods thought to cause GDM and found that these AGEs did not cause disease. Takahashi et al. (2014) conducted comprehensive protein and metabolic analyses to verify that coffee consumption leads to an ATP increase in conversion and demonstrate that coffee consumption can help prevent DM. Inulin has been reported to have a large number of diverse pharmaceutical and nutritional applications. A review by Tsurumaki et al. (2015) describes the current state of using omics techniques in elucidating the effect of inulin and inulin-containing prebiotics on transcriptome, proteome, metabolome, and gut levels to illustrate the complex beauty behind the relatively modest effect of food agents, such as inulin, on host health. Functional foods, according to Alkhatib et al. (2017), contain biologically active ingredients linked to physiological health benefits and the prevention and management of chronic diseases like T2D. Zhao et al. (2019) published a comprehensive study on glucose metabolism in T2D, as well as an investigation into the relationships between natural phytochemicals and glucose handling. Sébédio et al. (2017) proposed metabolism studies to discover new biomarkers of early metabolic dysfunction and predict biomarkers of developmental disease (e.g., obesity, metabolic syndrome, and T2D) but have focused on developing methods for identifying and validating biomarkers of nutrient exposure.

6.8 CONCLUSIONS

Nutrition is the study of health-promoting food ingredients as well as the science of human use and application of these ingredients. The main goal of nutrition research is to find ways to prevent diseases (especially metabolic diseases) and protect human health by eating a balanced diet on a daily basis. Nutritional growth has exploded as a result of the advancement of omics technology, and the word "precision medicine" has been coined. Precision medicine is a modern approach to disease prevention and treatment that considers a person's genetics, climate, and lifestyle choices. Precision medicine is a term that is gaining traction. Using large amounts of data, genomics, and other omics, such as metabolomics, proteomics, and transcriptomics, can make personalized medicine a reality in the near future (Mohan and Radha 2019). Furthermore, the Metabolomics Association claims that incorporating metabolomic data into precision medicine systems is timely and will provide highly useful new data to supplement existing data (Beger et al. 2016). This chapter summarized the findings of numerous researchers who used empirical omics approaches, and it serves as a resource for future study.

REFERENCES

Abdulwahab, R. A., Alaiya, A., Shinwari, Z., Allaith, A. A. A., and Giha, H. A. 2019. LC-MS/MS proteomic analysis revealed novel associations of 37 proteins with T2DM and notable upregulation of immunoglobulins. *International Journal of Molecular Medicine* 43:2118–32.

Alkhatib, A., Tsang, C., Tiss, A., et al. 2017. Functional foods and lifestyle approaches for diabetes prevention and management. *Nutrients* 9:1310.

Anderson, A. K., McDougald, D. M., and Steiner-Asiedu, M. 2010. Dietary trans fatty acid intake and maternal and infant adiposity. *European Journal of Clinical Nutrition* 64(11):1308–15.

Ashraf, A. P., Easson, N. B., Kabagambe, E. K., Haritha, J., Meleth, S., and McCormic, K. L. 2010. Dietary iron intake in the first 4 months of infancy and the development of type 1 diabetes: A pilot study. *Diabetology and Metabolic Syndrome* 2:58.

Aydin, Ö., Nieuwdorp, M., and Gerdes, V. 2018. The gut microbiome as a target for the treatment of type 2 diabetes. *Current Diabetes Reports* 18:55.

Baenas, N., and Wagner, A. E. 2019. *Drosophila melanogaster* as an alternative model organism in nutrigenomics. *Genes and Nutrition* 14:14.

Barroso, I., and McCarthy, M. I. 2019. The genetic basis of metabolic disease. *Cell* 177:146–61.

Beger, R. D., Dunn, W., Schmidt, M. A., et al. 2016. Metabolomics enables precision medicine: "A white paper, community perspective". *Metabolomics* 12:149.

Bernardo-Bermejo, S., Sánchez-López, E., Castro-Puyana, M., Benito, S., Lucio-Cazaña, F. J., and Marina, M. L. 2019. An untargeted metabolomic strategy based on liquid chromatography-mass spectrometry to study high glucose-induced changes in HK-2 cells. *Journal of Chromatography A* 1596:124–33.

Biagioni, C., D'Orazio, M., Lepore, G. O., d'Acapito, F., and Vezzoni, S. 2017. Thallium-rich rust scales in drinkable water distribution systems: A case study from northern Tuscany, Italy. *Science of the Total Environment* 587:491–501.

Bocarsly, M. E., Powell, E. S., Avena, N. M., and Hoebel, B. G. 2010. High fructose corn syrup causes characteristic obesity in rats: Increased body weight, body fat and triglyceride levels. *Pharmacology Biochemistry and Behavior* 97(1):101–6.

Brekke, H. K., and Ludvigsson, J. 2009. Daily vegetable intake during pregnancy negatively associated to islet autoimmunity in the offspring – the ABIS study. *Pediatrics Diabetes* 4:244–250.

Brostow, D. P., Odegaard, A. O., Koh, W. P., et al. 2011. Omega-3 fatty acids and incident type 2 diabetes: The Singapore Chinese Health Study. *American Journal of Clinical Nutrition* 94(2):520–6.

Caberlotto, L., Nguyen, T. P., Lauria, M., et al. 2019. Cross-disease analysis of Alzheimer's disease and type-2 Diabetes highlights the role of autophagy in the pathophysiology of two highly comorbid diseases. *Scientific Reports* 9:3965.

Chen, T., Liu, A. B., Sun, S., et al. 2019. Green tea polyphenols modify the gut microbiome in db/db Mice as co-abundance groups correlating with the blood glucose lowering effect. *Molecular Nutrition Food Research* 63:e1801064.

Chiang, S. Y., Tsai, M. L., Wang, C. Y., et al. 2012. Proteomic analysis and identification of aqueous humor proteins with a pathophysiological role in diabetic retinopathy. *Journal of Proteomics* 75:2950–9.

Cho, N. H., Shaw, J. E., Karuranga, S., et al. 2018. IDF diabetes atlas: Global estimates of diabetes prevalence for 2017 and projections for 2045. *Diabetes Research and Clinical Practice* 138:271–81.

Cifuentes, A. 2009. Food analysis and Foodomics. *Journal of Chromatography A* 1216:7109.

Colvin, R. 1997. Protease inhibitors and diabetes: A growing problem. *Common Factor* 11:8.

Cox, A. J., Lehtinen, A. B., Xu, J., et al. 2013. Polymorphisms in the Selenoprotein S gene and subclinical cardiovascular disease in the diabetes heart study. *Acta. Diabetologica* 50:391–9.

Czernichow, S., Vergnaud, A. C., Galan, P., et al. 2009. Effects of longterm antioxidant supplementation and association of serum antioxidant concentrations with risk of metabolic syndrome in adults. *American Journal of Clinical Nutrition* 90(2):329–35.

Defesche, J. C., Gidding, S. S., Harada-Shiba, M., Hegele, R. A., Santos, R. D., and Wierzbicki, A. S. 2017. Familial hypercholesterolaemia. *Nature Reviews Disease Primers* 3:17093.

Díaz-Rizzolo, D. A., Kostov, B., López-Siles, M., et al. 2020. Healthy dietary pattern and their corresponding gut microbiota profile are linked to a lower risk of type 2 diabetes, independent of the presence of obesity. *Clinical Nutrition* 39(2):524–32.

Djoussé, L., Biggs, M. L., Lemaitre, R. N., et al. 2011. Plasma omega-3 fatty acids and incident diabetes in older adults. *American Journal of Clinical Nutrition* 94(2):527–33.

Donahue, S. M., Rifas – Shiman, S. L., Gold, D R., Jouni, Z. E., Gillman, M. W., and Oken, E. 2011. Prenatal fatty acid status and child adiposity at age 3y: Results from a US pregnancy cohort. *American Journal of Clinical Nutrition* 93(4):780–8.

Dusaulcy, R., Handgraaf, S., Visentin, F., et al. 2019. High-fat diet impacts more changes in beta-cell compared to alpha-cell transcriptome. *PLoS One* 14:e0213299.

Ebrahimi, M., Ghanyour – Mobarhan, M., Rezaiean, S., et al. 2009. Omega-3 fatty acid supplements improve the cardiovascular risk profile of subjects with metabolic syndrome including markers of inflammation and autoimmunity. *Acta Cardiologica* 64(3):321–7.

Elliott, R. B., Pilcher, C. C., Fergusson, D. M., and Stewart, A. W. 1996. A population – based strategy to prevent insulin-dependent diabetes using nicotinamide. *Journal Pediatric Endocrinology and Metabolism* 9(5):501–9.

Fang, Z., Weng, C., Li, H., et al. 2019. Single-cell heterogeneity analysis and CRISPR screen identify key β-cell-specific disease genes. *Cell Reports* 26:3132–44.

Feskens, E. J. 2011. The prevention of type 2 diabetes. Should we recommend vegetable oils instead of fatty fish? *American Journal Clinical Nutrition* 94(2):369–70.

Fiehn, O. 2002. *Metabolomics – The Link between Genotypes and Phenotypes*, 155–71. Springer, Dordrecht, The Netherlands.

Ford, K. L., Anwar, M., Heys, R., et al. 2019. Optimisation of laboratory methods for whole transcriptomic RNA analyses in human left ventricular biopsies and blood samples of clinical relevance. *PLoS One* 14:e0213685.

Fronczak, C. M., Baron, A. E., Chase, H. P., et al. 2003. In utero dietary exposures and risk of islet autoimmunity in children. *Diabetes Care* 26(12):3237–42.

Gale, E. A., Bingley, P. J., Emmett, C. L., and Collier, T. 2004. European Nicotinamide Diabetes Intervention Trial (ENDIT): A randomized controlled trial of intervention before the onset of type 1 diabetes. *Lancet* 363(9413):925–31.

Gao, P., Uzun, Y., He, B., et al. 2019. Risk variants disrupting enhancers of TH1 and TREG cells in type 1 diabetes. *Proceedings of the National Academy of Sciences of the United States of America* 116:7581–90.

Gross, R. W., and Han, X. 2007. Lipidomics in diabetes and the metabolic syndrome. *Methods Enzymology* 433:73.

Haw, J. S., Galaviz, K. I., Straus, A. N., et al. 2017. Long-term sustainability of diabetes prevention approaches: A systematic review and meta-analysis of randomized clinical trials. *JAMA Internal Medicine* 177:1808–17.

He, Q., Zhu, S., Lin, M., et al. 2019. Increased GPR120 level is associated with gestational diabetes mellitus. *Biochemical and Biophysical Research Communication* 512:196–201.

Herrero, M., García-Cañas, V., Simo, C., and Cifuentes, A. 2010. Recent advances in the application of capillary electromigration methods for food analysis and foodomics. *Electrophoresis* 31:205–28.

Hong, Q., Zhang, L., Fu, J., et al. 2019. LRG1 promotes diabetic kidney disease progression by enhancing TGF-β-induced angiogenesis. *Journal of American Society of Nephrology* 30:54662.

Jain, C., Koren, S., Dilthey, A., Phillippy, A. M., and Aluru, S. 2018. A fast adaptive algorithm for computing whole-genome homology maps. *Bioinformatics* 34:i748–56.

Janšáková, K., Lengyelová, E., Pribulová, N., et al. 2019. Metabolic and renal effects of dietary advanced glycation end products in pregnant rats – a pilot study. *Physiology Research* 68:467–79.

Jenkins, D. J. A., Wolever, T. M. S., Jenkins, A. L., Josse, R., and Wong, G. S. 1984. Glycaemic response to carbohydrate foods. *Lancet* 2:388–91.

Jeong, K. H., Kim, J. S., Woo, J. T., et al. 2019. Genome-wide association study identifies new susceptibility loci for diabetic nephropathy in Korean patients with type 2 diabetes mellitus. *Clinical Genetics* 96:35–42.

Jimenez-Sanchez, G., Silva-Zolezzi, I., Hidalgo, A., and March, S. 2008. Genomic medicine in Mexico: Initial steps and the road ahead. *Genome Research* 18:11918.

Jorrin-Novo, J. V., Komatsu, S., Sanchez-Lucas, R., and Rodríguez de Francisco, L. E. 2018. Gel electrophoresis-based plant proteomics: Past, present, and future. *Journal of Proteomics* 198:1–10.

Kayode, J., Sola, A., Adelani, A., Adeyinka, A., Kolawole, O., and Bashiru, O. 2009. The role of carbohydrate in diabetic nutrition: A review. *Internet Journal of Laboratory Medicine* 3(2):1–18.

Kussmann, M., Affolter, M., and Fay, L. B. 2005. Proteomics in nutrition and health. *Combinatorial Chemistry and High Throughput Screening* 8:679–96.

Lamb, M. M., Yin, X., Barriga, K., et al. 2008. Dietary glycemic index, development of islet autoimmunity and subsequent progression to type 1 diabetes in young children. *Journal of Clinical Endocrinology Metabolism* 93(10):3936–42.

Lamichhane, S., Ahonen, L., Dyrlund, T. S., et al. 2018. A longitudinal plasma lipidomics dataset from children who developed islet autoimmunity and type 1 diabetes. *Science Data* 5:180250.

Lamichhane, S., Ahonen, L., Dyrlund, T. S., et al. 2019. Cord-blood lipidome in progression to islet autoimmunity and type 1 diabetes. *Biomolecules* 9:33.

Larsen, N., Vogensen, F. K., van den Berg, F. W., et al. 2010. Gut microbiota in human adults with type 2 diabetes differs from non-diabetic adults. *PLoS One* 5:e9085.

Lindeque, J. Z., Jansen van Rensburg, P. J., Louw, R., et al. 2015. Obesity and metabolomics: Metallothioneins protect against high-fat diet-induced consequences in metallothionein knockout mice. *Omics* 19:92–103.

Liu, F., Gan, P. P., Wu, H., Woo, W. S., Ong, E. S., and Li, S. F. 2012. A combination of metabolomics and metallomics studies of urine and serum from hypercholesterolaemic rats after berberine injection. *Analytical and Bioanalytical Chemistry* 403:847–56.

Loh, K., Deng, H., Fukushima, A., et al. 2009. Reactive oxygen species enhance insulin sensitivity. *Cell Membrane* 10(4):260–72.

Lopes, T. I., Geloneze, B., Pareja, J. C., Calixto, A. R., Ferreira, M. M., and Marsaioli, A. J. 2016. "Omics" prospective monitoring of bariatric surgery: Roux-En-Y gastric bypass outcomes using mixed-meal tolerance test and time-resolved ^{1}H NMR-based metabolomics. *Omics* 20:415–23.

Ludvigsson, J., Samuelsson, U., Johansson, C., and Sterhammar, L. 2001. Treatment with antioxidant at onset of type 1 diabetes in children: A randomised double-blind placebo-controlled study. *Diabetes Metabolism Research Review* 17(2):131–6.

Mahajan, A., Taliun, D., Thurner, M., et al. 2018. Fine-mapping type 2 diabetes loci to single-variant resolution using high-density imputation and islet-specific epigenome maps. *Natural Genetics* 50:1505–13.

Malik, V. S., Popkins, B. M., Bray, G. A., Pesprés, J. P., Willett, W. B., and Hu, F. B. 2010. Sugar-sweetened beverages and risk of metabolic syndrome and type 2 diabetes: A meta analysis. *Diabetes Care* 33(11):247783.

Malipatil, N., Fachim, H. A., Siddals, K., et al. 2019. Data independent acquisition mass spectrometry can identify circulating proteins that predict future weight loss with a diet and exercise programme. *Journal of Clinical Medicine* 8:141.

Massiera, F., Barbry, P., Guesnet, P., et al. 2010. A Western-like fat diet is sufficient to induce a gradual enhancement in fat mass over generations. *Journal Lipid Research* 51(8):2352–61.

Mericq, V., Piccardo, C., Cai, W., et al. 2010. Maternally transmitted and food derived glycotoxins: A factor preconditioning the young to diabetes? *Diabetes Care* 33(10):2232–7.

Miller, M. R., Yin, X., Seifert, J., et al. 2011. Erythrocyte membrane omega-3 fatty acid levels and omega-3 fatty acid intake are not associated with conversion to type 1 diabetes in children with autoimmunity: The diabetes autoimmunity study in the young (DAISY). *Pediatrics Diabetes* 12(8):669–5.

Mirza, Z., Ali, A., Ashraf, G. M., et al. 2014. Proteomics approaches to understand linkage between Alzheimer's disease and type 2 diabetes mellitus. *CNS and Neurological Disorder Drug Targets* 13:213–25.

Mohan, V., and Radha, V. 2019. Precision diabetes is slowly becoming a reality. *Medicinal Principal Practice* 8:1–9.

Moucheraud, C., Lenz, C., Latkovic, M., and Wirtz, V. J. 2019. The costs of diabetes treatment in low- and middle-income countries: A systematic review. *BMJ Global Health* 4:e001258.

Müller, M., and Kersten, S. 2003. Nutrigenomics: Goals and strategies. *Nature Review Genetics* 4:315–22.

Muralidharan, M., Bhat, V., Bindu, Y. S., and Mandal, A. K. 2019. Glycation profile of minor abundant erythrocyte proteome across varying glycemic index in diabetes mellitus. *Analytical Biochemistry* 573:37–43.

Murphy, R. C. 2018. Challenges in mass spectrometry-based lipidomics of neutral lipids. *Trends in Analytical Chemistry* 107:91–8.

Ng, S. F., Lin, R. C., Laybutt, D. R., Barres, R., Owens, J. A., and Morris, M. J. 2010. Chronic high-fat diet in fathers programs β-cell dysfunction in female rat offspring. *Nature* 467(7318):963–6.

Nicholson, J. K., Lindon, J. C., and Holmes, E. 1999. "Metabonomics": Understanding the metabolic responses of living systems to pathophysiological stimuli via multivariate statistical analysis of biological NMR spectroscopic data. *Xenobiotica* 29:1181–9.

Norris, J. M., Yin, X., Lamb, M. M., et al. 2007. Omega-3 polyunsaturated fatty acid intake and islet autoimmunity in children at increased risk for type 1 diabetes. *JAMA* 298(12):1420–8.

Ohtsu, A., Takeuchi, Y., Katagiri, S., et al. 2019. Influence of *Porphyromonas gingivalis* in gut microbiota of streptozotocin-induced diabetic mice. *Oral Diseases* 25:868–80.

Olivas-Aguirre, F. J., Rodrigo-García, J., Martínez-Ruiz, N. D., et al. 2016. Cyanidin-3-O-glucoside: Physical-chemistry, foodomics and health effects. *Molecules* 21:1264.

Osataphan, S., Macchi, C., Singhal, G., et al. 2019. SGLT2 inhibition reprograms systemic metabolism via FGF21-dependent and -independent mechanisms. *JCI Insight* 4(5):e123130.

Pape, J. A., Newey, C. R., Burrell, H. R., et al. 2018. Per-Arnt-Sim Kinase (PASK) Deficiency increases cellular respiration on a standard diet and decreases liver triglyceride accumulation on a Western high-fat high-sugar diet. *Nutrients* 10:1990.

Pasini, E., Corsetti, G., Assanelli, D., et al. 2019. Effects of chronic exercise on gut microbiota and intestinal barrier in human with type 2 diabetes. *Minerva Medicine* 110:3–11.

Pearson, T. A., and Manolio, T. A. 2008. How to interpret a genome-wide association study. *JAMA* 299:1335–44.

Prassad, M., Takkinen, H. M., Nevalainen, J., et al. 2011. Are serum α- and β- carotene concentrations associated with the development of advanced β-cell autoimmunity in children with increased genetic susceptibility to type 1 diabetes? *Diabetes Metabolism* 37(2):162–7.

Priyadarsini, S., Sarker-Nag, A., Allegood, J., Chalfant, C., and Karamichos, D. 2015. Description of the sphingolipid content and subspecies in the diabetic cornea. *Current Eye Research* 40:1204–10.

Qiao, Z., Han, J., Feng, H., et al. 2018. Fermentation Products of *Paenibacillus bovis* sp. nov. BD3526 alleviates the symptoms of type 2 diabetes mellitus in GK rats. *Front Microbiology* 9:3292.

Rao, P., Lu, X. M., Pattee, P., et al. 2007. Proteomic identification of urinary biomarkers of diabetic nephropathy. *Diabetes Care* 30:629–37.

Razquin, C., Toledo, E., Clish, C. B., et al. 2018. Plasma lipidomic profiling and risk of type 2 diabetes in the PREDIMED trial. *Diabetes Care* 41:2617–24.

Reddy, V. S., Palika, R., Ismail, A., Pullakhandam, R., and Reddy, G. B. 2018. Nutrigenomics: Opportunities and challenges for public health nutrition. *Indian Journal of Medical Research* 148:632–41.

Ricci, P., Magalhães, P., Krochmal, M., et al. 2019. Urinary proteome signature of renal cysts and diabetes syndrome in children. *Science Report* 9:2225.

Richa, S., Voight, B. F., Valeriya, L., et al. 2007. Genome-wide association analysis identifies loci for type 2 diabetes and triglyceride levels. *Science* 316:1331–6.

Roberts, M. A., Mutch, D. M., and German, J. B. 2001. Genomics: Food and nutrition. *Current Opinion Biotechnology* 12:516–22.

Ross, B. M., and Babgi, R. 2017. Volatile compounds in blood headspace and nasal breath. *Journal of Breath Research* 11:046001.

Roverso, M., Berté, C., Di Marco, V., et al. 2015. The metallome of the human placenta in gestational diabetes mellitus. *Metallomics* 7:1146–54.

Roverso, M., Di Marco, V., Badocco, D., et al. 2019. Maternal, placental and cordonal metallomic profiles in gestational diabetes mellitus. *Metallomics* 11:676–85.

Ruzzin, J., Petersen, R., Mengnier, E., et al. 2010. Persistent organic pollutant exposure leads to insulin resistance syndrome. *Environmental Health Perspectives* 18(4):465–71.

Sandovici, I., Smith, N. H., Nitert, M. D., et al. 2011. Maternal diet and aging alter the epigenetic control of a promoter enhancer interaction at the Hnf4a gene in rat pancreatic islet. *Proceedings of the National Academy of Sciences of the United States of America* 108(13):5449–54.

Santangelo, C., Zicari, A., Mandosi, E., et al. 2016. Could gestational diabetes mellitus be managed through dietary bioactive compounds? Current knowledge and future perspectives. *British Journal of Nutrition* 115:1129–44.

Saxena, A., Tiwari, P., Wahi, N., et al. 2019. Transcriptome profiling reveals association of peripheral adipose tissue pathology with type-2 diabetes in Asian Indians. *Adipocyte* 8:125–36.

Sébédio, J. L. 2017. Metabolomics, nutrition, and potential biomarkers of food quality, intake, and health status. *Advance Food Nutrition Research* 82:83–116.

Sims, E. K., and Evans-Molina, C. 2014. Urinary biomarkers for the early diagnosis of retinopathy and nephropathy in type 1 diabetes mellitus: A "steady stream" of information using proteomics. *Translation Research* 163:183–7.

Sonnenburg, E. D., and Sonnenburg, J. L. 2019. The ancestral and industrialized gut microbiota and implications for human health. *Nature Reviews Microbiology* 17:383–90.

Sramkova, V., Berend, S., Siklova, M., et al. 2019. Apolipoprotein M: A novel adipokine decreasing with obesity and upregulated by calorie restriction. *American Journal of Clinical Nutrition* 109:1499–510.

Steinbrenner, H., Speckmann, B., Pinto, A., and Sies, H. 2011. High selenium intake and increased diabetes risk: Experimental evidence for interplay between selenium and carbohydrate metabolism. *Journal of Clinical Biochemistry and Nutrition* 48:40–5.

Stene, L. C., Hongve, D., Magnus, P., RØnningen, K. S., and Joner, G. 2002. Acidic drinking water and risk of childhood – onset type 1 diabetes. *Diabetes Care* 25(9):1534–8.

Stene, L. C., Ulriksen, J., Magnus, P., and Joner, G. 2000. Use of cod liver oil during pregnancy associated with lower risk of type 1 diabetes in the offspring. *Diabetologia* 43(9):1093–8.

Takahashi, S., Saito, K., Jia, H., and Kato, H. 2014. An integrated multi-omics study revealed metabolic alterations underlying the effects of coffee consumption. *PLoS One* 9:e91134.

Trujillo, E., Davis, C., and Milner, J. 2006. Nutrigenomics, proteomics, metabolomics, and the practice of dietetics. *Journal of American Dietetic Association Science* 106:403–13.

Tsurumaki, M., Kotake, M., Iwasaki, M., et al. 2015. The application of omics technologies in the functional evaluation of inulin and inulin-containing prebiotics dietary supplementation. *Nutrition Diabetes* 5:e185.

Ulf, S., Oikarinen, S., Hyöty, H., and Ludvigsson, J. 2011. Low Zinc in drinking water is associated with the risk of type 1 diabetes in children. *Pediatrics Diabetes* 12(3–1):156–64.

US National Institutes of Health. 2019. A review of 10 years of human microbiome research activities, Fiscal Years 2007–2016. *Microbiome* 7:31.

Uusitalo, L., Kenward, M. G., Virtanen, S. M., et al. 2008. Intake of antioxidant vitamins and trace elements during pregnancy and risk of advanced beta cell autoimmunity in the child. *American Journal of Clinical Nutrition* 88(2):458–64.

VanBuren, C., Imrhan, V., Vijayagopal, P., et al. 2018. "Omics" education in dietetic curricula: A comparison between two institutions in the USA and Mexico. *Lifestyle Genomics* 11:136–46.

Vangipurapu, J., Stancáková, A., Smith, U., Kuusisto, J., and Laakso, M. 2019. Nine amino acids are associated with decreased insulin secretion and elevated glucose levels in a 4.6-year follow-up study of 5181 Finnish men. *Diabetes* 68:1353–8.

Villegas, R., Xiang, Y. B., Elasy, T., et al. 2011. Fish, shellfish, and long-chain n-3 fatty acid consumption and risk of incident type 2 diabetes in middle-aged Chinese men and women. *American Journal of Clinical Nutrition* 94(2):543–51.

Virtanen, S. M., Niisisto, S., Nevalainen, J., et al. 2010. Serum fatty acids and risk of advanced β-cell autoimmunity: A nested case-control study among children with HLA-conferred susceptibility to type 1 diabetes. *European Journal of Clinical Nutrition* 64(8):792–9.

Virtanen, S. M., Uusitalo, L., Kenwaed, M. G., et al. 2011. Maternal food consumption during pregnancy and risk of advanced β-cell autoimmunity in the offspring. *Pediatrics Diabetes* 12(2):95–9.

Wang, J., Zhang, L., Xiao, R., et al. 2019. Plasma lipidomic signatures of spontaneous obese rhesus monkeys. *Lipids Health Disease* 18:8.

Wen, H., Gris, D., Lei, Y., et al. 2011. Fatty acid-induced NLRP3-ASC inflammation activation interferes with insulin signalling. *Nature Immunology* 12(5):408–15.

Whang, A., Nagpal, R., and Yadav, H. 2018. Bi-directional drug-microbiome interactions of anti-diabetics. *EBioMedicine* 39:591.

Wieczorek, G., Bigaud, M., Pfister, S., et al. 2019. Blockade of CD40-CD154 pathway interactions suppresses ectopic lymphoid structures and inhibits pathology in the NOD/ShiLtJ mouse model of Sjögren's syndrome. *Annals of the Rheumatics Disease* 78:974–8.

Yang, Q., Vijayakumar, A., and Kahn, B. B. 2018. Metabolites as regulators of insulin sensitivity and metabolism. *Natural Reviews Molecular Cell Biology* 19:654–72.

Yazdanpanah, S., Rabiee, M., Tahriri, M., et al. 2017. Evaluation of glycated albumin (GA) and GA/HbA1c ratio for diagnosis of diabetes and glycemic control: A comprehensive review. *Critical Review Clinical Laboratory Science* 54:219–32.

Yu, Y., Ping, J., Chen, H., et al. 2010. A comparative analysis of liver transcriptome suggests divergent liver function among human, mouse and rat. *Genomics* 96:281–9.

Zhai, L., Ning, Z. W., Huang, T., et al. 2018. *Cyclocarya paliurus* tea leaves improves dyslipidemia in diabetic mice: A lipidomics-based network pharmacology study. *Frontiers in Pharmacology* 9:973.

Zhang, W., Zhang, D., Chen, Q., Wu, J., Ouyang, Z., and Xia, Y. 2019. Online photochemical derivatization enables comprehensive mass spectrometric analysis of unsaturated phospholipid isomers. *Nature Communication* 10:79.

Zhang, X., Wen, F., Zuo, C., Li, M., Chen, H., and Wu, K. 2011. Association of genetic variation on chromosome 9p21 with polypoidal choroidal vasculopathy and neovascular age-related macular degeneration. *Investigative Ophthalmology and Visual science* 52:8063–7.

Zhang, Y., Ying, H., and Xu, Y. 2019. Comparative genomics and metagenomics of the metallomes. *Metallomics* 11:1026–43.

Zhao, C., Yang, C., Wai, S. T. C., et al. 2019. Regulation of glucose metabolism by bioactive phytochemicals for the management of type 2 diabetes mellitus. *Critical Reviews in Food Science and Nutrition* 59:830–47.

Zhao, H. X., Mold, M. D., Stenhouse, E. A., et al. 2001. Drinking water composition and childhood-onset type 1 diabetes mellitus in Devon and Cornwall England. *Diabetic Medicine* 18(9):709–17.

Zoccali, C., and Mallamaci, F. 2019. Nonproteinuric progressive diabetic kidney disease. *Current Opinion in Nephrology and Hypertension* 28:227–32.

7 Dietary Control of the Resolution Response to Optimize Inflammation

Genetic, Clinical, and Omics Perspectives

Barry Sears and Asish K. Saha*

CONTENTS

7.1 INTRODUCTION TO INFLAMMATION AND RESOLUTION

There are two distinct phases to the body's response to any injury: the initiation of inflammation and its resolution. Although the molecular biology of the initiation of inflammation is well understood, the detailed knowledge of the molecular biology of the resolution remains an emerging field (Serhan 2014). Successful healing of any

* Corresponding author emails: bsears@drsears.com, bsears@zoneliving.com, asaha@zoneliving.com

DOI: 10.1201/9781003142195-7

inflammation-induced injury requires the coordinated reduction of the initial inflammation, resolving residual inflammation, and finally repairing the damaged tissue leading to a return to homeostasis. We term this complex process that leads to healing as the resolution response (Sears et al. 2021).

If the resolution response is not sufficiently robust to balance the initial acute inflammation induced by an injury, there will be a buildup of chronic low-level unresolved inflammation. Although this type of resulting unresolved inflammation is below the perception of pain, it is also a major driving factor for developing a wide variety of age-related chronic diseases ranging from diabetes, cardiovascular disease, cancer, and autoimmune and neurological conditions.

The resolution response is an evolutionarily conserved mechanism to protect the organism from unresolved injury-induced inflammation. Although microbial invasions will generate an inflammatory response, there are a far greater number of other potential causes of injury-induced inflammation (e.g., physical injuries [internal and external]; diet-induced, oxidative stress-induced, surgery-induced, drug-induced, and stressor-induced [physical, emotional, and environmental] inflammation).

While there are diverse types of injuries that can induce an initial inflammatory response, the components of the resolution response that control the healing of the damage caused by the injury are ancient and highly conserved mechanisms that are under robust dietary control.

The resolution response's molecular components that can be directly affected by the diet fall into two separate broad classes of signaling agents. One class is hormones consisting of eicosanoids and specialized pro-resolving mediators or SPMs. Eicosanoids would include prostaglandins and leukotrienes, whereas SPMs would include resolvins, protectins, and maresins. The other class of signaling agents is gene modulators. These include NF-κB that is the genetic switch to initiate inflammation, and 5'-adenosine monophosphate–activated protein kinase (AMPK) that is the master switch of metabolism that ultimately not only reduces NF-κB activity but is necessary to repair the damaged tissue. A graphical depiction of those signaling agents is shown in Figure 7.1.

These signaling agents of the resolution response represent on-demand responses and must be continually balanced to maintain homeostasis. In particular, acute inflammation is only activated by injury, and the onset of inflammation triggers resolution. The initial acute inflammatory response is protective as it alerts the immune system to respond to the injury. However, if unresolved, it leads to tissue damage that transforms the otherwise protective initial inflammatory response into chronic low-level inflammation associated with many disease conditions. To successfully heal from any injury-induced inflammation, one must increase those diet-controlled nutrients or their metabolites that activate AMPK and enhance SPM formation. Simultaneously, one also has to decrease the intake of those diet-controlled nutrients that promote excessive NF-κB activity and increased eicosanoid formation. Thus, rather than concentrating on any one dietary component of the resolution response, one must focus on the broader vision of maintaining all of the diet-controlled factors of the resolution response within appropriate operating ranges. Thus, the resolution response can be best understood from a dynamic systems-based biology viewpoint consisting of complex, interrelated systems necessary for successful healing.

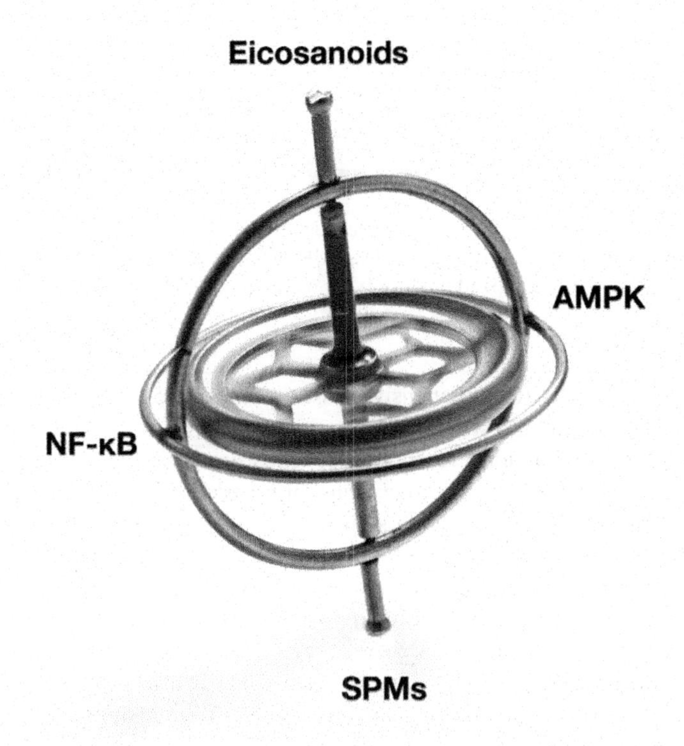

FIGURE 7.1 Illustration of the balancing of the signaling agents involved in the resolution response. Abbreviations: AMPK (5' adenosine monophosphate–activated protein kinase); NF-κB (nuclear factor kappa-B); SPMs (specialized pro-resolving meditators).

7.2 GENERAL DESCRIPTION OF THE DIETARY IMPACT ON EACH PHASE OF THE RESOLUTION RESPONSE

The three distinct phases of the resolution response can be summarized as (1) reducing injury-induced inflammation, (2) resolving the inflammation, and (3) repairing the tissue damage caused by injury-induced inflammation, as shown in Figure 7.2.

7.2.1 Reducing Inflammation

The most obvious way to reduce existing inflammation is following a highly defined anti-inflammatory diet. The problem is how to describe such a diet. The most important consideration for any anti-inflammatory diet is calorie restriction. Any reduction of excess calorie intake will lead to a decrease in systemic oxidative stress. Calorie restriction has been the most successful therapeutic intervention to improve healthspan (defined as longevity minus years of disability) in virtually every species studied (Most et al. 2017). Significant metabolic benefits were achieved by calorie restriction in both healthy overweight and normal-weight individuals who participated in

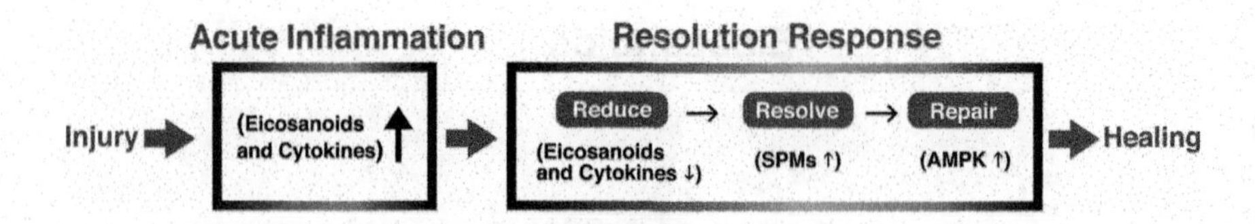

FIGURE 7.2 A graphic illustration of the sequential events for a successful resolution response to injury-induced inflammation. Abbreviations: AMPK (5'-adenosine monophosphate–activated protein kinase); SPMs (specialized pro-resolving meditators).

the various CALERIE (Comprehensive Assessment of the Long-Term Effects of Reducing Intake of Energy) studies (Martin et al. 2011; Das et al. 2017).

Successful lifetime calorie restriction depends on the ability of such a diet to reduce hunger. From this perspective, consuming adequate protein levels at each meal may represent a necessary first step. This concept is known as protein leveraging (Simpson and Raubenheimer 2005; Gosby et al. 2014). Potential protein-leveraging mechanisms may include increasing glucagon levels to stabilize blood glucose levels in the blood and the increased release of satiety hormones such as PYY and GLP-1 from the gut (Ludwig et al. 1999; Ven der Klaauw et al. 2013). The intake of fermentable fiber in a calorie-restricted diet is also essential for generating short-chain fatty acids (SCFA) that further enhance the signaling intensity of PYY and GLP-1 release, which is governed by protein intake at a meal (Chambers et al. 2015).

An anti-inflammatory diet should also substantially reduce the reservoir of the omega-6 fatty acid arachidonic acid (AA) in the plasma membrane. AA is the primary building block of eicosanoids. The vast majority of eicosanoids derived from AA are pro-inflammatory hormones that can significantly intensify any initial inflammatory response, making it more challenging to resolve the initial acute inflammation. A specific AA level in the plasma membrane is required to generate the necessary eicosanoids to create an acute inflammatory response. This begins with the activation of phospholipase A_2 that releases AA from the plasma membrane phospholipids. This free AA is immediately metabolized into eicosanoids. However, excess AA levels in the plasma membrane will cause increased amplification of the initial inflammatory response. Although reducing the dietary intake of AA is one possible way to achieve this goal, it should be emphasized that much of the AA in the body (and especially in the plasma membrane) comes from the metabolism of the omega-6 fatty acid linoleic acid into AA (Sears 1995). This metabolic conversion of linoleic acid to AA is accelerated by elevated insulin levels generated either by a consistently high glycemic load of the diet or by existing insulin resistance. In either case, elevated insulin levels will activate the rate-limiting enzymes (delta-6-desaturase and delta-5-desaturase), leading to increased AA formation from dietary intake of linoleic acid (Brenner 2003).

On the other hand, the hormone glucagon, induced by the diet's protein content, will inhibit the same desaturase enzymes (Christophersen et al. 1982; Brenner 2003). Thus, the balance of the protein-to-glycemic load of an anti-inflammatory diet is essential in reducing excess formation of AA that can result in excessive eicosanoid-driven inflammation (Sears 1995). Furthermore, an anti-inflammatory diet should also be low in linoleic acid, which will further decrease AA levels by the abovementioned metabolic pathways.

The development of insulin resistance can also increase AA formation. Insulin resistance appears to be strongly influenced by the levels of cytokines (especially TNFα) often induced by activation of NF-κB (Hotamisligil et al. 1993; Borst 2004; Akash et al. 2018).

NF-κB is also activated by high levels of saturated fatty acids (primarily palmitic acid) in the blood that can interact with the toll-like receptors TLR-2 and TLR-4. The result of this activation of NF-κB is the increased production of cytokines (Schaeffler et al. 2009; Hwang et al. 2016). Thus, an additional dietary requirement for an anti-inflammatory diet is low intakes of both linoleic acid and saturated fats, especially palmitic acid.

Increased insulin resistance eventually leads to elevated blood glucose levels if beta-cell function in the pancreas begins to fail (Taylor et al. 2019). The combination of high blood glucose levels and oxidative stress generated by excess calorie intake can lead to increased production of advanced glycosylated end products, or AGEs (Moldogazieva et al. 2019). These glycosylated proteins can interact with specific receptors (RAGE) on the cell surface, providing another diet-related pathway to increase cytokine production by activating NF-κB (Ott et al. 2014).

Just as it is necessary to reduce the dietary intake of omega-6 and saturated fatty acids, it is also essential to increase the omega-3 fatty acid intake, especially of the long-chain omega-3 fatty acids eicosapentaenoic acid (EPA) and docosahexaenoic acid (DHA). EPA is a feedback inhibitor of the delta-5-desaturase enzyme that is the rate-limiting step in the production of AA (Dias and Parsons 1995). Thus, the higher the levels of EPA in the diet, the less AA is generated.

Eicosanoids can be generated from EPA but not DHA (Calder 2017). The eicosanoids generated from the EPA are approximately 100–1,000 times lower in their inflammatory intensity than the same eicosanoids derived from AA. Thus, the eicosanoids derived from EPA are not strictly anti-inflammatory hormones but are weakly pro-inflammatory hormones compared to those derived from AA. The net result is a reduction in the intensity of the inflammatory response.

Another reason for increasing the omega-3 levels in an anti-inflammatory diet is the reduction of inflammasome activation in response to microbe-derived pathogen-associated molecular patterns (PAMPs) or danger-associated molecular patterns (DAMPs) sensed within the cell, which will cause the generation of IL-1β and IL-18 (Man and Kanneganti 2015). The NLRP3 inflammasome is the most investigated of the various inflammasomes (Sutterwala et al. 2014). Omega-3 fatty acids, such as EPA and DHA, can inhibit the activation of inflammasomes (Yan et al. 2013). However, it appears that DHA may be more effective than EPA in this regard (Lee et al. 2019).

Finally, the inflammatory effects of metabolic endotoxemia can be significantly reduced following an anti-inflammatory diet by ensuring an intact mucosal barrier in the gut (Cani et al. 2007). This improvement in the integrity of the gut's tight junctions appears to be related to the increased production of *Akkermansia muciniphila*, which can be improved with an increased dietary combination of omega-3 fatty acids and polyphenols (Kaliannan et al. 2015; Roopchand et al. 2015).

The dietary foundation for reducing diet-induced inflammation would consist of the following nutritional composition: calorie restriction with adequate protein coupled with a moderate level of low glycemic-load carbohydrates to reduce excess glucose intake. Furthermore, the diet should be low in total fat (especially omega-6 and saturated fatty acids) yet with sufficient levels of fermentable fiber, omega-3 fatty acids, and polyphenols.

7.2.2 Increasing Resolution

Reducing the inflammation caused by an injury is only the first step toward the ultimate healing of any damage caused by an injury. The second obligatory step of the resolution response is resolving any residual inflammation (Loftus and Finlay 2016). Unlike the variety of dietary interventions that help reduce inflammation, increasing resolution of any residual inflammation is purely a function of omega-3 fatty acids in the diet that are the building blocks to produce levels of adequate specialized pro-resolving mediators (SPMs). These hormones control the resolution of residual inflammation. SPMs represent a diverse superfamily of hormones consisting of three primary families: resolvins, marseins, and protectins. These SPMs are biosynthesized from EPA, docosapentaenoic acid (DPA), and docosahexaenoic acid (DHA) (Serhan 2014; Serhan and Levy 2018).

SPMs are critical for several distinct stages of resolution, including (1) stopping neutrophil swarming to the injury site, (2) causing the transition of pro-inflammatory macrophages (M1) to pro-resolution macrophages (M2) to remove cell debris from the injury site, and (3) increasing efferocytosis to remove apoptotic cells (Dalli and Serhan 2017).

The levels of omega-3 fatty acids required to achieve these goals can be estimated by the ratio of leukotrienes to SPMs (Fredman et al. 2016; Rymut et al. 2020). Unfortunately, such a determination requires highly sophisticated instrumentation. Leukotrienes are derived from AA, and many SPMs (such as the E-series resolvins) are derived from EPA. Consequently, the ratio of AA/EPA in the blood can serve as an upstream surrogate marker to determine whether a therapeutic level of omega-3 fatty acids is being maintained to generate sufficient levels of SPMs to complete the resolution phase of the resolution response. The production of SPMs, such as resolvins, may also be a critical factor in preventing the priming of the inflammasome (Yin et al. 2017; Lopategi et al. 2019).

7.2.3 Altering Gene Expression

The final and most complex phase of the resolution response is the activation of the master switch of metabolism, AMPK (Sears 2019; Sears et al. 2021). AMPK is a highly conserved sensor of energy that senses the levels of ATP and AMP. As the AMP/ATP ratio is increased as happens with calorie restriction, AMPK is activated, which sets in motion a broad cascade of gene transcription factors that switch metabolism from anabolic to catabolic to restore ATP levels (Jeon 2016; Day et al. 2017; Hardie 2018; Herzig and Shaw 2018). Figure 7.3 indicates just a few of the many metabolic effects that take place once AMPK is activated.

While all these actions will significantly affect metabolism, perhaps the most critical benefit of AMPK activation is inhibiting NF-κB activity (Acquisto et al. 2002; Salminen et al. 2011; Chen J et al. 2018; Chen X et al. 2018). This inhibition of NF-κB leads to a substantial reduction of both excess eicosanoid and cytokine levels. The activation of AMPK thus reduces inflammation induced by NF-κB activation. This essential metabolic control of NF-κB by AMPK is obligatory for the successful repair of damaged tissue.

This repair process starts with increased autophagy to supply the molecular building blocks for tissue repair and increased mitophagy to replace damaged mitochondria to provide the energy required for tissue repair (Li and Chen 2019). These

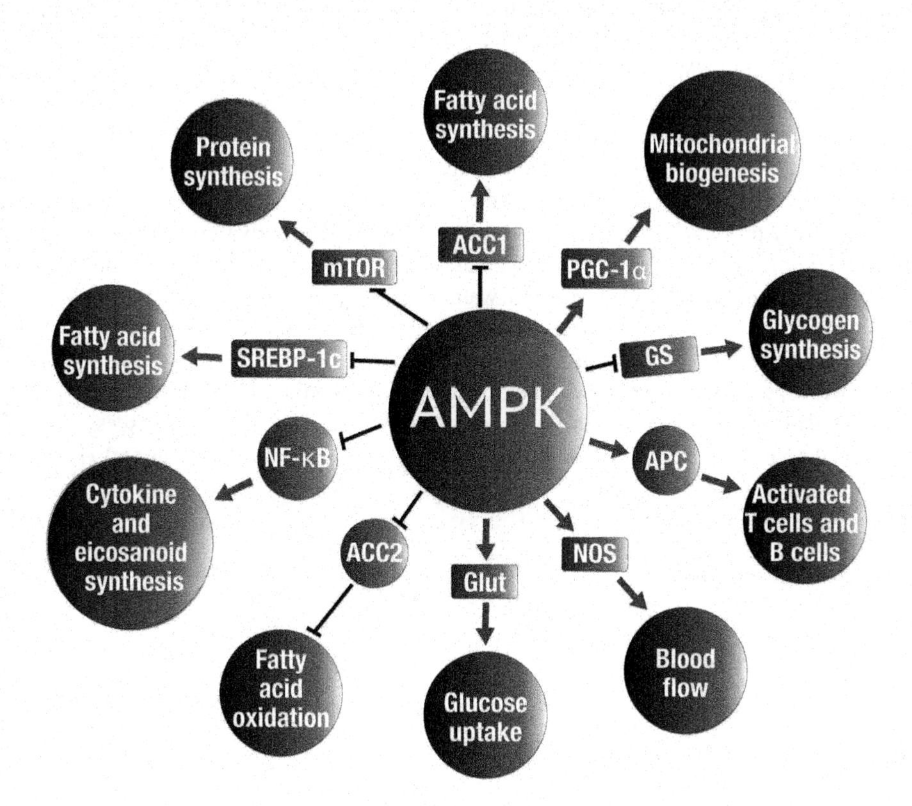

FIGURE 7.3 Metabolic effects of AMPK activation. Arrows on the "spokes" indicate activation; lines with a bar at the end indicate inhibition. Abbreviations: ACC 1 and ACC2 (acetyl-CoA carboxylase 1 and 2); AMPK (5'-adenosine monophosphate–activated protein kinase); FOXO-antigen-presenting cell; Glut (glucose transporter protein); GS (glycogen synthetase); mTOR (mammalian target of rapamycin); NF-κB (nuclear factor kappa-B); NOS (nitrogen oxide synthetase); PGC-1α (peroxisome proliferator-activated receptor gamma coactivator 1-alpha); SREBP-1c (sterol regulatory element-binding protein 1c).

processes are controlled by AMPK via activation of ULK-1, which is the first step to increase mitophagy (Li and Chen 2019).

A potential link between increased SPM formation and increased AMPK activity appears to be mediated by receptors for various SPMs. One well-characterized receptor is FPR2/ALX, a receptor for lipoxin A_4 and the anti-inflammatory/pro-resolution protein annexin (McArthur et al. 2020). FPR2/ALX is also a receptor for the Resolvin D1 (RvD1) derived from DHA (Norling et al. 2012). Thus, it is quite likely that RvD1 and other SPMs signaling through similar receptors may also be instrumental for increased AMPK activation (Hellmann et al. 2011; Park et al. 2020).

However, the most potent dietary effector of AMPK may be polyphenols. Polyphenols activate AMPK indirectly by binding to various sirtuins (SIRT) that are deacetylating enzymes dependent on NAD^+ (Chung et al. 2010; Rahnasto-Rilla 2018). One of the various SIRT targets is liver kinase B1 (LKB1). Once LKB1 is deacetylated, it activates AMPK, which in turn inhibits NF-κB (Shackelford and Shaw 2009; Alexander and Walker 2011). In addition, AMPK activates the rate-limiting enzyme (nicotinamide phosphoribosyltransferase, or NAMPT) of the salvage pathway that regenerates NAD^+, needed for the deacetylating activity of various SIRT proteins. This crosstalk between SIRT and AMPK creates a positive feedback loop for AMPK activation (Ruderman et al. 2010; Liu et al. 2012; Price et al. 2012; Brandauer et al. 2013). This is shown in Figure 7.4.

The only problem with dietary polyphenols as AMPK activators is their limited water-solubility. However, specific subclasses of polyphenols such as anthocyanins (particularly delphinidins) have high water-solubility making it possible to obtain adequate blood levels to increase AMPK activity (Lizuka et al. 2018; Schon et al. 2018; Lai et al. 2019; Park et al. 2019).

AMPK activity is under robust dietary control. It is activated by calorie restriction, resolvins, and polyphenols. On the other hand, AMPK is inhibited by excess calorie intake and elevated blood glucose levels (Coughlan et al. 2014; Lin and Hardie

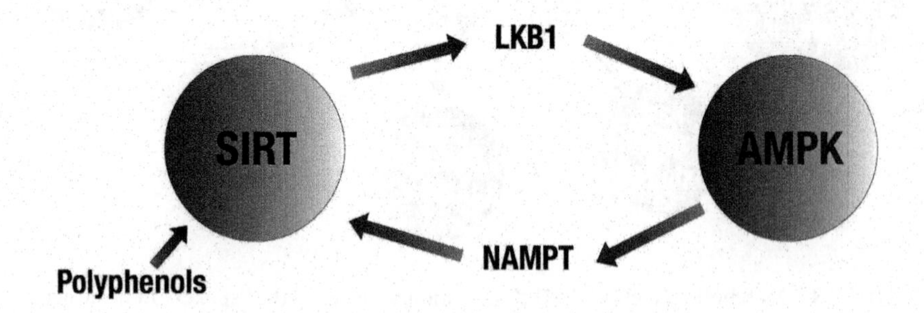

FIGURE 7.4 Crosstalk between SIRT and AMPK. Any decrease in the cell's energy state measured by an increased AMP/ATP ratio will activate AMPK. This activation of AMPK leads to increasing NAMPT activity that produces NAD^+ required for SIRT deacetylation activity. SIRT then deacetylates LKB1, which activates AMPK. Abbreviations: AMPK (5'-adenosine monophosphate–activated protein kinase); LKB1 (liver kinase B1); NAMPT (nicotinamide phosphoribosyltransferase); SIRT (sirtuins).

2018). Thus, one can obtain the maximum dietary activation of AMPK activity by following a calorie-restricted diet with a low glycemic index with adequate levels of omega-3 fatty acids and water-soluble polyphenols such as anthocyanins, especially bioavailable delphinidins (Schon et al. 2018; Lappi et al. 2021).

7.3 SPECIFIC DIETARY GUIDELINES TO OPTIMIZE THE RESOLUTION RESPONSE

Optimizing the resolution response requires viewing dietary nutrients as pro-drugs to generate signaling agents, as shown in Table 7.1.

7.3.1 Protein

Adequate protein intake plays a critical role in the long-term use of calorie restriction necessary to activate AMPK by controlling satiety via protein leveraging (Simpson and Raubenheimer 2005; Gosby et al. 2014). Protein leveraging is based upon the hypothesis that the protein levels at each meal determine the degree of appetite suppression of that meal. Without adequate appetite suppression between meals, long-term success for calorie restriction is highly unlikely. There are two potential mechanisms of protein leveraging. The first mechanism is to have adequate dietary protein at any meal to release sufficient levels of hormones such as PYY and GLP-1 from the small intestine that goes directly to the brain via the vagal nerve to reach the hypothalamus to reduce hunger (Batterham et al. 2006; Westerterp-Plantenga 2008). The less protein consumed in a meal, the more likely excess calories will be needed to be consumed at that meal to cause sufficient appetite suppression by alternative pathways. The second mechanism is the increase in glucagon levels in the blood stimulated by dietary protein (Ludwig et al. 1999). Glucagon will release stored glycogen from the liver to maintain stable blood glucose levels, thereby reducing hunger. Clinical data suggest that weight regain after controlled purposeful weight loss is better preserved with a higher protein percentage in the diet. It appears that approximately 25% of the total calories as protein at each meal may be a threshold for this effect (Ludwig et al. 1999; Hochstenbach-Waelen et al. 2009). For a 400-calorie meal, this would mean consuming approximately 25 grams of

TABLE 7.1
Dietary Nutrients and Their Signaling Agents in the Resolution Response

Nutrient	Signaling agent
Protein	Glucagon, PYY, and GLP-1
Carbohydrates	Insulin
Fats	Eicosanoids and SPMs
Fermentable fiber	Short-chain fatty acids
Polyphenols	AMPK

protein. However, the actual amount of daily dietary protein required is based on the individual's lean body mass and physical activity (Sears 1995). For the average female, this will be approximately 75 grams of protein per day. For the average male, the protein level will be about 100 grams of protein per day. Because of the requirement of calorie restriction for an anti-inflammatory diet, these recommended levels of daily protein are slightly higher than the recommended minimum daily protein intake to prevent loss of lean body mass, especially when combined with resistance training (Amamou et al. 2017). Furthermore, the total protein should be spread evenly throughout the day for improved hormonal control (Sears 1995, 1997). However, these protein intake levels for an anti-inflammatory diet are typical for the US population (Fulgoni 2008).

Another nuance of protein leveraging is the timing of protein consumption during a meal. Eating protein before consuming carbohydrates generates more significant glycemic control in T2D subjects than consuming carbohydrates first before protein (Shukla et al. 2017, 2019). One potential reason may be that protein requires a longer transit time in the small intestine to reach the L-cells that secrete PYY and GLP-1. These gut hormones go directly via the vagal nerve to the brain's appetite center in the hypothalamus to generate satiety. This timing factor suggests that the blood levels of amino acids needed to stimulate glucagon will rise more slowly than glucose levels (especially high-glycemic load carbohydrates rich in glucose) required to stimulate insulin release. Thus, consuming protein first in a meal should generate a more favorable postprandial glucagon-to insulin balance after the meal. Clinical data suggests an improved balance of glucagon-to-insulin leads to a substantial reduction in consumed calories under *ad libitum* conditions after consuming two consecutive balanced meals compared to isocaloric meals with a lower protein-to-carbohydrate ratio (Ludwig et al. 1999).

7.3.2 Carbohydrates

Since excess dietary glucose is an inhibitor of AMPK, consideration of the glucose content in a meal and its entry rate into the bloodstream will be essential for optimizing the resolution response. The rate of entry of glucose into the blood is measured by its glycemic index. However, a more relevant parameter is the glycemic load. The glycemic load takes into account how rapidly the total carbohydrate of a meal raises blood glucose levels. (Ludwig 2002). Meals consisting of a high glycemic load will inhibit AMPK activity. The highest glycemic load comes from having grains and starches as the primary carbohydrates in a meal. Therefore, for minimum inhibition of AMPK, the carbohydrate content of a meal should consist primarily of carbohydrates with a low glycemic impact. These carbohydrates would mainly consist of primarily non-starchy vegetables and limited amounts of fruits (mostly berries). Epidemiology studies have indicated that individuals consuming ten servings per day of non-starchy vegetables and fruits have lower mortality and morbidity than those consuming fewer servings of these low glycemic impact carbohydrates (Aune et al. 2017). This epidemiological observation would be consistent with decreased inhibition of AMPK activity.

7.3.3 Fats

Total fat content should remain low for maintaining calorie restriction. However, one must also consider the composition of that total fat intake. The balance of omega-6 to omega-3 fatty acids should be no greater than 2:1. A lower omega-6 to omega-3 fatty acid ratio will ensure a better balance of their bioactive biosynthetic products (eicosanoids coming from omega-6 fatty acids and SPMs coming from omega-3 fatty acids) to help improve the resolution of any injury-induced inflammation. The omega-6 to omega-3 fatty acid balance in the United States was approximately 10:1 in 1999 (Blasbalg et al. 2011; Guyenet and Carlson 2015). The levels of saturated fats (principally palmitic acid) should also remain low because of their potential generation of inflammation in the hypothalamus (Tse et al. 2018). This increased hypothalamic inflammation can also potentially attenuate satiety signals from the gut and the blood (Cheng et al. 2015). As discussed earlier, high levels of palmitic acid can interact with the TLR-2 and TLR-4 receptors to activate NF-κB to generate cytokines (Schaeffler et al. 2009; Hwang et al. 2016). Thus, the bulk of the limited fat content for an anti-inflammatory diet should come from monounsaturated fatty acids.

7.3.4 Macronutrient Balance

The macronutrient balance of the diet at every meal can also further control hormonal responses. Ideally, the level of low-glycemic-load carbohydrates should be approximately one-third more than the protein content in a meal (Sears 1995). This is the same balance of protein and carbohydrate was also estimated for a Paleolithic diet (Kuipers et al. 2010). Furthermore, this balance of protein and carbohydrate should be consistent for each meal. It is known from clinical experiments that the protein-to-carbohydrate ratio profoundly affects the blood's resulting insulin-to-glucagon balance under isocaloric conditions (Ludwig et al. 1999). This hormonal balance is essential since the delta-6 and delta-5 desaturase enzymes that convert the omega-6 fatty acid linoleic acid into AA are activated by insulin (Brenner 2003). In contrast, glucagon inhibits these same enzymes, decreasing the potential excess formation of AA, thereby reducing possible excess eicosanoid formation (Christophersen et al. 1982; Brenner 2003).

Finally, to maintain appropriate calorie restriction, the total fat content of the diet should be less than 50 grams per day. Thus, the macronutrient composition of an anti-inflammatory diet should be approximately one gram of fat for every two grams of protein and every three grams of carbohydrate at every meal. This macronutrient balance is also consistent with estimates of Paleolithic diets (Kuipers et al. 2010). A diet with such a macronutrient composition has been shown to be both anti-inflammatory and non-ketogenic (Johnston et al. 2006).

7.3.5 Fermentable Fiber

Gut bacteria require the dietary intake of fermentable fiber to generate short-chain fatty acids (SCFAs). SCFAs act as signaling agents to maintain the gut barrier's integrity by decreasing inflammation in the gut wall (Parada Venegas et al. 2019; Sitolo et al. 2020).

The improvement of the gut wall's integrity will reduce metabolic endotoxemia as a significant source of gut-induced inflammation (Cani et al. 2007). SCFAs produced in the gut can also significantly affect neurological function via the vagus nerve (Silva et al. 2020). Finally, SCFAs have a significant role in maintaining satiety by enhancing the secretion of PYY and GLP-1 from the gut (Kaji et al. 2014; Larraufie et al. 2018).

7.3.6 Polyphenols

Polyphenols constitute a large group of more than 8,000 compounds that can be potentially metabolized into less complex phenolic compounds that can also act as signaling agents (Luca et al. 2020). It is challenging to measure polyphenols in the blood. However, the metabolites of those polyphenols that were absorbed can be found in the urine.

Studies have suggested that it is the increased levels of polyphenols in the urine, which are associated with reduced frailty and mortality as opposed to the estimated dietary intake of polyphenols from food diaries (Zamora-Ros et al. 2013; Urpi-Sarda et al. 2015).

Only certain polyphenol structures appear to be maximally useful as allosteric agents to increase the sirtuins' deacetylating activity, as described earlier. Those polyphenols with the most significant potential to cause an allosteric activation of the various sirtuins to appear to require an intact flavonoid structure and a net positive charge to enhance their water solubility (Rahnasto-Rilla et al. 2018). The subgroup of polyphenols that has both structural characteristics is anthocyanins. Berries are a rich source of anthocyanins. It should be noted that increased anthocyanin intake is associated with decreased incidence of cardiovascular disease, although the effect appears to be stronger in women than men (Cassidy et al. 2013; Zamora-Ros et al. 2013; Cassidy et al. 2016).

7.4 CLINICAL MARKERS TO DETERMINE AN OPTIMAL RESOLUTION RESPONSE

The ultimate approach to healing is to optimize the resolution response. Success requires reducing, resolving, and repairing inflammatory damage caused by any injury. Successful dietary management of the resolution response can be determined by the extent to which each of the clinical markers is maintained within their desired ranges. Such blood markers must be highly validated and easily obtained and provide clear guidelines to personalize the individual's diet. The three clinical markers that meet these criteria are the following:

1. *Reducing insulin resistance:* The TG/HDL ratio (measured in mg/dL) should be less than one for controlling insulin resistance (McLaughlin et al. 2004; Fan et al. 2011; Gonzalez-Chavez et al. 2011; Murguia-Romero et al.

2013; Quispe et al. 2016; Salazar et al. 2017; Lind et al. 2018; Pantoja-Torres et al. 2019).

2. *Increasing resolution:* The AA/EPA ratio should be maintained between 1.5 and 3 to maintain an appropriate balance of precursors for a balanced formation of eicosanoids and SPMs (Kondo et al. 1986; Endres et al. 1989; Adams et al. 1996; Germano et al. 2007; Sorgi et al. 2007; Yokoyama et al. 2007; Oikawa et al. 2009; Rizzo et al. 2010; Kashiyama et al. 2011; Caspar-Bauguil et al. 2012; Rizzo et al. 2012; Sekikawa et al. 2012; Fujihara et al. 2013; Harris et al. 2013; Inoue et al. 2013; Ninomiya et al. 2013; Ohnishi and Saito 2013; Sears et al. 2013; Fukuda et al. 2014; Georgiou 2014; Ito et al. 2014; Ikeya et al. 2015; Ishitobi et al. 2015; Nagai et al. 2015; Pareja-Galeano 2015; Wakabayashi et al. 2015; Yamano et al. 2015; Nagahara et al. 2016). It should be noted that the average AA/EPA ratio in the US is greater than 20 (Harris et al. 2012; Harris et al. 2013) indicative of a highly unbalanced ratio of potential eicosanoid to SPM formation.
3. *Increasing AMPK activation:* The HbA1c level should be between 4.9 and 5.1%, indicating the lack of glucose inhibition of AMPK activity (Lin and Hardie 2018).

The recommended appropriate ranges for these markers are lower than the typical average levels for healthy individuals, but they are still within normal ranges. Only when all three of these three clinical markers are in their assigned ranges can the resolution response be optimized for an individual.

Furthermore, each of the markers can be modulated by specific dietary interventions. For example, the level of insulin resistance can be significantly reduced by following an anti-inflammatory diet. The dietary intake of omega-3 fatty acids strongly influences the AA/EPA ratio. Finally, the dietary intake of polyphenols to activate AMPK will strongly affect the HbA1c levels. It should be noted that AMPK can also be activated (although to a lesser extent) by increased SPM synthesis and calorie restriction that is the foundation for an anti-inflammatory diet. This illustrates the significant crosstalk of the various dietary components discussed above.

7.5 POTENTIAL NEED FOR SUPPLEMENTATION

In principle, an appropriate anti-inflammatory diet should be sufficient to optimize the resolution response. In reality, the diet will often require supplementation with omega-3 fatty acids and polyphenols to reach the target ranges of the clinical markers described above. This need for potential supplementation is because the omega-3 fatty acids levels required to effectively resolve the residual inflammation caused by the injury are often beyond the intake provided by the best anti-inflammatory diet. This is also true for the amounts of polyphenols needed to activate AMPK to repair damaged tissue.

In particular, supplementation with EPA and DHA concentrates may be required to increase the biosynthesis of the SPMs needed to resolve residual inflammation and reduce inflammasome formation (Yan et al. 2013; Martínez-Micaelo et al. 2016;

Williams-Bey et al. 2014; Lin et al. 2017; Yin et al. 2017; Lopategi et al. 2019). The best sources of polyphenols to enhance AMPK activity will come from polyphenol concentrates of the anthocyanin family. These polyphenols can enhance the allosteric activation of sirtuins to indirectly activate AMPK (Rahnasto-Rilla 2018) and inhibit inflammasome formation (Zhu et al. 2018; Fan et al. 2020). Such polyphenol concentrates should also be devoid of glucose that would otherwise impede the activation of AMPK.

The amounts of supplementation can be determined by titration to the appropriate ranges described above. The AA/EPA ratio will determine the optimal amount of omega-3 fatty acid supplementation, and reaching the target HbA1c range determines the amount of optimal level of polyphenol supplementation required.

7.6 SUMMARY

The dietary control of the resolution response based upon systems-based biology can provide new insights into the role of specific nutrients to optimize the body's internal ability to heal from injury-induced inflammation. Maintaining constant dietary optimization of the resolution response is fundamental for maintaining organ homeostasis. This complex interaction can be optimized using validated blood markers, thus placing diet into the realm of translational medicine. Reaching the appropriate ranges of those clinical markers that define the optimization of the resolution response can be translated into an increased healthspan using diet as if it were a drug to alter the complex systems-based biology of healing.

ACKNOWLEDGMENTS

This study was supported by the Inflammation Research Foundation, Peabody, MA, USA.

REFERENCES

Acquisto, F. D., May, M. J., and Ghosh, S. 2002. Inhibition of nuclear factor kappa B (NF-κB): An emerging theme in anti-inflammatory therapies. *Molecular Interventions* 2(1):22–35.

Adams, P. B., Lawson, S., Sanigorski, A., and Sinclair, A. J. 1996. Arachidonic acid to eicosapentaenoic acid ratio in blood correlates positively with clinical symptoms of depression. *Lipids* 31:S157–61S.

Akash, M. S. H., Rehman, K., and Liaqat, A. 2018. Tumor necrosis factor-alpha: Role in development of insulin resistance and pathogenesis of type 2 diabetes mellitus. *Journal of Cell Biochemistry* 119(1):105–10.

Alexander, A., and Walker, C. L. 2011. The role of LKB1 and AMPK in cellular responses to stress and damage. *FEBS Letters* 585(7):952–7.

Amamou, T., Normandin, E., Pouliot, J., Dionne, I. J., Brochu, M., and Riesco, E. 2017. Effect of a high-protein energy-restricted diet combined with resistance training on metabolic profile in older individuals with metabolic impairments. *Journal of Nutrition, Health and Aging* 21(1):67–74.

Aune, D., Giovannucci, E., Boffetta, P., et al. 2017. Fruit and vegetable intake and the risk of cardiovascular disease, total cancer and all-cause mortality – a systematic review and dose-response meta-analysis of prospective studies. *International Journal of Epidemiology* 46(3):1029–56.

Batterham, R. L., Heffron, H., Kapoor, S., et al. 2006. Critical role for peptide YY in protein-mediated satiation and body-weight regulation. *Cell Metabolism* 4(3):223–33.
Blasbalg, T. L., Hibbeln, J. R., Ramsden, C. E., Majchrzak, S. F., and Rawlings, R. R. 2011. Changes in consumption of omega-3 and omega-6 fatty acids in the United States during the 20th Century. *American Journal of Clinical Nutrition* 93(5):950–62.
Borst, S. E. 2004. The role of TNF-alpha in insulin resistance. *Endocrinology* 23(2–3):177–82.
Brandauer, J., Vienberg, S. G., Andersen, M. A., et al. 2013. AMP-activated protein kinase regulates nicotinamide phosphoribosyl transferase expression in skeletal muscle. *Journal of Physiology* 591(20):5207–20.
Brenner, R. R. 2003. Hormonal modulation of delta-6 and delta-5 desaturases: Case of diabetes. *Prostaglandins Leukortiense Essential Fatty Acids* 68(2):151–62.
Calder, P. C. 2017. Omega-3 fatty acids and inflammatory processes: From molecules to man. *Biochemical Society Transactions* 45(5):1105–15.
Cani, P. D., Amar, J., Iglesias, M. A., et al. 2007. Metabolic endotoxemia initiates obesity and insulin resistance. *Diabetes* 56(7):1761–72.
Caspar-Bauguil, S., Fioroni, A., Galinier, A., et al. 2012. Pro-inflammatory phospholipid arachidonic acid/eicosapentaenoic acid ratio of dysmetabolic severely obese women. *Obesity Surgery* 22(6):935–44.
Cassidy, A., Bertoia, M., Chiuve, S., Flint, A., Forman, J., and Rimm, E. B. 2016. Habitual intake of anthocyanins and flavanones and risk of cardiovascular disease in men. *American Journal of Clinical Nutrition* 104(3):587–94.
Cassidy, A., Mukamal, K. J., Liu, L., Franz, M., Eliassen, A. H., and Rimm, E. B. 2013. High anthocyanin intake is associated with a reduced risk of myocardial infarction in young and middle-aged women. *Circulation* 127(2):188–96.
Chambers, E. S., Morrison, D. J., and Frost, G. 2015. Control of appetite and energy intake by SCFA: What are the potential underlying mechanisms? *Proceedings of the Nutrition Society* 74(3):328–36.
Chen, J., Zhu, Y., Zhang, Y., et al. 2018. Delphinidin induced protective autophagy via mTOR pathway suppression and AMPK pathway activation in HER-2 positive breast cancer cells. *BMC Cancer* 18(1):342.
Chen, X., Li, X., Zhang, W., et al. 2018. Activation of AMPK inhibits inflammatory response during hypoxia and reoxygenation through modulating JNK-mediated NF-kappaB pathway. *Metabolism* 83:256–70.
Cheng, L., Yu, Y., Szabo, A., et al. 2015. Palmitic acid induces central leptin resistance and impairs hepatic glucose and lipid metabolism in male mice. *Journal of Nutritional Biochemistry* 26(5):541–8.
Christophersen, B. O., Hagve, T. A., and Norseth, A. 1982. Studies on the regulation of arachidonic acid synthesis in isolated rat liver cells. *Biochimica et Biophysica Acta* 712(2):305–14.
Chung, S., Yao, H., Caito, S., Hwang, J. W., Arunachalam, G., and Rahman, I. 2010. Regulation of SIRT1 in cellular functions: Role of polyphenols. *Archives of Biochemistry and Biophysics* 501(1):79–90.
Coughlan, K. A., Valentine, R. J., Ruderman, N. B., and Saha, A. K. 2014. AMPK activation: A therapeutic target for type 2 diabetes? *Diabetes Metabolism Syndrome Obesity* 7:241–53.
Dalli, J., and Serhan, C. N. 2017. Pro-resolving mediators in regulating and conferring macrophage function. *Frontiers in Immunology* 8:1400.
Das, S. K., Roberts, S. B., Bhapkar, M. V., Villareal, D. T., Fontana, L., and Martin, C. K. 2017. CALERIE-2 study group. Body-composition changes in the comprehensive assessment of long-term effects of reducing intake of energy (CALERIE)-2 study: A 2-y randomized controlled trial of calorie restriction in nonobese humans. *American Journal of Clinical Nutrition* 105(4):913–27.

Day, E. A., Ford, R. J., and Steinberg, G. R. 2017. AMPK as a therapeutic target for treating metabolic diseases. *Trends in Endocrinology and Metabolism* 28(8):545–60.

Dias, V. C., and Parsons, H. G. 1995. Modulation in delta 9, delta 6, and delta 5 fatty acid desaturase activity in the human intestinal CaCo-2 cell line. *Journal of Lipid Research* 36(3):552–63.

Endres, S., Ghorbani, R., Kelley, V. E., et al. 1989. The effect of dietary supplementation with n-3 polyunsaturated fatty acids on the synthesis of interleukin-1 and tumor necrosis factor by mononuclear cells. *New England Journal of Medicine* 320(5):265–71.

Fan, R., You, M., Toney, A. M., et al. 2020. Red raspberry polyphenols attenuate high-fat diet-driven activation of NLRP3 inflammasome and its paracrine suppression of adipogenesis via histone modifications. *Molecular Nutrition and Food Research* 64(15):e1900995.

Fan, X., Liu, E. Y., Hoffman, V. P., Potts, A. J., Sharma, B., and Henderson, D. C. 2011. Triglyceride/high-density lipoprotein cholesterol ratio: A surrogate to predict insulin resistance and low-density lipoprotein cholesterol particle size in nondiabetic patients with schizophrenia. *Journal of Clinical Psychiatry* 72(6):806–12.

Fredman, G., Hellmann, J., Proto, J. D., et al. 2016. An imbalance between specialized pro-resolving lipid mediators and pro-inflammatory leukotrienes promotes instability of atherosclerotic plaques. *Nature Communication* 7:12859.

Fujihara, M., Fukata, M., Odashiro, K., Maruyama, T., Akashi, K., and Yokoi, Y. 2013. Reduced plasma eicosapentaenoic acid-arachidonic acid ratio in peripheral artery disease. *Angiology* 64(2):112–8.

Fukuda, S., Fujioka, S., Hosaka, S., et al. 2014. Mizoue, T. Relationship between arteriosclerosis obliterans and the ratio of serum eicosapentaenoic acid to arachidonic acid. *Annals of Thoracic and Cardiovascular Surgery* 20(1):44–7.

Fulgoni, V. L. 2008. Current protein intake in America: Analysis of the National Health and Nutrition Examination Survey, 2003–2004. *American Journal of Clinical Nutrition* 87(5):1554S–7S.

Georgiou, T., Neokleous, A., Nikolaou, D., and Sears, B. 2014. Pilot study for treating dry age-related macular degeneration (AMD) with high-dose omega-3 fatty acids. *Pharma Nutrition* 2:8–11.

Germano, M., Meleleo, D., Montorfano, G., et al. 2007. Plasma, red blood cells phospholipids and clinical evaluation after long chain omega-3 supplementation in children with attention deficit hyperactivity disorder (ADHD). *Nutrition Neuroscience* 10(1–2):1–9.

Gonzalez-Chavez, A., Simental-Mendia, L. E., and Elizondo-Argueta, S. 2011. Elevated triglycerides/HDL-cholesterol ratio associated with insulin resistance. *Cirugia Cirujanos* 79(2):126–31.

Gosby, A. K., Conigrave, A. D., Raubenheimer, D., and Simpson, S. J. 2014. Protein leverage and energy intake. *Obesity Review* 15(3):183–91.

Guyenet, S. J., and Carlson, S. E. 2015. Increase in adipose tissue linoleic acid of US adults in the last half century. *Advances in Nutrition* 6(6):660–4.

Hardie, D. G. 2018. Keeping the home fires burning: AMP-activated protein kinase. *Journal of Royal Society of Interface* 15(138):20170774.

Harris, W. S., Pottala, J. V., Lacey, S. M., Vasan, R. G, Larson, M. G., and Robins, S. J. 2012. Clinical correlates and heritability of erythrocyte eicosapentaenoic and docosahexaenoic acid content in the Framingham Heart Study. *Atherosclerosis* 225(2):425–31.

Harris, W. S., Pottala, J. V., Varvel, S. A., Borowski, J. J., Ward, J. N., and McConnell, J. P. 2013. Erythrocyte omega-3 fatty acids increase and linoleic acid decreases with age: Observations from 160,000 patients. *Prostaglandins Leukotrienes Essential Fatty Acid* 88(4):257–63.

Hellmann, J., Tang, Y., Kosuri, M., Bhatnagar, A., and Spite, M. 2011. Resolvin D1 decreases adipose tissue macrophage accumulation and improves insulin sensitivity in obese-diabetic mice. *Federation of American Societies for Experimental Biology Journal* 25(7):2399–407.

Herzig, S., and Shaw, R. J. 2018. AMPK: Guardian of metabolism and mitochondrial homeostasis. *Nature Reviews Molecular and Cellular Biology* 19(2):121–35.

Hochstenbach-Waelen, A., Veldhorst, M. A., Nieuwenhuizen, A. G., Westerterp-Plantenga, M. S., and Westerterp, K. R. 2009. Comparison of 2 diets with either 25% or 10% of energy as casein on energy expenditure, substrate balance, and appetite profile. *American Journal of Clinical Nutrition* 89(3):831–8.

Hotamisligil, G. S., Shargill, N. S., and Spiegelman, B. M. 1993. Adipose expression of tumor necrosis factor-alpha: Direct role in obesity-linked insulin resistance. *Science* 259(5091):87–91.

Hwang, D. H., Kim, J. A., and Lee, J. Y. 2016. Mechanisms for the activation of Toll-like receptor 2/4 by saturated fatty acids and inhibition by docosahexaenoic acid. *European Journal of Pharmacology* 785:24–35.

Ikeya, Y., Fukuyama, N., and Mori, H. 2015. Low plasma eicosapentaenoic acid concentration as a possible risk factor for intracerebral hemorrhage. *Nutrition Research* 35(3):214–20.

Inoue, K., Kishida, K., Hirata, A., Funahashi, T., and Shimomura, I. 2013. Low serum eicosapentaenoic acid/arachidonic acid ratio in male subjects with visceral obesity. *Nutrition and Metabolism* 10(1):25.

Ishitobi, T., Hyogo, H., Kan, H., Hiramatsu, A., Arihiro, K., and Aikata, H. 2015. Eicosapentaenoic acid/arachidonic acid ratio as a possible link between non-alcoholic fatty liver disease and cardiovascular disease. *Hepatology Research* 45(5):533–9.

Ito, R., Satoh-Asahara, N., Yamakage, H., Sasaki, Y., Odori, S., and Kono, S. 2014. An increase in the EPA/AA ratio is associated with improved arterial stiffness in obese patients with dyslipidemia. *Journal of Atherosclerosis and Thrombosis* 21(3):248–60.

Jeon, S. M. 2016. Regulation and function of AMPK in physiology and diseases. *Experimental and Molecular Medicine* 48(7):e245.

Johnston, C. S., Tjonn, S. L., Swan, P. D., White, A., Hutchins, H., and Sears, B. 2006. Ketogenic low-carbohydrate diets have no metabolic advantage over non-ketogenic low-carbohydrate diets. *American Journal of Clinical Nutrition* 83(5):1055–61.

Kaji, I., Karaki, S., and Kuwahara, A. 2014. Short-chain fatty acid receptor and its contribution to glucagon-like peptide-1 release. *Digestion* 89(1):31–6.

Kaliannan, K., Wang, BF, Li, X. Y., Kim, K. J., and Kang, J. X. 2015. A host-microbiome interaction mediates the opposing effects of omega-6 and omega-3 fatty acids on metabolic endotoxemia. *Science Report* 5:11276.

Kashiyama, T., Ueda, Y., Nemoto, T., Wada, M., Masumura, Y., and Matsuo, K. 2011. Relationship between coronary plaque vulnerability and serum n-3/n-6 polyunsaturated fatty acid ratio. *Circulation Journal* 75(10):2432–8.

Kondo, T., Ogawa, K., Satake, T., et al. 1986. Plasma-free eicosapentaenoic acid/arachidonic acid ratio: A possible new coronary risk factor. *Clinical Cardiology* 9(9):413–16.

Kuipers, R. S., Luxwolda, M. F., Dijck-Brouwer, D. A., et al. 2010. Estimated macronutrient and fatty acid intakes from an East African Paleolithic diet. *British Journal of Nutrition* 104(11):1666–87.

Lai, D., Huang, M., Zhao, L., et al. 2019. Delphinidin-induced autophagy protects pancreatic beta cells against apoptosis resulting from high-glucose stress via AMPK signaling pathway. *Acta Biochimica Biophysica Sinica* 51(12):1242–9.

Lappi, J., Raninen, K., Väkeväinen, K., Kårlund, A., Törrönen, R., and Kolehmainen, M. 2021. Blackcurrant (*Ribes nigrum*) lowers sugar-induced postprandial glycaemia independently and in a product with fermented quinoa: A randomized crossover trial. *British Journal of Nutrition* 126(5):708–17.

Larraufie, P., Martin-Gallausiaux, C., Lapaque, N., et al. 2018. SCFAs strongly stimulate PYY production in human enteroendocrine cells. *Science Report* 8(1):74.

Lee, K. R., Midgette, Y., and Shah, R. 2019. Fish oil derived omega 3 fatty acids suppress adipose NLRP3 inflammasome signaling in human obesity. *Journal of the Endocrinology Society* 3(3):504–15.

Li, Y., and Chen, Y. 2019. AMPK and autophagy. *Advances in Experimental Medicine and Biology* 1206:85–108.

Lin, C., Chao, H., Li, Z., et al. 2017. Omega-3 fatty acids regulate NLRP3 inflammasome activation and prevent behavior deficits after traumatic brain injury. *Experimental Neurology* 290:115–22.

Lin, S. C., and Hardie, D. G. 2018. AMPK: Sensing glucose as well as cellular energy status. *Cell Metabolism* 27(2):299–313.

Lind, L., Ingelsson, E., Arnlov, J., Sundström, J., Zethelius, B., and Reaven, G M. 2018. Can the plasma concentration ratio of triglyceride/high-density lipoprotein cholesterol identify individuals at high risk of cardiovascular disease during 40-year follow-up? *Metabolic Syndrome Related Disorder* 16(8):433–9.

Liu, T. F., Brown, C. M., El Gazzar, M., McPhail, L., Millet, P., and Rao, A. 2012. Fueling the flame: Bioenergy couples metabolism and inflammation. *Journal of Leukocyte Biology* 92(3):499–507.

Lizuka, Y., Ozeki, A., Tani, T., and Tsuda, T. 2018. Blackcurrant extract ameliorates hyperglycemia in type 2 diabetic mice in association with increased basal secretion of glucagon-like peptide-1 and activation of AMP-activated protein kinase. *Journal of Nutritional Science and Vitaminology* 64(4):258–64.

Loftus, R. M., and Finlay, D. K. 2016. Immunometabolism: Cellular metabolism turns immune regulator. *Journal of Biological Chemistry* 291(1):1–10.

Lopategi, A., Flores-Costa, R., Rius, B. E., et al. 2019. Specialized pro-resolving lipid mediators inhibit the priming and activation of the macrophage NLRP3 inflammasome. *Journal of Leukocyte Biology* 105(1):25–36.

Luca, S. V., Macovei, I., Bujor, A., Miron, A., Skalicka-Wozniak, K., and Aprotosoaie, A. C. 2020. Bioactivity of dietary polyphenols: The role of metabolites. *Critical Review of Food Science and Nutrition* 60(4):626–59.

Ludwig, D. S. 2002. The glycemic index: Physiological mechanisms relating to obesity, diabetes, and cardiovascular disease. *The Journal of the American Medical Association* 287(18):2414–23.

Ludwig, D. S., Majzoub, J. A., Al-Zahrani, A., Dallal, G. E., Blanco, I., and Roberts, S. B. 1999. High glycemic index foods, overeating, and obesity. *Pediatrics* 103(3):E26.

Man, S. M., and Kanneganti, T. D. 2015. Regulation of inflammasome activation. *Immunological Reviews* 265(1):6–21.

Martin, C. K., Das, S. K., Lindblad, L., Racette, S. B., McCrory, M. A., and Weiss, E. P. 2011. Effect of calorie restriction on the free-living physical activity levels of non-obese humans: Results of three randomized trials. *Journal of Applied Physiology* 110(4):956–63.

Martínez-Micaelo, N., González-Abuín, N., Pinent, M., Ardévol, A., and Blay, M. 2016. Dietary fatty acid composition is sensed by the NLRP3 inflammasome: Omega-3 fatty acid (DHA) prevents NLRP3 activation in human macrophages. *Food and Function* 7(8):3480–7.

McArthur, S., Juban, G., Gobbetti, T., et al. 2020. Annexin A1 drives macrophage skewing to accelerate muscle regeneration through AMPK activation. *Journal of Clinical Investigation* 130(3):1156–67.

McLaughlin, T., Allison, G., Abbasi, F., Lamendola, C., and Reaven, G. M. 2004. Prevalence of insulin resistance and associated cardiovascular disease risk factors among normal weight, overweight, and obese individuals. *Metabolism* 53(4):495–9.

Moldogazieva, N. T., Mokhosoev, I. M., Melnikova, T. I., Porozov, Y. B., and Terentiev, A. A. 2019. Oxidative stress and advanced lipo-oxidation and glycation end products (ALEs and AGEs) in aging and age-related diseases. *Oxidative Medicine and Cellular Longevity* 2019:3085756.

Most, J., Tosti, V., Redman, L. M., and Fontana, L. 2017. Calorie restriction in humans: An update. *Ageing Research Reviews* 39:36–45.

Murguia-Romero, M., Jimenez-Flores, J. R., Sigrist-Flores, S. C., et al. 2013. Plasma triglyceride/HDL-cholesterol ratio, insulin resistance, and cardiometabolic risk in young adults. *Journal of Lipid Research* 54(10):2795–9.

Nagahara, Y., Motoyama, S., Sarai, M., Ito, H., Kawai, H., and Takakuwa, Y. 2016. Eicosapentaenoic acid to arachidonic acid (EPA/AA) ratio as an associated factor of high-risk plaque on coronary computed tomography in patients without coronary artery disease. *Atherosclerosis* 250:30–7.

Nagai, K., Koshiba, H., Shibata, S., Matsui, T., and Kozaki, K. 2015. Correlation between the serum eicosapentanoic acid-to-arachidonic acid ratio and the severity of cerebral white matter hyperintensities in older adults with memory disorder. *Geriatrics Gerontology International* 15(S1):48–52.

Ninomiya, T., Nagata, M., Hata, J., Hirakawa, Y., Ozawa, M., and Yoshida, D. 2013. Association between ratio of serum eicosapentaenoic acid to arachidonic acid and risk of cardiovascular disease: The Hisayama Study. *Atherosclerosis* 231(2):261–7.

Norling, L. V., Dalli, J., Flower, R. J, Serhan, C. N., and Perretti, M. 2012. Resolvin D1 limits polymorphonuclear leukocyte recruitment to inflammatory loci: Receptor-dependent actions. *Arteriosclerosis Thromboasis Vascular Biology* 32(8):1970–8.

Ohnishi, H., and Saito, Y. 2013. Eicosapentaenoic acid (EPA) reduces cardiovascular events: Relationship with the EPA/arachidonic acid ratio. *Journal of Atherosclerosis and Thrombosis* 20(12):861–77.

Oikawa, S., Yokoyama, M., Origasa, H., Matsuzaki, M., Matsuzawa, Y., and Saito, Y. 2009. Suppressive effect of EPA on the incidence of coronary events in hypercholesterolemia with impaired glucose metabolism: Sub-analysis of the Japan EPA Lipid Intervention Study (JELIS). *Atherosclerosis* 206(2):535–9.

Ott, C., Jacobs, K., Haucke, E., Navarrete Santos, A., Grune, T., and Simm, A. 2014. Role of advanced glycation end products in cellular signaling. *Redox Biology* 2:411–29.

Pantoja-Torres, B., Toro-Huamanchumo, C. J., Urrunaga-Pastor, D., Guarnizo-Poma, M., Lazaro-Alcantara, H., and Paico-Palacios, S. 2019. A high triglyceride to HDL-cholesterol ratio is associated with insulin resistance in normal-weight healthy adults. *Diabetes and Metabolic Syndrome* 13(1):382–8.

Parada Venegas, D., De la Fuente, M. K., Landskron, G., González, M. J., Quera, R., and Dijkstra, G. 2019. Mediated gut epithelial and immune regulation and its relevance for inflammatory bowel diseases. *Frontier Immunology* 10:277.

Pareja-Galeano, H., Sanchis-Goma, R. F., Santos-Lozano, A., Garatachea, N., Fiuza-Luces, C., and Lucia, A. 2015. Serum eicosapentaenoic acid to arachidonic acid ratio is associated with cardio-healthy exceptional longevity. *International Journal of Cardiology* 184:655–6.

Park, J., Langmead, C. J., and Riddy, D. M. 2020. New advances in targeting the resolution of inflammation: Implications for specialized pro-resolving mediator GPCR drug discovery. *ACS Pharmacology and Translation Science* 3(1):88–106.

Park, M., Sharma, A., and Lee, H. J. 2019. Anti-adipogenic effects of delphinidin-3-O-beta-glucoside in 3T3-L1 preadipocytes and primary white adipocytes. *Molecule* 24(10):1848.

Price, N. L., Gomes, A. P., Ling, A. J., Duarte, F. V., Martin-Montalvo, A., and North, B. J. 2012. SIRT1 is required for AMPK activation and the beneficial effects of resveratrol on mitochondrial function. *Cell Metabolism* 15(5):675–90.

Quispe, R., Martin, S. S., and Jones, S. R. 2016. Triglycerides to high-density lipoprotein-cholesterol ratio, glycemic control and cardiovascular risk in obese patients with type 2 diabetes. *Current Opinion of Endocrinology Diabetes and Obesity* 23(2):150–6.

Rahnasto-Rilla, M., Tyni, J., Huovinen, M., et al. 2018. Natural polyphenols as sirtuin 6 modulators. *Science Report* 8(1):4163.

Rizzo, A. M., Corsetto, P. A., Montorfano, G., et al. 2012. Comparison between the AA/EPA ratio in depressed and non-depressed elderly females: Omega-3 fatty acid supplementation correlates with improved symptoms but does not change immunological parameters. *Nutrition Journal* 11:82.

Rizzo, A. M., Montorfano, G., Negroni, M., et al. 2010. A rapid method for determining arachidonic: Eicosapentaenoic acid ratios in whole blood lipids: Correlation with erythrocyte membrane ratios and validation in a large Italian population of various ages and pathologies. *Lipid Health Disease* 9:7.

Roopchand, D. E., Carmody, R. N., Kuhn, P., et al. 2015. Dietary polyphenols promote growth of the gut bacterium *Akkermansia muciniphila* and attenuate high-fat diet-induced metabolic syndrome. *Diabetes* 64(8):2847–58.

Ruderman, N. B., Xu, X. J., Nelson, L., et al. 2010. AMPK and SIRT1: A long-standing partnership? *American Journal of Physiology and Endocrinology Metabolism* 298(4):E751–60E.

Rymut, N., Heinz, J., Sadhu, S., Hosseini, Z., Riley, C. O., and Marinello, M. 2020. Resolvin D1 promotes efferocytosis in aging by limiting senescent cell-induced MerTK cleavage. *Federation of American Society of Experimental Biology Journal* 34(1):597–609.

Salazar, M. R., Carbajal, H. A., Espeche, W. G., Aizpurúa, M., Marillet, A. G., and Leiva Sisnieguez, C. E. 2017. Use of the triglyceride/high-density lipoprotein cholesterol ratio to identify cardiometabolic risk: Impact of obesity? *Journal of Investigative Medicine* 65(2):323–7.

Salminen, A., Hyttinen, J. M. T., and Kaarniranta, K. 2011. AMP-activated protein kinase inhibits NF-κB signaling and inflammation: Impact on healthspan and lifespan. *Journal of Molecular Medicine* 89(7):667–76.

Schaeffler, A., Gross, P., Buettner, R., et al. 2009. Fatty acid-induced induction of Toll-like receptor-4/nuclear factor-kappaB pathway in adipocytes links nutritional signaling with innate immunity. *Immunology* 126(2):233–45.

Schon, C., Wacker, R., Micka, A., Steudle, J., Lang, S., and Bonnlander, B. 2018. Bioavailability study of maqui berry extract in healthy subjects. *Nutrient* 10(11):1720.

Sears, B. 1995. *The Zone*. Regan Books, 356. HarperCollins Publishers Inc, New York, NY.

Sears, B. 1997. *Mastering the Zone*, 367. Regan Books, New York, NY.

Sears, B. 2019. *The Resolution Zone*, 243. Zone Press, Palm City, FL.

Sears, B., Bailes, J., and Asselin, B. 2013. Therapeutic uses of high-dose omega-3 fatty acids to treat comatose patients with severe brain injury. *PharmaNutrition* 1:86–9.

Sears, B., Perry, M., and Saha, A. K. 2021. Dietary technologies to optimize healing from injury-induced inflammation. *Antiinflammatory Antiallergy Agents in Medicinal Chemistry* 20(2):123–31.

Sekikawa, A., Steingrimsdottir, L., Ueshima, H., et al. 2012. Serum levels of marine-derived n-3 fatty acids in Icelanders, Japanese, Koreans, and Americans – a descriptive epidemiologic study. *Prostaglandins, Leukotrienes and Essential Fatty Acids* 87(1):11–6.

Serhan, C. N. 2014. Pro-resolving lipid mediators are leads for resolution physiology. *Nature* 510(7503):92–101.

Serhan, C. N., and Levy, B. D. 2018. Resolvins in inflammation: Emergence of the pro-resolving superfamily of mediators. *Journal of Clinical Investigation* 128(7):2657–69.

Shackelford, D. B., and Shaw, R. J. 2009. The LKB1-AMPK pathway: Metabolism and growth control in tumour suppression. *Nature Reviews Cancer* 9(8):563–75.

Shukla, A. P., Andono, J., Touhamy, S. H., et al. 2017. Carbohydrate-last meal pattern lowers postprandial glucose and insulin excursions in type 2 diabetes. *BMJ Open Diabetes Research and Care* 5(1):e000440.

Shukla, A. P., Dickison, M., Coughlin, N., Karan, A., Mauer, E., and Truong, W. 2019. The impact of food order on postprandial glycaemic excursions in prediabetes. *Diabetes Obesity Metabolism* 21(2):377–81.

Silva, Y. P., Bernardi, A., and Frozza, R. L. 2020. The role of short-chain fatty acids from gut microbiota in gut-brain communication. *Frontiers in Endocrinology* 11:25.
Simpson, S. J., and Raubenheimer, D. 2005. Obesity: The protein leverage hypothesis. *Obesity Reviews* 6(2):133–42.
Sitolo, G. C., Mitarai, A., Adesina, P. A., Yamamoto, Y., and Suzuki, T. 2020. Fermentable fibers upregulate suppressor of cytokine signaling1 in the colon of mice and intestinal Caco-2 cells through butyrate production. *Bioscience, Biotechnology and Biochemistry* 84(11):2337–46.
Sorgi, P. J., Hallowell, E. M., Hutchins, H. L., and Sears, B. 2007. Effects of an open-label pilot study with high-dose EPA/DHA concentrates on plasma phospholipids and behavior in children with attention deficit hyperactivity disorder. *Nutritional Journal* 6:16.
Sutterwala, F. S., Haasken, S., and Cassel, S. L. 2014. Mechanism of NLRP3 inflammasome activation. *Annals New York Academy of Science* 1319(1):82–95.
Taylor, R., Al-Mrabeh, A., and Sattar, N. 2019. Understanding the mechanisms of reversal of type 2 diabetes. *Lancet Diabetes Endocrinology* 7(9):726–36.
Tse, E. K., Salehi, A., Clemenzi, M. N., and Belsham, D. D. 2018. Role of the saturated fatty acid palmitate in the interconnected hypothalamic control of energy homeostasis and biological rhythms. *American Journal of Physiology and Endocrinology Metabolism* 315(2):E133–40.
Urpi-Sarda, M., Andres-Lacueva, C., Rabassa, M., et al. 2015. The relationship between urinary total polyphenols and the frailty phenotype in a community-dwelling older population: The InCHIANTI Study. *The Journals of Gerontology. Series A, Biological Sciences and Medical Sciences* 70(9):1141–7.
van der Klaauw, A. A., Keogh, J. M., Henning, E., et al. 2013. High protein intake stimulates postprandial GLP1 and PYY release. *Obesity* 21(8):1602–7.
Wakabayashi, Y., Funayama, H., Ugata, Y., et al. 2015. Low eicosapentaenoic acid to arachidonic acid ratio is associated with thin cap fibroatheroma determined by optical coherence tomography. *Journal of Cardiology* 66(6):482–8.
Westerterp-Plantenga, M. S. 2008. Protein intake and energy balance. *Regulatory Peptides* 149(1–3):67–9.
Williams-Bey, Y., Boularan, C., Vural, A., et al. 2014. Omega-3 free fatty acids suppress macrophage inflammasome activation by inhibiting NF-κB activation and enhancing autophagy. *PLoS One* 9(6):e97957.
Yamano, T., Kubo, T., Shiono, Y., et al. 2015. Impact of eicosapentaenoic acid treatment on the fibrous cap thickness in patients with coronary atherosclerotic plaque: An optical coherence tomography study. *Journal of Atherosclerosis Thrombosis* 22(1)52–61.
Yan, Y., Jiang, W., Spinetti, T., et al. 2013. Omega-3 fatty acids prevent inflammation and metabolic disorder through inhibition of NLRP3 inflammasome activation. *Immunity* 38(6):1154–63.
Yin, Y., Chen, F., Wang, W., Wang, H., and Zhang, X. 2017. Resolvin D1 inhibits inflammatory response in STZ-induced diabetic retinopathy rats: Possible involvement of NLRP3 inflammasome and NF-kappaB signaling pathway. *Molecular Vision* 23:242–50.
Yokoyama, M, Origasa, H, Matsuzaki, M., et al. 2007. Effects of eicosapentaenoic acid on major coronary events in hypercholesterolaemic patients (JELIS): A randomized open-label, blinded endpoint analysis. *Lancet* 369(9567):1090–8.
Zamora-Ros, R., Rabassa, M., Cherubini, A., et al. 2013. High concentrations of a urinary biomarker of polyphenol intake are associated with decreased mortality in older adults. *Journal of Nutrition* 143(9):1445–50.
Zhu, M. J., Kang, Y., Xue, Y., et al. 2018. Red raspberries suppress NLRP3 inflammasome and attenuate metabolic abnormalities in diet-induced obese mice. *Journal of Nutritional Biochemistry* 53:96–103.

8 Customized Nutritional Practices and Dietary Recommendations through Integrative High-Throughput Omics Approaches

Ramachandran Chelliah, Inamul Hasan Madar, Khanita Suman Chinnanai, Ghazala Sultan, Pravitha Kasu Sivanandan, Bandana Pahi, Mahamuda Begum, Syeda Mahvish Zahra, Iftikhar Aslam Tayubi, and Deog-Hwan Oh*

CONTENTS

* Corresponding author email: ramachandran865@gmail.com

DOI: 10.1201/9781003142195-8

8.1 INTRODUCTION

In the modern era of advancement in science, technology, health, and economics, the elevating population and ecological problems fetch novel trials to the contemporary world. Developments in analytical technologies are the foremost innovations for chief deriving foods and concerned thriftily comprehensive consumers to have food with the healthier nutrient distribution; advancements of several foodstuffs primarily target consumers of distinct age bunches and financial status and health. Encroachment in omics technologies has provided massive prospects to research the gene-diet interface.

The ability of diet to influence genetic information flow may occur at a variety of regulatory sites. Advances in genomics, transcriptomics, proteomics, and metabolomics have made it possible to understand how bioactive substances impact human health more rapidly and comprehensively (Fenech et al. 2011). Because of the swift progression and assortment in propitious diagnostic platforms and computational analysis, exploration in food sciences and nutrition is likely to be altered using omics applications in the future (Alfaro and Young 2018). The collection of technologies to analyze the function, structure, and intermolecular interactions of several biological molecules in biological samples is called omics (Coughlin 2014). These high-throughput technologies result in manifold evaluations instantaneously and estimate overall gene products like proteins, expressed genes, and metabolites in studied samples. Genomics, transcriptomics, proteomics, and metabolomics are the main high-throughput omics. The omics technologies provide vast prospects for understanding diet's effect at a molecular level (Figure 8.1). The ultimate aim of omics technologies is to recognize the molecular key signatures of dietary food nutrients and non-nutrient that contribute to a particular phenotype and provide tailored nutritional suggestions for maintaining health and disease prevention (Zhang et al. 2008). Technological invention is essential for augmenting the capacity and efficacy

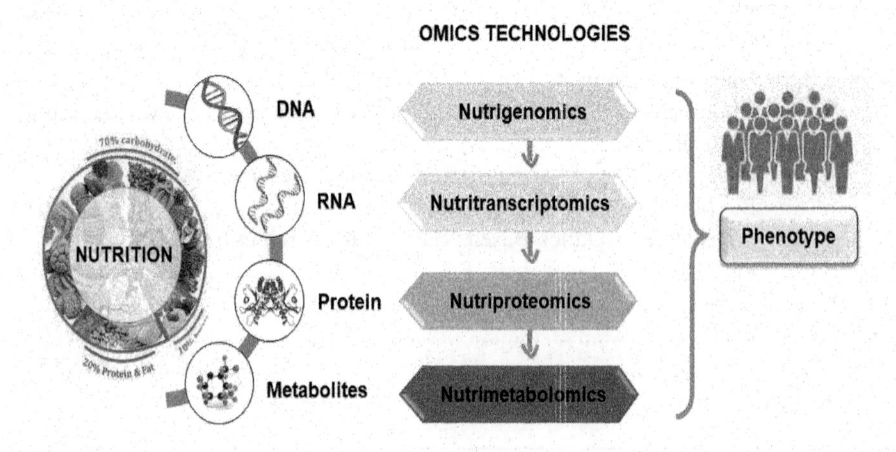

FIGURE 8.1 Role of omics technologies in nutritional research.

of diagnostics of innumerable diseases, immunology, and nutritional preparation to determine food safety and quality.

8.2 PRESENT ADVANCES AND POTENTIAL LIMITATIONS OF OMICS TECHNOLOGIES IN NUTRITION RESEARCH

8.2.1 Nutritional Transcriptomics

Many new insights into diet-gene interactions have come from transcriptomic approaches. The technology has progressed to the point that it can now be used as a routine tool by all researchers who want to generate high-quality data. To ensure that data can be used to its full potential, uniform standards and infrastructures for microarray data collection, storage, and sharing must be created. The potential for human nutritional intervention studies that use transcriptomic analysis of accessible tissues, while not yet thoroughly studied, appears to be very promising. This form of research opens up new possibilities for the development of unique nutritional biomarkers.

At present, DNA microarrays are the extensively used tool for transcriptomics, which permits an estimation of the expression levels up to 50,000 transcripts concurrently. To assess cellular reactions to dietary elements and their target molecules, DNA microarrays are used in cell culture or laboratory animals. Vitamins D and E (Johnson and Manor 2004), green tea catechins (McLoughlin et al. 2004), and polyunsaturated fatty acids (Kitajka et al. 2004) are some examples.

In recent times, DNA microarray had been used to determine the impact of quercetin on gene expression in COIIS, human colon cancer cell lines, and discovered around 5,000 to 7,000 DEGs (differentially expressed genes) – that is, quercetin possibly utilizes an extensive modulatory impact on gene expression levels in colon carcinoma (Murtaza et al. 2006). The microarray technique had used to determine hepatic gene expression in tumor and cancer cells. Fifty-six genes responsive to arginine in normal liver cells and 162 from the tumor cells were recognized (Leong et al. 2006). Microarray gene expression profiling of human adipocytes reacted with anthocyanins, a group of significant pigments that repressed the progression of obesity (Murtaza et al. 2006). The substantial changes in adipocytokine expression and the genes involved in lipid metabolism had confirmed through the results. It demonstrates that anthocyanins could predict to enhance the adipocyte function of diabetes and obesity.

Furthermore, DNA microarrays scrutinize the functionality and security of hypoallergenic wheat flour (HWF). Hypoallergenic wheat flour is formed from wheat flour with actinase and cellulose that avoids wheat allergy (Narasaka et al. 2006). Rats were fed with a diet consisting of regular flour and HWF and were compared individually for the liver and intestines gene expression profiles. About 30 genes were upregulated and downregulated after HWF consumption (one week/one month). These results demonstrate that microarray analysis of DNA is also a proficient methodology to estimate food safety. This gene expression analysis determines the molecular pathways reactively to dietary configuration and caloric constraints within the adipose tissue (Mangravite et al. 2007). More than 1,000 transcripts had ominously downregulated expression. This outcome has proven that in the adipose tissue, stearoyl-coenzyme A desaturase (SCD) expression is independently regulated by carbohydrate and saturated fat consumption, weight loss, and so on. DGAT2 (diacylglycerol transferase 2) and SCD expression might be involved in systemic triacylglycerol metabolism regulation. We can undoubtedly say that there will be advancements in similar findings that investigate the functionality and welfare of specific food elements in the upcoming future.

However, there are few restrictions for nutritranscriptiomics in human nutrition. One of the limitations is that expression analysis needs substantial amounts of tissue material to segregate the required RNA. In contrast, the availability of human tissues is limited, though it is unbearable to attain biopsies from control subjects in nutrition research. On the contrary, a vast inter-individual discrepancy happens in healthy persons' gene expression profiles (Cobb et al. 2005). Another limitation is cost expensive. The analysis needs to be recurrent to determine the actual measurements, mainly when lesser expression-distinctive requirements are observed, and consequently, research becomes relatively costly.

8.2.2 Nutriproteomics

The proteome is a highly complex system that is continuously evolving in response to external factors such as diet. Nutritional proteomics has a lot of potential for (1) profiling and characterizing body and dietary proteins, as well as digestion and absorption; (2) identification of potential biomarkers of nutritional status and health/disease conditions; and (3) understanding the roles of nutrients and other numerous dietary factors involved in growth, reproduction, metabolism, and health (Sénéchal and Kussmann 2011). Nutriproteomics is a promising research zone that needs proteomic tools to depict cellular and molecular changes in protein expression and their interactions with nutrients. The functions and bioavailability of nutrients, bioactive proteins, and peptides can be influenced by other compounds/nutrients. Nutriproteomics is the authenticated tool in personalized nutrition (Table 8.1). It aids in the characterization and quantification of bioactive proteins and peptides from the food devious from determining the biomarkers for explaining their action and efficacy mechanism (Kussmann 2010). To monitor physiological responses at an individual range, endogenously expressed human peptides and proteins also serve as biomarkers. The food has bioactive peptides and proteins that provide extensive information on homeostatic regulation, growth, and antagonistic allergic reactions (Sauer and Luge 2015). Proteomics is core to nutrigenomic research and defines how the genome expresses itself as a reaction to diet. In nutrition research, proteomics can determine and quantify bioactive peptides and proteins and also provides their nutritional bio-efficiency (Kussmann and Affolter 2009). Proteomic techniques are used for estimating the quality of food, especially about personalized nutrition, primarily through evaluating the whole proteome or metabolome of foods (Werf et al. 2001). This approach had used in the post-marketing surveillance of foods from genetically modified crops. It may aid as a powerful tool in the upcoming future (Kuiper et al. 2001) for the determination of bioactive compounds in functional foods and nutraceuticals (Galvani et al. 2001).

TABLE 8.1
Application of Proteomic Techniques in Nutrition Research

Proteomic techniques	Nutriproteomic applications
SELDI-TOF-MS	Identification of new biomarkers
LC-ESI-Q-TOF-MS/MS	Identification, characterization, and quantification
ICAT	Peptide quantification
DIGE	Protein separation and quantification
iTRAQ	Examination of differentially expressed proteins
MALDI-MS/MS	Visualization of small metabolites to identify nutritional content

Currently, only a few studies on the use of MS-based proteomics in nutrition research are available. SELDI-TOF-MS analysis of plasma samples from retinol-sufficient and retinol-deficient rats revealed three possible biomarkers of vitamin A deficiency. This tool may be encouraging to determine changes in nutrition research (Linke et al. 2004). Furthermore, the MS-based method selects prime allergens in processed peanuts by combining capillary LC with nano-ESI-Q-TOF-MS/MS (Chassaigne et al. 2007). Five peptides have been discovered as biomarkers for peanut allergens based on the study of roasted and raw peanuts.

Recently, several quantitative protein and peptide analysis techniques like ICAT (isotope-coded affinity tag), DIGE (difference gel electrophoresis), and iTRAQ (isobaric tags for relative and absolute quantification) have been developed (Chen, Sun, Yu et al. 2007). A DIGE, ICAT, and iTRAQ comparative analysis was carried out (Wu et al. 2006). The results showed that all three methods produced reasonably accurate quantitative results, even though iTRAQ has higher sensitivity compared to ICAT and DIGE. Nevertheless, some potential issues occur, like the protein configuration issue for DIGE, the cysteine-content effect for ICAT, and vulnerability to faults in ancestor ion separation for iTRAQ. The respective information gained from different approaches can enhance the understanding of the biological effects of food intervention as these techniques have shown a limited overlap between the observed proteins. The proteomics variation approach has been carried out between different strawberry diversities by MALDI-MS/MS and DIGE (Alm et al. 2007). They discovered that the natural changes were more pretentious by other growth circumstances than by other diversities. The quantity of strawberry allergens was different between strawberry varieties. The allergen is colorless (white) and is inferior to that in the red ones. The three proteins are identical between the proteins interrelated with the allergen and the color (i.e., possible to strain a strawberry with less allergen). Therefore, a proteomic approach was utilized for the various enhancement of fruits or vegetables.

8.2.3 Nutrimetabolomics

Nutrimetabolomics, a relatively new area of research, offers fascinating insights into the metabolic responses of humans and animals to dietary interventions. MS-based metabolomics has enormous potential for high-throughput screening of lower molecular mass metabolites in biological conditions, given the rapid progress of MS approaches. The main advantage of the MS method is the high sensitivity and speed at which structure/mass data can be determined. MS in conjunction with chromatographic technologies such as CE, GC, and LC are the most widely used MS instruments. HPLC systems are also being used in metabolomics, with sub-2 m packing columns combined with UPLC technology (high-operating technology). The UPLC-TOF-MS system is faster, has better sensitivity, and has a higher peak ability than HPLC-TOF-MS systems with 3–5 m packing columns. This method assists in high-throughput metabolomics MS screening. These technologies are effective in the discovery of cancer biomarkers (Zhang et al. 2007). Only a small amount of nutrimetabolomic research is conducted in support of the MS method. HPLC-TOF-MS, for example, can be used to investigate changes in endogenous urinary metabolites in rats as they age. For a broad understanding of systems reactions to aristolochic acid interference in rats, a combination of GC-MS and LC-MS metabolic profiling was used (Ni et al. 2007) and an ESI-Q-TOF-MS for the diversity of quality and maturity of bananas, grapes, and strawberries (Chen, Sun, Wortmann et al. 2007).

One of the crucial concerns in nutrimetabolomics, gut microflora–host metabolism interaction, is that humans' microbiome interaction becomes a superorganism (Goodacre 2007). Because of the large-bowel microflora's significant metabolic signals (more than 400 microbial species in healthy humans), simple metabolomic signals of nutrients in diet may be jumbled and biofluids' metabolome human nutrition may be altered. The metabolic relationship between gut microflora and host co-metabolic phenotypes was determined using plasma and urinary NMR analysis in mice (Dumas, Barton et al. 2006). They discovered that methylamines from the precursor choline were excreted in the urine, suggesting a direct correlation between microbiota metabolism, mammalian host metabolism, and microflora metabolism. Proton NMR technology is a widely used technique in nutrition research for metabolomic trials. For example, the classification of metabolic inconsistency in different populations (for example, Americans, the Chinese, and the Japanese [Dumas, Barton et al. 2006] or Swedish and British people [Lenz et al. 2004]) and the evaluation of biochemical effects of soy isoflavones in the diet of five stable premenopausal women (Solanky et al. 2003). Also, the high- and low-meat diets (Stella et al. 2006); the metabolic outcome of supplementing vitamin E to a mouse model for motor neuron degeneration (Griffin et al. 2002) and the discovery of human biological responses to different diets (e.g., chamomile tea or vegetarian) (Wang et al. 2005). The metabolic reactions of rats fed with whole-grain flour (WGF) and refined wheat flour (RF) have recently been studied using an NMR-based metabolomic methodology. The results revealed that in the urine of rats fed the WGF diet, certain aromatic amino acids, tricarboxylic acid intermediates (cycle), and hippurate had dangerously increased (Fardet et al. 2007).

8.2.4 Bioinformatics

Bioinformatics, an interdisciplinary area, is an essential scientific discipline that conveys a prototype swing in several fields like biotechnology, genetic evolution, molecular medicine, comparative genomics, drug development, and microbial genome applications (Can 2014). Several bioinformatic methodologies have recognized the potential for a significant impact in the nutrition field. Bioinformatics aids in imagining and assessing the expected and unintended effects of microbes on food, conducting research to meet food production requirements, food processing, genomics, proteomics, and refining the quality and nutrient rate of food sources, among many other things. Aside from yield potential and disease resistance, bioinformatic methodologies can also generate a decent crop quality. Meat and its elements, nutritional value, chemistry, and biology are all protected by numerous databases. Bioinformatics is essential in various flavor complexes for new product development based on perceptions, tastes, and consumer needs (Mengjin Liu et al. 2008).

Bioinformatics experts have developed a method for identifying and categorizing bacterial food pathogens. The Food and Drug Administration designed the device for molecular classification of bacterial foodborne pathogens using gene expression analysis such as microarrays (Fang et al. 2010).

Food allergen studies may benefit from bioinformatics. Allergens have similar sequences and structural similarities in general. Homology analyses and structural bioinformatics may be used to assess protein cross-reactivity and allergenicity. This method reassures the WHO that sequence similarity search should be included in the rules for estimating allergenicity in GM foods (genetically modified foods) (Jenkins et al. 2005). Food allergens are covered by a few databases, including AllerMatch (Fiers et al. 2004), Informall FARRP Allergen database, and SDAP (Mari et al. 2006).

Bioinformatics recently revealed the techniques for the detection of bioactive peptides (Walther and Sieber 2011). Protein sequences from UniProtKB, SwissProt, and TreMBL are one way to find bioactive peptides. The frequency of bioactive peptides crypt in primary structures of food proteins has been determined using the formula a/N, where a represents the number of peptides demonstrating bioactivity of a particular kind present in sequence and N represents the total number of amino acid residues present within the proteins. This approach reduces the time required to test for bioactive peptides in food using traditional methods. It makes it possible to find new and established bioactive peptides. As a result of the stimulation of proteolytic specificities of various enzymes, some software has been produced to produce profiles for in silico peptides (Udenigwe 2014).

8.3 FUTURE APPLICATIONS

8.3.1 Integrative Use of Various Omics Technologies and Systems Biology Technology

Understanding how diet affects metabolic control and how it has changed to improve health is a key systemic goal in nutritional research. To achieve this goal, we must transition from a single omics medium to incorporating multiple omics media or integromics and finally to systems biology (Thomas and Ganji 2006). Initial findings in this area show that systems biology can be applied to nutrition research with great success. Orotic acid therapy was used to diagnose disconcerted metabolic pathways using a combination of reverse functional genomic and metabolic process (Griffin et al. 2004). The 60 most differentially expressed genes and the most modified metabolite trimethylamine-N-oxide were investigated using statistical bootstrapping. Stearyl-CoA desaturase one has identified the most significant negative association in the relationship between transcripts and metabolites in lipid pathways. Proteome and transcriptome analysis of human colon cancer cells treated with flavone was completed in one of the studies (Herzog et al. 2004). The results show that around 488 mRNA targets had been identified regulated by flavone no less than twofold.

On the other hand, flavone acquaintance transformed many proteins associated with gene regulation, detoxification, and intermediate metabolism. They are annexin II and apolipoprotein A1. The main molecular variations in hepatocellular lipid metabolism in zinc-deficient rats were determined using transcriptome and proteome analysis (Dieck et al. 2005). The findings suggest that an unstable gene transcription regulation mediated by PPAR, thyroid hormone, and SREBP could account for the majority of the implications of zinc deficiency on hepatic fat metabolism. Integrative transcriptome and lipid-metabolome methods provide a basis for understanding the molecular processes affected by PUFA consumption (Mutch et al. 2005). Stearoyl-CoA desaturase was identified as a priority of an arachidonate-rich diet. They discovered a previously unknown and distinct function for arachidonate in the regulation of hepatic lipid metabolism. The combined use of different omics technologies improves our understanding of metabolic control in response to dietary changes.

8.3.2 Translation of Omics-Based Nutrition Research into Clinical Practice

The omics-based nutrition research serves as a platform to comprehend the relationship between disease and diet and between health and diet and transform these investigational results into clinical practice. This will lead to the approval for personalized nutrition. Individual biochemical variability has defined individual biochemical variability for individualized food based on the environmental factors, genetic variation, and dietary behaviors linked to civilizations, beliefs, and life routines. Because of this biochemical diversity, different people have different reactions to the same nutritional intervention. Some foods are known to induce significant changes in some people's urine; for example, beetroot causes red urine in some people, while asparagus causes foul urine in many others (Mitchell 2001). As a result, nutrition researchers and dietetics practitioners can integrate multiple omics technologies and systems biology approaches to calculate, model, and imagine biological reactions and responses of individuals to nutritional modifications, allowing personalized nutrition to become a reality. The mechanism of identification of biomarkers of particular nutrients, shown in Figure 8.2.

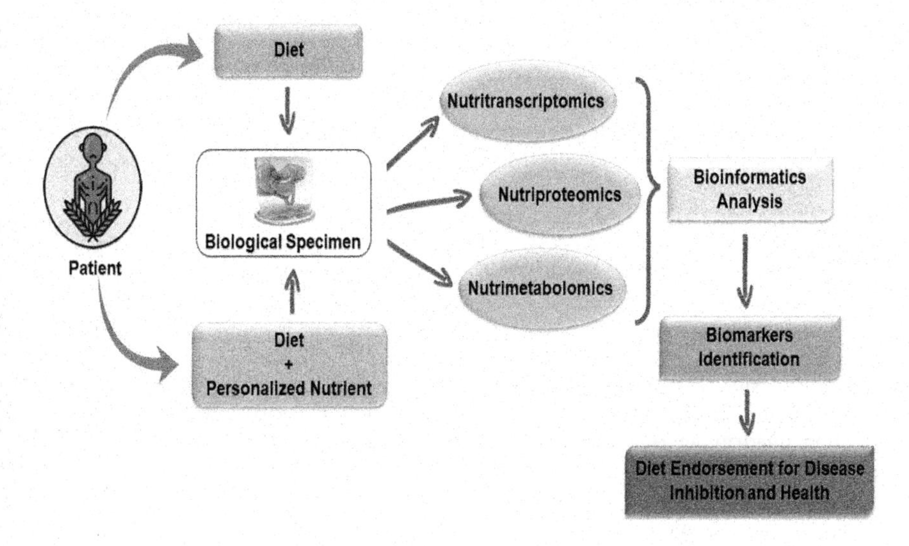

FIGURE 8.2 Process of biomarker identification of nutrients in omics-based nutrition research.

8.4 CONCLUSION

In most cases, omics-based nutrition research has been accomplished on animals using omics technologies exclusively MS-based nutrimetabolomics/nutriproteomics in nutritional analysis. High-throughput omics technologies produce enormous quantities of data, which necessitate curation and analysis. Bioinformatics is a key field in the food industry because it allows to effectively manage large quantities of data produced by different projects. Combining multiple omics technologies would make it much easier to identify new biomarkers linked to particular nutrients or other dietary factors. Systems biology amalgamates several omics technologies to comprehend the biological behavior response to external signals. It also shows the precise direction of nutrient complex interface linkage in biological systems between nutrients and molecules. Ideally, future omics-based human nutrition studies will create the most appropriate dietary guidelines for the entire planet, avoiding chronic diseases, such as cancer, metabolic syndromes, T2D, cardiovascular disease, and obesity.

ACKNOWLEDGMENTS

The authors gratefully acknowledge Inamul Hasan Madar, Ghazala Sultan, and Deog-Hwan Oh for their expert technical support and helpful discussions. This work was funded by the National Research Foundation of Korea (NRF), grant number 2018007551, and Brain Korea (BK) 21 Plus Project, grant number 4299990913942.

REFERENCES

Alfaro, A. C., and Young, T. 2018. Showcasing metabolomic applications in aquaculture: A review. *Review in Aquaculture* 10:135–52.

Alm, R., Ekefjard, A., Krogh, M., Hakkinen, J., and Emanuelsson, C. 2007. Proteomic variation is as large within as between strawberry varieties. *Journal of Proteome Research* 6(8):3011–20.

Can, T. 2014. Introduction to Bioinformatics. In: *Mirnomics: MicroRNA Biology and Computational Analysis. Methods in Molecular Biology (Methods and Protocols)*, eds. M. Yousef and J. Allmer, Vol. 1107. Humana Press, Totowa, NJ.

Chassaigne, H., Norgaard, J. V., and van Hengel, A. J. 2007. Proteomics-based approach to detect and identify major allergens in processed peanuts by capillary LC-QTOF (MS/MS). *Journal of Agricultural and Food Chemistry* 55(11):4461–73.

Chen, H. W., Sun, Y. P., Wortmann, A., Gu, H. W., and Zenobi, R. 2007. Differentiation of maturity and quality of fruit using noninvasive extractive electrospray ionization quadrupole time-of-flight mass spectrometry. *Analytical Chemistry* 79(4): 1447–55.

Chen, X., Sun, L. W., Yu, Y. B., Xue, Y., and Yang, P. Y. 2007. Amino acid-coded tagging approaches in quantitative proteomics. *Expert Review of Proteomics* 4(1):25–37.

Cobb, J. P., Mindrinos, M. N., Miller-Graziano, C., et al. 2005. Application of genome-wide expression analysis to human health and disease. *Proceedings of the National Academy of Sciences United States of America* 102:4801–6.

Coughlin, S. S. 2014. Toward a road map for global-omics: A primer on-omic technologies. *American Journal of Epidemiology* 180:1188–95.

Dieck, H. T., Doring, F., Fuchs, D., Roth, H. P., and Daniel, H. 2005. Transcriptome and proteome analysis identifies the pathways that increase hepatic lipid accumulation in zinc-deficient rats. *Journal of Nutrition* 135(2):199–205.

Dumas, M. E., Barton, R. H., Toye, A., et al. 2006. Metabolic profiling reveals a contribution of gut microbiota to fatty liver phenotype in insulin-resistant mice. *Proceedings of the National Academy of Sciences United States of America* 103(33):12511–6.

Fang, H., Xu, J., Ding, D., et al. 2010. An FDA bioinformatics tool for microbial genomics research on molecular characterization of bacterial foodborne pathogens using microarrays. *BMC Bioinformatics* 11:S4.

Fardet, A., Canlet, C., Gottardi, G., et al. 2007. Whole-grain and refined wheat flours show distinct metabolic profiles in rats as assessed by a ^{1}H NMR-based metabonomic approach. *Journal of Nutrition* 137(4):923–9.

Fenech, M., El-Sohemy, A., Cahill, L., et al. 2011. Nutrigenetics and nutrigenomics: Viewpoints on the current status and applications in nutrition research and practice. *Journal of Nutrigenetics and Nutrigenomics* 4(2):69–89.

Fiers, M. W., Kleter, G. A., Nijland, H., et al. 2004. Allermatch™, a webtool for the prediction of potential allergenicity according to current FAO/WHO Codex alimentarius guidelines. *BMC Bioinformatics* 5:133.

Galvani, M., Hamdan, M., and Righetti, P. G. 2001. Two-dimensional gel electrophoresis/matrix-assisted laser desorption/ionisation mass spectrometry of commercial bovine milk. *Rapid Communications in Mass Spectrometry* 15:258–64.

Goodacre, R. 2007. Metabolomics of a superorganism. *Journal of Nutrition* 137(1):259S–66S.

Griffin, J. L., Bonney, S. A., Mann, C., et al. 2004. An integrated reverse functional genomic and metabolic approach to understanding orotic acid-induced fatty liver. *Physiological Genomics* 17(2):140–9.

Griffin, J. L., Muller, D., Woograsingh, R., et al. 2002. Vitamin E deficiency and metabolic deficits in neuronal ceroid lipofuscinosis described by bioinformatics. *Physioogical. Genomics* 11(3):195–203.

Herzog, A., Kindermann, B., Döring, F., Daniel, H., and Wenzel, U. 2004. Pleiotropic molecular effects of the pro-apoptotic dietary constituent flavone in human colon cancer cells identified by protein and mRNA expression profiling. *Proteomics* 4:2455–64.

Jenkins, J. A., Griffiths-Jones, S., Shewry, P. R., Breiteneder, H., and Mills, E. C. 2005. Structural relatedness of plant food allergens with specific reference to cross-reactive allergens: An in silico analysis. *Journal of Allergy and Clinical Immunology* 115:163–70.

Johnson, A., and Manor, D. 2004. The transcriptional signature of vitamin E. *Annals of the New York Academy of Sciences* 1031:337–8.

Kitajka, K., Sinclair, A. J., Weisinger, R. S., et al. 2004. Effects of dietary omega-3 polyunsaturated fatty acids on brain gene expression. *Proceedings of the National Academy of Sciences of the United States of America* 101(30):10931–36.

Kuiper, H. A., Kleter, G. A., Noteborn, H. P., Kok, E. J. 2001. Assessment of the food safety issues related to genetically modified foods. *Plant Journal* 27:503–28.

Kussmann, M. 2010. Nutriproteomics-linking proteomics variation with personalized nutrition. *Current Pharmacogenomics and Personalized Medicine* 8:245–56.

Kussmann, M., and Affolter, M. 2009. Proteomics at the center of nutrigenomics: Comprehensive molecular understanding of dietary health effects. *Nutrition* 25:1085–93.

Lenz, E. M., Bright, J., Wilson, I. D., et al. 2004. A metabonomics, dietary influences and cultural differences: A ^{1}H NMR based study of urine samples obtained from healthy British and Swedish subjects. *Journal of Pharmaceutical and Biomedical Analysis* 36(4):841–9.

Leong, H. X., Simkevich, C., Lesieur-Brooks, A., et al. 2006. Short-term arginine deprivation results in large-scale modulation of hepatic gene expression in both normal and tumor cells: Microarray bioinformatic analysis. *Nutrition, and Metabolism* 3:37.

Linke, T., Ross, A. C., and Harrison, E. H. 2004. Profiling of rat plasma by surface-enhanced laser desorption/ionization time-of-flight mass spectrometry, a novel tool for biomarker discovery in nutrition research. *Journal of Chromatography A* 1043(1):65–71.

Liu, M., Nauta, A., Francke, C., and Siezen, R. J. 2008. Comparative genomics of enzymes in flavor-forming pathways from amino acids in lactic acid bacteria. *Applied and Environmental Microbiology* 74(15):4590–600.

Mangravite, L. M., Dawson, K., Davis, R. R., and Gregg, J. P. 2007. Krauss fatty acid desaturase regulation in adipose tissue by dietary composition is independent of weight loss and is correlated with the plasma triacylglycerol response. *American Journal of Clinical Nutrition* 86(3):759–67.

Mari, A., Scala, E., Palazzo, P., et al. 2006. Bioinformatics applied to allergy: Allergen databases, from collecting sequence information to data integration. The Allergome platform as a model. *Cellular Immune* 244:97–100.

McLoughlin, P., Roengvoraphoj, M., Gissel, C., Hescheler, J., Certa, U., and Sachinidis, A. 2004. Transcriptional responses to epigallocatechin-3 gallate in HT 29 colon carcinoma spheroids. *Genes Cells* 9(7):661–9.

Mitchell, S. C. 2001. Food idiosyncrasies: Beetroot and asparagus. *Drug Metabolism and Disposition* 29(4):539–43.

Murtaza, L., Marra, G., Schlapbach, R., et al. 2006. A preliminary investigation demonstrating the effect of quercetin on the expression of genes related to cell-cycle arrest, apoptosis and xenobiotic metabolism in human COIIScolon-adenocarcinoma cells using DNA microarray. *Biotechnology and Applied Biochemistry* 45:29–36.

Mutch, D. M., Grigorov, M., Berger, A., et al. 2005. An integrative metabolism approach identifies stearoyl-CoA desaturase as a target for an arachidonate-enriched diet. *FASEB Journal* 19(1):599.

Narasaka, S., Endo, Y., Fu, Z. W., et al. 2006. Safety evaluation of hypoallergenic wheat flour by using a DNA microarray. *Bioscience, Biotechnology, and Biochemistry* 70(6):1464–70.

Ni, Y., Su, M. M., Qiu, Y. P., et al. 2007. Metabolic profiling using combined GC-MS and LC-MS provides a systems understanding of aristolochic acid-induced nephrotoxicity in rat. *FEBS Letters* 581(4):707–11.

Plowman, J. E., Bryson, W. G., and Jordan, T. W. 2000. Application of proteomics for determining protein markers for wool quality traits. *Electrophoresis* 21:1899–906.

Sauer, S., and Luge, T. 2015. Nutriproteomics: Facts, concepts and perspectives. *Proteomics* 15:997–1013.

Sénéchal, S., and Kussmann, M. 2011. Nutriproteomics: Technologies and applications for identification and quantification of biomarkers and ingredients. *The Proceedings of the Nutrition Society* 70(3):351–64.

Solanky, K. S., Bailey, N. J, C., Beckwith-Hall, B. M., et al. 2003. Application of biofluid ^{1}H nuclear magnetic resonance-based metabonomic techniques for the analysis of the biochemical effects of dietary isoflavones on human plasma profile. *Anal. Biochem.* 323(2):197–204.

Stella, C., Beckwith-Hall, B., Cloarec, O., et al. 2006. Susceptibility of human metabolic phenotypes to dietary modulation. *J. Proteome. Res.* 5:2780–88.

Thomas, C. E., and Ganji, G. 2006. Integration of genomic and metabonomic data in systems biology – are we "there" yet? *Current Opinion in Drug Discovery & Development* 9(1):92–100.

Udenigwe, C. C. 2014. Bioinformatics approaches, prospects and challenges of food bioactive peptide research. *Trends in Food Science and Technology* 36:137–43.

Walther, B., and Sieber, R. 2011. Bioactive proteins and peptides in foods. *International Journal for Vitamin and Nutrition Research* 81:181.

Wang, Y. L., Tang, H. R., Nicholson, J. K., Hylands, P. J., Sampson, J., and Holmes, E. A. 2005. Metabonomic strategy for the detection of the metabolic effects of chamomile (*Matricaria recutita* L.) ingestion. *Journal of Agricultural and Food Chemistry* 53(2):191–6.

Werf, M., Schuren, F., Bijlsma, S., Tas, A., van Ommen, B. 2001. Nutrigenomics: Application of genomics technologies in nutritional sciences and food technology. *Journal of Food Science* 66:772–80.

Wu, W. W., Wang, G. H., Baek, S. J., and Shen, R. F. 2006. Comparative study of three proteomic quantitative methods, DIGE, cICAT and iTRAQ, using 2D gel- or LC MALDI TOF/TOF. *Journal of Proteome Research* 5(3):651–8.

Zhang, X. W., Wei, D., Yap, Y. L., Li, L., Guo, S. Y., and Chen, F. 2007. Mass spectrometry-based "omics" technologies in cancer diagnostics. *Mass Spectrometry Reviews* 26:403–13.

Zhang, X. W., Yap, Y., Wei, D., Chen, G., and Chen, F. 2008. Novel omics technologies in nutrition research. *Biotechnology Advances* 26(2):169–76.

9 Omics for Natural Products as Adjunct Nutrition

*Yeannie Hui-Yeng Yap and Shin-Yee Fung**

CONTENTS

9.1 INTRODUCTION

Omics is defined as the analysis of large amounts of data representing an entire set of molecules, such as proteins, lipids, or metabolites, in a cell, organ, or organism (American Heritage Dictionary 2007). Genomics refers to the study of a genome and the interactions of genes within the organism as well as with the environment. It includes scientific investigation into complex diseases to understand the effect of the combination of genetic and environmental factors and looks into possible treatment and diagnostic methods. DNA found in the genome, when transcribed, results in RNA, which can be analyzed to determine if genes are being turned on or off in the cells and tissues of an organism. A number of transcripts can be used to determine the amount of gene activity (gene expression) in a certain cell or tissue. Comparative studies of gene expressions may allow the understanding of the functional behaviors of cells/tissues under normal or altered circumstances. In essence, transcriptomic studies may enable researchers to generate a comprehensive knowledge of the function of the genome. Proteomics (protein level) and metabolomics (metabolic

* Corresponding author emails: syfung@um.edu.my, syfung@ummc.edu.my

DOI: 10.1201/9781003142195-9

level) are branches of genomics looking into the proteins and metabolites, which are chemical fingerprints of an organism. Both proteomics and metabolomics gain the limelight for playing significant roles in the areas of disease diagnostics, especially in giving insights into cell signaling, protein synthesis, and degradation, as well as post-translational modifications.

The subclassifications of application for genomics, transcriptomics, proteomics, and metabolomics into other fields of sciences have then led to areas of work, such as epigenomics, lipidomics, glycomics, foodomics, and nutriomics.

A revolution in the methodologies of science has brought about large-scale omics datasets. Integrative analyses of these datasets can reveal interesting information, taking into account developing methods of the techniques involved in order to understand the complexity and limitations of each dataset.

9.2 OMICS TECHNOLOGIES IN NUTRITION RESEARCH

The role of diet in health improvement has been the focus of many researchers and consumers alike in recent years. The omics platforms and various software in bioinformatics are potentially useful in shedding light on the complex relationship between nutrition and metabolism (Zhang et al. 2008). An individual's genetic makeup can contribute to differential responses to diversified dietary habits, termed as nutrigenetic effects. Different components found in food that is consumed in daily diet can also affect one's genetic expression and subsequently the distribution and bioactivity of proteins and other metabolites in the bodily system (nutritional transcriptomic, epigenomic, proteomic, and metabolomic effects, respectively) (Davis and Milner 2004).

In the last ten years or so, many studies that investigated the nutrigenetic effects of different foods/diets have been reported, describing linkages of those foods/diets with diseases. For example, the Mediterranean diet shows inverse associations with metabolic diseases, cardiovascular pathologies, and various types of cancer (Divella et al. 2020). Nutrition has also been looked into as one of the factors leading to brain disorders, including mental health problems, autism, eating disorders, Alzheimer's disease, schizophrenia, Parkinson's disease, and brain tumors (Dauncey 2013; Endreffy et al. 2016; Thaler and Steiger 2017). Diet dominated by increased intake of animal and partially hydrogenated fats and lower intakes of fiber and increased access to fast food are also linked to metabolic diseases (Allum and Grundberg 2020).

Whilst the integration of omics reveals much about the linkages with diseases and how dietary habits can cause diseases, a therapeutic outlook using food as medicine was coined. In 1989, Stephen DeFelice coined the term "nutraceutical" (Kalra 2003), which is a combination of "nutrition" and "pharmaceutical" and is defined as "a food (or part of a food) that provides medical or health benefits, including the prevention and/or treatment of a disease" (Brower 1998). Nutraceuticals not only supplement the diet but also aid in the prevention and/or treatment of disease and/or disorder (Kalra 2003). Many scientific pieces of evidence point to the use of food as an imperative to wellness and as an alternative to modern medicines. Natural products that contain many bioactive components have a good potential to be developed as nutraceuticals, and with the assistance of omics technology, many discoveries are possible by looking into the synergistic effects of these bioactive components with the genetics of the biological systems and the interaction of the components with the microenvironment within the system. These components can also form a foundation for drugs discovery in the pharmaceutical industry.

9.3 OMICS STUDIES OF NATURAL PRODUCTS

Natural products are products from living organisms and mainly comprise primary and secondary metabolites. The former comprises nucleic acids, amino acids, sugars, and fatty acids, which are required to make the respective macromolecules, including DNA, RNA, proteins, carbohydrates, and lipids that are important to sustain life. Primary metabolites are directly involved in normal growth, development, and reproduction, and thus, it has often been found in many organisms or cells. In a recent report, Zaynab et al. (2019) further highlight the startling role of primary metabolites in plant defense against pathogens.

On the other hand, secondary metabolites are compounds not essential for organism growth and/or reproduction but confer selective advantages to them. For instance, allelochemicals play a major role in plant defense against herbivores by influencing the behavior, growth, or survival of these herbivores – an inhibitory action against core biological processes. Examples of secondary metabolite classes include phenolics, alkaloids, saponins, terpenes, lipids, and carbohydrates (Hussein and El-Anssary 2018).

Various omics studies have been applied to mine the underlying compounds. Data mining via omics often comes in handy when the genome database of the investigated organisms is readily available. Herein, we will look into current research of omics studies pertaining to natural products.

9.3.1 Omics-Based Approaches: Recent Advances in Natural Products Study

Various combinations of omics approaches – that is, multi-omics and meta-analysis approaches – have been used for near-novel natural products discoveries and mining of bioactive compounds relevant to biological disease markers, treatment, and pharmacological mechanism.

9.3.1.1 Bioactive Compounds Discovery

Owing to the recent advances of omics studies, many research teams have been producing genome sequences and/or other omics datasets for a wide range of organisms with various degrees of bioactivities, including but not limited to microalgae, fungi, and plants.

Marine microorganisms such as microalgae are capable of producing secondary metabolites with beneficial biological activities, such as antipredator, allelopathic, antiproliferative, cytotoxic, anticancer, photoprotective, anti-infective, and antifouling activities due to their diversity and unique metabolic pathways with high adaptability (Lauritano et al. 2019). Therefore, research drive is high for novel bioactive metabolites exploration in marine microorganisms with potential biotechnological and biomedical applications. Leão et al. (2021) employed a multi-omics phylum-wide analysis to characterize the natural product potential of tropical filamentous marine cyanobacteria. In the study, they used the license-free antiSMASH (Blin et al. 2019) to annotate the major classes of biosynthetic gene clusters (BGCs) from 24 tropical filamentous marine cyanobacteria genome which were further networked via BiG-SCAPE (https://bigscape-corason.secondarymetabolites.org/index.html) by pairwise similarity scores between the BGCs to reveal the most promising strains for natural product discovery. Often, abundance is key to distinguishing molecules and molecular classes of interest. To do that, the team performed LCMS/MS-based metabolomics using Global Natural Products Social Molecular Networking (GNPS) (Wang et al. 2016), a multi-tool automatic annotation platform with built-in MolNetENhancer. Molecular work, including heterologous expression, isolation and structural characterization of novel natural products, and pharmacological description, was then possible for targeted secondary metabolite BGCs, such as peptides (non-ribosomal peptides [NRPs], bacteriocins, and cyanobactins), terpenes, lipids (type 1 polyketide synthase [T1PKS]) and lipopeptides (NRPS-T1PKS hybrids).

Mutually beneficial symbiotic partners, fungi comprise eukaryotic organisms that include microorganisms such as yeasts and molds, as well as the more familiar mushrooms. Mushroom proteins have been reported to possess pharmaceutical activities ranging from antifungal, antimicrobial, antiviral, antiproliferative, antimitogenic, immunomodulatory, and hypotensive effects (Chaturvedi et al. 2018). For the past decade, the Medicinal Mushroom Research Group (MMRG) from the University of Malaya has been working on the cultivar of a novel species, namely *Lignosus rhinocerus* TM02, or more commonly known by its local name tiger milk mushroom. It was first described in 1920 by mycologists Curtis Gates Lloyd and Camille Torrend and has a long history of ethnobotanical uses. The novel cultivar strain was introduced in 2009 (Tan 2009), and due to limited literature and resources available, a genome-wide sequencing analysis was performed, and this was further followed by transcriptomics and proteomics using its genome as a reference database. The genome of *L. rhinocerus* TM02 encodes a repertoire of enzymes engaged in carbohydrate and glycoconjugate metabolism, along with cytochrome P450s, putative bioactive proteins (lectins and fungal immunomodulatory proteins), laccases, and several BCGs responsible for secondary metabolite biosynthesis (Yap et al. 2014). Further transcriptomic studies revealed a plethora of highly expressed genes encoding the cysteine-rich cerato-platanin, hydrophobins, and sugar-binding lectins. Genes encoding enzymes involved in the biosynthesis of glucans, six gene clusters encoding four terpene synthases, and one each of non-ribosomal peptide synthetase and polyketide synthase were also identified (Yap, Chooi et al. 2015). The expression of some of these bioactive proteins was further confirmed by LCMS/MS-based proteomics. Total proteins from the mushroom sclerotia were extracted with Tris-buffered phenol (Yap, Fung et al. 2015). It is interesting to note that the work done is only possible with the existence of the mushroom's genome database, as earlier trials with commercially available databases did not yield desirable results. The MMRG researchers managed to link these reported bioactive proteins to their respective biopharmacological properties in later studies.

To a certain extent, investigators also mined for established bioactive proteins from natural resources, and to do this, a combination of methods utilizing an integrated omics dataset is often employed in order to achieve a more comprehensive coverage. The ribosomally synthesized and post-translationally modified peptides (RiPPs) are a highly versatile family of ribosome-originated natural products and are actively expanding. RiPP precursors have huge sequence diversity and are modifiable, thus making them excellent targets for new drugs discovery such as nisin A, lyciumin A, gymnopeptide B, and freyrasin, just to mention but a few (Berridge et al. 1952; Kersten and Weng 2018; Hudson et al. 2019). Kloosterman et al. (2021) reviewed a series of omics-based strategies for novel RiPP discovery. Various genome-mining methodologies that contribute toward the discovery of novel RiPP classes were highlighted (e.g., antiSMASH, BAGEL, RiPP-PRISM, RODEO, RiPPer, decRIPPter, and DEREPLICATOR). Some of these methods prioritize novel BGCs based on shared modifications between RiPP classes, while others identify RiPP precursors using machine-learning classifiers.

9.3.1.2 Disease-Related Biomarkers and Pharmacological Applications

Large-scale omics analysis advanced the medical research revolution where integrative tactics have been used for disease-related marker discoveries and potential treatment applications.

Traditional Chinese medicine (TCM) is tradition-based medical practice of various forms, including herbal medicine. It is often prepared as a concoction consisting of a mixture of natural products from medicinal plants, animals, and/or minerals with more than one active ingredient (Keith et al. 2005). It is believed that these ingredients work synergistically to achieve an ideal therapeutic outcome, and in fact, TCM has been associated with the treatment of various complex diseases, such as cardiovascular, infectious, metabolic, and neurodegenerative diseases (Guo et al. 2020). In order to explain the pathogenesis and medicinal mechanisms of how such multicomponent preparations work, integrated informatics and experimental pipeline via molecular approach is necessary.

For instance, Yinchenhao Tang (YCHT) is an effective formulation consisting of *Rheum palmatum* L., *Gardenia jasminoides* Ellis, and *Artemisia annua* L., which have been used for treating liver disorders. Wang et al. (2013) conducted a systematic analysis of the therapeutic effects of the active components namely 6,7-dimethylesculetin (D), geniposide (G), and rhein (R) in YCHT using immunohistochemistry, biochemistry, metabolomics (UPLC-HDMS), and proteomics (MALDI-TOF-MS/MS)–gene ontology (GO) mapping. It was found that a combination of DGR exerts the most robust therapeutic effect by hitting multiple targets in a rat model of hepatic injury. It intensified dynamic changes in metabolic biomarkers, regulates molecular networks through target proteins, has a synergistic/additive effect, and activates both intrinsic and extrinsic pathways (Wang et al. 2013). In their work, a network pharmacology approach was employed to find the connection between the active components to a network of disease pathways. This approach is getting more attention recently, and thus, the development of relevant tools is on the rise; for example, precision-modification metabolomics (PMM) and Chinmedomics (the integrative method of the serum pharmacochemistry of TCM with metabolomics to investigate the effectiveness and safety aspects of TCM) were designed for identification of drug targets and functional compounds and mechanisms of action annotation (Guo et al. 2020).

A more advanced example of network pharmacology study can be seen in a more recent investigation by Zhang, Chao et al. (2021) on Guchang Zhixie Wan (GZW). As with other TCM, GZW is also a multi-compound herb preparation used for the treatment of ulcerative colitis (UC). The group retrieved the active ingredients, potential targets, and UC-related genes of GZW from available public databases, such as Traditional Chinese Medicine Database at Taiwan (http://tcm.cmu.edu.tw/zh-tw/) (Chen et al. 2014), Traditional Chinese Medicine Systems Pharmacology (TCMSP) database (http://lsp.nwu.edu.cn/tcmsp.php) (Ru et al. 2014), and Bioinformatics Analysis Tool for Molecular Mechanism of Traditional Chinese Medicine (BATMAN-TCM) (http://bionet.ncpsb.org/batman-tcm/) (Liu et al. 2016). Bioinformatics analysis was then employed to determine the pharmacological mechanisms of GZW by first key components analysis, followed by potential targeting and signaling pathway mapping. Their analysis revealed that GZW consists of 26 active compounds (quercetin, kaempferol, and β-sitosterol among them), which can be related to 148 potential target proteins associated with UC. Further, GO and KEGG enrichment analysis showed that these target proteins (e.g., IFNG, IL-1A, IL-1B, JUN, RELA, and STAT1) are highly enriched in inflammatory, immune, and oxidative-stress-related pathways. Verification of the findings was further done by virtual molecular docking and cell experiments in which it is indicated that the protective effects of GZW on the inflammatory bowel disease pathway were through the STAT3/NF-κB/IL-6 pathway (Zhang, Chao et al. 2021).

To date, public databases have been shown to be advantageous for network pharmacology for molecular mechanism exploration. A study by Wang and team used KEGG to determine the potential molecular mechanism of the key genes regulated by *Carthamus tinctorius* L. (safflower) and *Salvia miltiorrhiza* Burge (salvia) for the treatment of cardio-cerebrovascular disease (Wang et al. 2020). These plant products have been found to consist of a wide range of secondary metabolites of lipophilic and hydrophilic nature, which are important for circulation improvement and blood stasis prevention (Su et al. 2015; Pang et al. 2016). The methodology and pipeline adapted by the team are almost similar to Zhang, Chao et al. (2021), where firstly, compounds and targets for *C. tinctorius* and *S. miltiorrhiza* were retrieved from TCMSP, and the known therapeutic targets for myocardial infarction (MI) and cerebral infarction (CI) were from DrugBank (www.drugbank.ca/), TTD (https://db.idrblab.org/ttd/), and DisGeNET (www.disgenet.org/) databases. A disease-target-drug network analysis was then established using Cytoscape software (https://cytoscape.org/), and databases from Kyoto Encyclopedia of Genes and Genomes (KEGG; www.genome.jp/kegg/) and Gene Ontology (Ashburner et al. 2000; Gene Ontology Consortium 2020) were used for functional characterization. Verification of findings was conducted in rat middle cerebral artery occlusion model, and a total of 247 genes targeted by 52 compounds from *C. tinctorius* and 119 genes targeted by 48 compounds from *S. miltiorrhiza* with 23 common targets between the plants' active compounds and MI and CI were reported (Wang et al. 2020).

There is always an important aspect of investigation when it comes to natural products analysis for treatment potential, especially their biopharmacological effects upon prescription. Gonulalan and team used metabolomic and proteomic strategies in addition to correlation analyses to find the relation between brain-derived neurotrophic factor (BDNF) activity and the metabolomic and proteomic profiles of several plant extracts (*Valeriana officinalis* L., *Melissa officinalis* L., *Hypericum perforatum* L., and *Passiflora incarnata* L.) used in sedative anxiolytic and sleep disorders. Among the investigated plants, *M. officinalis* exhibited the most significant increase of BDNF expression in SH-SY5Y cells with dysregulation of 117 metabolites and 30 proteins.

Some of the primary metabolites are from the Krebs cycle, while secondary metabolites are mainly flavonoids, xanthones, coumarins, tannins, naphthalenes, terpenoids, and carotenoids. Some of the proteins identified were from the cytochrome P450 family (Gonulalan et al. 2020). This study demonstrated that metabolomic and proteomic studies based on MS have high sensitivity and thus allow multiple components detection even at very low concentrations.

9.4 COMPARATIVE OMICS IN FOOD RESEARCH

Nutriomics is a branch of food sciences and nutritional studies that aims for consumers' well-being and health improvement. Innovative solutions through omics (e.g., genetics and molecular approaches) were employed to improve plant nutrient efficiency and crop productivity in the mode of comparison to gauge the supremacy of one over another. This section summarizes current efforts and progress in comparative nutriomic research from several research studies.

Fruit, vegetables, and legumes are nutrient-rich foods that provide minerals, vitamins, fiber, and secondary metabolites, such as polyphenols, flavonoids, and carotenoids. There are ongoing debates relating to food quality of wild-type (natural) versus cultivated strains (including genetically modified organisms [GMOs]) where advances in nutrition science can aid in the comparative work of food quality via omics approaches.

For example, watermelons belong to the Cucurbitaceae family along with cantaloupe, honeydew, and cucumber, which have been known to provide hydration and are good sources of essential nutrients, including vitamins, minerals, and antioxidants (Edwards et al. 2003). The nutritional compositions vary with genotype and environment. Yuan et al. (2021) investigated the metabolomic profile of the fruit flesh of wild and cultivated watermelons (*Citrullus* sp.) via LC-MS, and the MWDB database from Wuhan Metware Biotechnology Co., Ltd. was used for metabolite identification. Several secondary metabolites were found to diverge among the compared species (e.g., the apigenin 6-C-glucoside, luteolin 6-C-glucoside, chrysoeriol C-hexoside, naringenin C-hexoside, C-pentosyl-chrysoeriol O-hexoside, and sucrose). In particular, flavonoids – which are important for plant growth but have bad taste – are highly associated with the divergence. The group further inferred that the *C. lanatus* edible-seed watermelon (cultivar) had the closest relation to *C. mucosospermus* (wild) due to comparable metabolic profiles and phenotypic traits. Thus, this suggests that the edible-seed watermelon may be a relative of wild species and a relatively primitive differentiation type of cultivated watermelon (Yuan et al.

2021). The findings from this study provide a deeper understanding of the evolution of domestication and breeding history of watermelon.

Terfeziaceae, or more commonly known as desert truffles, are local to Kuwait and some other Mediterranean regions. They belong to the hypogeous fungi kingdom, although they have a resemblance to potatoes. Farag et al. (2021) compared the metabolome of desert truffles *Terfezia claveryi* and *Terfezia boudieri* based on their aroma and nutrients profile using GC-MS coupled with headspace solid-phase microextraction (HS-SPME), where the latter was used to reveal the distinct aroma of the truffles. The truffles were found to contain sugars, sugar alcohols, and amino acids as primary metabolites with nutrition benefits, while a total of 106 volatiles were annotated belonging to alcohols, ketones, aldehydes, esters, ethers, and furans. The team conducted a multivariate analysis (MVA) and found that 1-octen-3-ol and 3-octanone were among the significant discriminators between *T. claveryi* and *T. boudieri*. Further, *T. claveryi* also has more essential amino acid content and a better sugar diet composition as compared to *T. boudieri* (Farag et al. 2021).

Milk, a natural product from humans or any other living organism, has also been analyzed using omics methodologies. It is well understood that breastfeeding is recommended for babies from birth (World Health Organization 2021). However, on certain occasions where breastfeeding and/or breast milk consumption is not possible, infant formula is used. Infant/baby formula is designed and marketed for up to 12 months of age, and it is industrially produced to mimic the nutritional composition of breast milk. In Zhang, Liu et al. (2021) study, a comparison of the lipidome and fatty acid composition between breast milk and infant formula of animal and/or plant origin was made. UHPLC-Q-TOF-MS analysis using positive and negative ionization modes revealed 48 and 71 common lipid species, respectively. The group further reported that the triacylglycerol-rich breast milk contains linoleic acid, α-linolenic acid, arachidonic acid, and docosahexaenoic acid. Its sphingomyelin content is comparable to plant-based infant formula. Univariate and MVA discovered 37, 34, 31, and 36 lipid species as key discriminators between breast milk and infant formula, which will be useful in designing new milk formulas that more closely resemble breast milk (Zhang, Liu et al. 2021).

9.5 POSSIBLE FUTURE APPLICATION OF OMICS DATA

To date, there is no single platform to integrate the large datasets from the various omics methodologies. Each model organism (test/control) used in the various reported studies poses different challenges in the analysis due to the uniqueness of metabolite abundance, gene expression, epigenetic regulation, and cell-type specificity of a given omics dataset (Misra et al. 2019). It is beyond doubt that despite the advancement of omics technology, the integration of these data can be tedious.

The future for the application of omics in nutrition may be one that includes personalized nutrition, which is formulated based on a systems biology approach – that is, to measure, model, and predict biological responses based on individual genetics and individualistic responses to nutritional modulations (Zhang et al. 2008).

ACKNOWLEDGMENTS

We thank the Fundamental Research Grant (FRGS/1/2019/SKK08/MAHSA/03/1) for its support.

REFERENCES

Allum, F., and Grundberg, E. 2020. Capturing functional epigenomes for insight into metabolic diseases. *Molecular Metabolism* 38:100936.

American Heritage Dictionary. 2007. *The American Heritage Medical Dictionary*, 909. Houghton Mifflin Company, MA, Harper reference; Updated edition (March 1, 2007).

Ashburner, M., Ball, C. A., Blake, J. A., et al. 2000. Gene ontology: Tool for the unification of biology. The gene ontology consortium. *Nature Genetics* 25(1):25–9.

Berridge, N. J., Newton, G. G. F., and Abraham, E. P. 1952. Purification and nature of the antibiotic nisin. *The Biochemical Journal* 52(4):529–35.

Blin, K., Shaw, S., Steinke, K., et al. 2019. antiSMASH 5.0: Updates to the secondary metabolite genome mining pipeline. *Nucleic Acids Research* 47(W1):W81–W7.

Brower, V. 1998. Nutraceuticals: Poised for a healthy slice of the healthcare market? *Nature Biotechnology* 16(8):728–31.

Chaturvedi, V. K., Agarwal, S., Gupta, K. K., Ramteke, P. W., and Singh, M. P. 2018. Medicinal mushroom: Boon for therapeutic applications. *3 Biotech* 8(8):334.

Chen, F. P., Chang, C. M., Hwang, S. J., Chen, Y. C., and Chen, F. J. 2014. Chinese herbal prescriptions for osteoarthritis in Taiwan: Analysis of national health insurance dataset. *BMC Complementary and Alternative Medicine* 14:91.

Dauncey, M. J. 2013. Genomic and epigenomic insights into nutrition and brain disorders. *Nutrients* 5(3):887–914.

Davis, C. D., and Milner, J. 2004. Frontiers in nutrigenomics, proteomics, metabolomics and cancer prevention. *Mutation Research* 551(1–2):51–64.

Divella, R., Daniele, A., Savino, E., and Paradiso, A. 2020. Anticancer effects of nutraceuticals in the mediterranean diet: An epigenetic diet model. *Cancer Genomics and Proteomics* 17(4):335–50.

Edwards, A. J., Vinyard, B. T., Wiley, E. R., et al. 2003. Consumption of watermelon juice increases plasma concentrations of lycopene and β-carotene in humans. *Journal of Nutrition* 133(4):1043–50.

Endreffy, I., Bjørklund, G., Dicső, F., Urbina, M. A., and Endreffy, E. 2016. Acid glycosaminoglycan (aGAG) excretion is increased in children with autism spectrum disorder, and it can be controlled by diet. *Metabolic Brain Disease* 31(2):273–8.

Farag, M. A., Fathi, D., Shamma, S., et al. 2021. Comparative metabolome classification of desert truffles *Terfezia claveryi* and *Terfezia boudieri* via its aroma and nutrients profile. *LWT – Food Science and Technology* 142:111046.

Gene Ontology Consortium. 2020. The Gene Ontology resource: Enriching a GOld mine. *Nucleic Acids Research* 49(D1):D325–34.

Gonulalan, E. M., Nemutlu, E., Bayazeid, O., Koçak, E., Yalçın, F. N., and Demirezer, L. O. 2020. Metabolomics and proteomics profiles of some medicinal plants and correlation with BDNF activity. *Phytomedicine* 74:152920.

Guo, R., Luo, X., Liu, J., Liu, L., Wang, X., and Lu, H. 2020. Omics strategies decipher therapeutic discoveries of traditional Chinese medicine against different diseases at multiple layers molecular-level. *Pharmacological Research* 152:104627.

Hudson, G. A., Burkhart, B. J., DiCaprio, A. J., et al. 2019. Bioinformatic mapping of radical S-adenosylmethionine-dependent ribosomally synthesized and post-translationally modified peptides identifies new Cα, Cβ, and Cγ-linked thioether-containing peptides. *Journal of the American Chemical Society* 141(20):8228–38.

Hussein, R. A., and El-Anssary, A. A. 2018. Plants secondary metabolites: The key drivers of the pharmacological actions of medicinal plants. In: *Herbal Medicine*, ed. P. F. Builders. IntechOpen, London.

Kalra, E. K. 2003. Nutraceutical – definition and introduction. *AAPS Pharm Science* 5(3):E25.

Keith, C. T., Borisy, A. A., and Stockwell, B. R. 2005. Multicomponent therapeutics for networked systems. *Nature Reviews Drug Discovery* 4(1):71–8.

Kersten, R. D., and Weng, J. K. 2018. Gene-guided discovery and engineering of branched cyclic peptides in plants. *Proceedings of the National Academy of Sciences of the United States of America* 115(46):E10961–9.

Kloosterman, A. M., Medema, M. H., and van Wezel, G. P. 2021. Omics-based strategies to discover novel classes of RiPP natural products. *Current Opinion in Biotechnology* 69:60–7.

Lauritano, C., Ferrante, M. I., and Rogato, A. 2019. Marine natural products from microalgae: An omics overview. *Marine Drugs* 17(5):269.

Leão, T., Wang, M., Moss, N., et al. 2021. A multi-omics characterization of the natural product potential of tropical filamentous marine cyanobacteria. *Marine Drugs* 19(1):20.

Liu, Z., Guo, F., Wang, Y., et al. 2016. BATMAN-TCM: A bioinformatics analysis tool for molecular mechanism of traditional chinese medicine. *Scientific Reports* 6:21146.

Misra, B. B., Langefeld, C., Olivier, M., and Cox, L. A. 2019. Integrated omics: Tools, advances and future approaches. *Journal of Molecular Endocrinology* 62:R21.

Pang, H., Wu, L., Tang, Y., Zhou, G., Qu, C., and Duan, J. A. 2016. Chemical analysis of the herbal medicine *Salviae miltiorrhizae* Radix et Rhizoma (Danshen). *Molecules* 21(1):51.

Ru, J., Li, P., Wang, J., et al. 2014. TCMSP: A database of systems pharmacology for drug discovery from herbal medicines. *Journal of Cheminformatics* 6:13.

Su, C. Y., Ming, Q. L., Rahman, K., Han, T., and Qin, L. P. 2015. *Salvia miltiorrhiza*: Traditional medicinal uses, chemistry, and pharmacology. *Chinese Journal of Natural Medicines* 13(3):163–82.

Tan, C. S. 2009. Setting-up pilot-plant for up-scaling production of "Tiger-Milk"-mushroom as dietary functional food. Technical Report MOA TF0109M004, Government of Malaysia.

Thaler, L., and Steiger, H. 2017. Eating disorders and epigenetics. In *Neuroepigenomics in Aging and Disease*, ed. R. Delgado-Morales, 93–103. Springer International Publishing, Cham, Switzerland.

Wang, M., Carver, J. J., Phelan, V. V., et al. 2016. Sharing and community curation of mass spectrometry data with global natural products social molecular networking. *Nature Biotechnology* 34(8):828–37.

Wang, X., Zhang, A., Wang, P., et al. 2013. Metabolomics coupled with proteomics advancing drug discovery toward more agile development of targeted combination therapies. *Molecular and Cellular Proteomics* 12(5):1226–38.

Wang, Y., Shi, Y., Zou, J., et al. 2020. Network pharmacology exploration reveals a common mechanism in the treatment of cardio-cerebrovascular disease with *Salvia miltiorrhiza* Burge. and *Carthamus tinctorius* L. *BMC Complementary Medicine and Therapies* 20(1):351.

World Health Organization. 2021. Breastfeeding. Available from: www.who.int/health-topics/breastfeeding#tab=tab_1.

Yap, H. Y. Y., Chooi, Y. H., Firdaus-Raih, M., et al. 2014. The genome of the Tiger Milk mushroom, *Lignosus rhinocerotis*, provides insights into the genetic basis of its medicinal properties. *BMC Genomics* 15(1):635.

Yap, H. Y. Y., Chooi, Y. H., Fung, S. Y., Ng, S. T., Tan, C. S., and Tan, N. H. 2015. Transcriptome analysis revealed highly expressed genes encoding secondary metabolite pathways and small cysteine-rich proteins in the sclerotium of *Lignosus rhinocerotis*. *PLoS One* 10(11):e0143549.

Yap, H. Y. Y., Fung, S. Y., Ng, S. T., Tan, C. S., and Tan, N. H. 2015. Genome-based proteomic analysis of *Lignosus rhinocerotis* (Cooke) Ryvarden sclerotium. *International Journal of Medical Sciences* 12(1):23–31.

Yuan, P., He, N., Umer, M. J., et al. 2021. Comparative metabolomic profiling of *Citrullus* spp. fruits provides evidence for metabolomic divergence during domestication. *Metabolites* 11(2):78.

Zaynab, M., Fatima, M., Sharif, Y., Zafar, M. H., Ali, H., and Khan, K. A. 2019. Role of primary metabolites in plant defense against pathogens. *Microbial Pathogenesis* 137:103728.

Zhang, W., Chao, X., Wu, J. Q., et al. 2021. Exploring the potential mechanism of Guchang Zhixie Wan for treating ulcerative colitis by comprehensive network pharmacological approaches and molecular docking validation as well as cell experiments. *Chemistry and Biodiversity* 18(1):e2000810.

Zhang, X., Liu, L., Wang, L., et al. 2021. Comparative lipidomics analysis of human milk and infant formulas using UHPLC-Q-TOF-MS. *Journal of Agricultural and Food Chemistry* 69(3):1146–55.

Zhang, X., Yap, Y., Wei, D., Chen, G., and Chen, F. 2008. Novel omics technologies in nutrition research. *Biotechnology Advances* 26(2):169–76.

10 Nutrigenomics, Olive Polyphenols, and Human Health

Maria Antónia da Mota Nunes, Maria Beatriz Prior Pinto Oliveira, and Rita Carneiro Alves*

CONTENTS

10.1 INTRODUCTION

The dynamic interaction between humans and the environment occurs at several levels, from immediate and short-term responses to the environment to long-term ones, such as natural selection through gene modifications (Raubenheimer and Simpson 2016).

Diet is a critical environmental factor since individuals are exposed to dietary components, able to modulate genes expression (Peña-Romero et al. 2018). In addition, foods are composed of several nutrients, bioactive compounds, and sometimes

* Corresponding author email: antonianunes.maria@gmail.com

DOI: 10.1201/9781003142195-10

anti-nutrients and toxins, involved in a matrix, and each compound has different bioactions and targets. Currently, most of the consumed products come from a process that comprises collecting, packaging, and distribution or increasingly often come from extensive processing, leading to a profound modification of the initial nutritional profile (Raubenheimer and Simpson 2016).

For good maintenance of human health, nutrients are required at a particular level, which changes according to age, physical activity, diseases, and reproductive state. However, general recommendations comprise macro- and micronutrients but not compounds such as polyphenols, known for their role in diseases prevention (Durazzo et al. 2019). Finally, the intestinal microbiota differs among individuals and changes during the life cycle and is strongly related to the host and diet (Ferguson et al. 2016).

Regarding the olive fruit, the quantity and type of polyphenols may be dependent on the olive cultivar, edaphoclimatic conditions, agricultural practices, and maturation degree. Moreover, olive processing can likewise modify the profile and amount of compounds of the final products obtained. For example, the extraction process used to produce olive oil can influence the polyphenols profile of the virgin olive oil obtained (Klen and Vodopivec 2012).

Virgin olive oil is considered a simple, pressed, and cold-treated juice, as olives are only milled, and the obtained paste is mixed and centrifuged. Despite not being used in any technological adjuvant or biological, chemical, or thermal processing, the olive's bioactive compounds suffer natural modifications and partition during processing. Therefore, olive oil polyphenols include those initially present in the drupe and others that are newly formed by enzymatic and chemical reactions (Klen et al. 2015). Moreover, polyphenols fractioning between the olive oil and the by-products generated occurs. Most of the polyphenols are retained in the olive pomace or extracted with the olive mill wastewaters (~98%), and only a lower amount is transferred (1–2%) to olive oil (Rodis et al. 2002).

Therefore, olive products and by-products have been largely explored as sources of polyphenols that impact human health. Moreover, their potential as food products/ingredients, food supplements, and nutraceuticals have been increasingly recognized (Gorzynik-Debicka et al. 2018; Rodríguez-López et al. 2020). Nutrition sciences have arisen over the last years and successfully treated, and even made disappear, some diseases associated with micronutrient deficiencies, such as scurvy, beriberi, and rickets. In spite of that evolutive impact on public health, some chronic diseases present high prevalence and are still increasing despite all the health public measures and recommendations. Obesity and cancer are some examples. As we look at non-communicable chronic diseases, it is even more relevant to contextualize each person's environment and genetic background. Thus, the role of the biology-environment interface for humans is complex and currently a great challenge (Raubenheimer and Simpson 2016).

Hydroxytyrosol, tyrosol, and oleuropein are phenolic compounds almost exclusively from olives, being rare to find them in other plants. Consequently, olive products and by-products are also sources of those polyphenols with human health benefits.

This chapter presents a comprehensive overview of the polyphenols of the olive fruit and their derived products and by-products, focusing on their classic uses in human nutrition as foods (olive oil, olive leaves, and table olives) and upcycled by-products (olive mill wastewaters and olive pomace). The analysis of the interaction gene-olive polyphenols will explore how these products can lead to known health outcomes under the focus of nutrigenomics.

10.2 OLIVE POLYPHENOLS: CLASSIFICATION AND BIOACTIVITY

Polyphenols are secondary plant metabolites with strong antioxidant activity. They are widely distributed in nature in vegetables, fruits, nuts, seeds, roots, bark, plant leaves, herbs, and whole-grain products. More than 8,000 phenolics were identified with a variable chemical structure. They are the response of plants to pests, bacterial infections, and environmental stressors and are involved in the growth, lignification, pollination, and pigmentation processes (Fraga et al. 2010; Gorzynik-Debicka et al. 2018). Phenolics present an aromatic ring linked to one hydroxyl group, whereas polyphenols are characterized by having at minimum two phenyl rings and one or more hydroxyl groups. In fact, "polyphenols" is a collective denomination for numerous subgroups of compounds that should be strict to the structures presenting at least two phenolic moieties. Nevertheless, the denominations "phenolic" and "polyphenol" are often found in scientific literature as a similar designation for the same compound (Durazzo et al. 2019). In this chapter, the term "polyphenol" will be recurrent throughout the text. Also, the classification of polyphenols in different groups is controversial. A more straightforward classification divides polyphenols into flavonoids and non-flavonoid polyphenols (Durazzo et al. 2019). Other often-used classifications group polyphenols with phenolic acids (hydroxycinnamic and hydroxybenzoic acids) and flavonoids (isoflavones, flavanones, flavanols, flavones, anthocyanins), curcuminoids, lignans, and stilbenes (Milenkovic et al. 2013). Oxidation is a naturally occurring process in the human body, which originates reactive oxygen species (ROS), reactive sulfur species (RSS), and reactive nitrogen species (RNS), as superoxide, hydrogen peroxide, singlet oxygen, and nitric oxide (NO) radicals. In physiological conditions, the endogenous antioxidant system, which includes enzymatic (catalase, glutathione peroxidase, and superoxide dismutase) and non-enzymatic compounds (bilirubin and albumin), can scavenge radicals and maintain homeostasis (Santos-Sánchez et al. 2019). However, when the antioxidant enzyme system cannot efficiently eliminate radical overproduction, oxidative stress occurs, leading to chronic and degenerative diseases (Ji et al. 2020). In this case, dietary sources are crucial to providing sufficient antioxidant compounds, such as polyphenols, to complement the endogenous system.

The accumulation of reactive species in the body is deleterious and can lead to pathologies as cardiovascular diseases and cancer. Superoxide is one of the most reactive radical species. It contains at least one unpaired electron and is generated by the one-electron reduction of oxygen by transition metals, reducing radicals, or UV radiation. Superoxide is produced by endogenous biological sources purposely or as an outcome of metabolic processes in mitochondria, multiprotein complexes (e.g., nicotinamide adenine dinucleotide phosphate [NADPH] oxidases) or enzymes (e.g., xanthine oxidase) (Winterbourn 2020). Autoxidation reactions are also responsible for superoxide generation. For example, hemoglobin (Hb) in erythrocytes constantly undergoes autoxidation, leading to a considerable presence of superoxide in these cells (Nishida et al. 2016). Indeed, aerobic human conditions demand oxygen to maintain cell metabolism and life. Partially oxidized intermediates, like ROS, are formed and present high reactivity (Santos-Sánchez et al. 2019). Superoxide is, hence, the result of physiological functions (Winterbourn 2020). ROS and RSS are chemically similar. RSS, produced from sequential one-electron oxidations, are described as even more reactive than ROS and have been mainly studied lately (Kolluru et al. 2020; Olson 2020). RSS can result from the oxidation of sulfite or sulfate molecules or a by-product of major thiols and can damage cellular components (Bora et al. 2018). NO is the most active radical of the RNS resultant from L-arginine through the NO synthase enzyme. Other RNS are nitrogen dioxide, nitrosoperoxycarbonate, nitronium ions, peroxynitrite, peroxynitrous acid, and dinitrogen trioxide. NO at physiological levels contributes to the blood vessels' smooth muscle relaxation (Santos-Sánchez et al. 2019). Excessive free radicals can act as biological oxidants and deleteriously by damaging cells. When the human body's response is not sufficient to oxidative stress, several pathophysiological processes are triggered. Among them, cell aging, inflammation, atherosclerosis, mutagenesis, and cancer are prevalent (Santos-Sánchez et al. 2019).

However, not only physiological conditions are linked to the generation of radicals. Current lifestyle habits, pollution, and stress can contribute increasingly to radical production. Therefore, it is important to reinforce the natural endogenous antioxidant system with exogenous antioxidants such as carotenoids vitamin C, minerals (selenium and zinc), and polyphenols. Because of their chemical structure, polyphenols act as antioxidants by reactive-free radicals scavenging and metal sequestration activities (Santos-Sánchez et al. 2019). The interactions of polyphenols with membrane components as lipids and proteins can also mediate some biological effects by modifying the plasma membrane structure and the electrical and fluidity properties resulting in occurrences, such as enzyme activity, interactions between ligand and receptor, ion and/or metabolite fluxes, and modulation of signal transduction. Hence, polyphenols also provide antioxidant protection through mechanisms besides free radical scavenging or metal-chelating activities (Fraga et al. 2010).

10.2.1 Olive Fruit, Virgin Olive Oil, and Table Olives

The olive tree is an evergreen tree belonging to the family Oleaceae (*Olea europaea* L.), and its fruit is the olive. The fruit is classified as a drupe. It is a fleshy fruit with a central stone containing the seed. Compared to other drupes, olive contains less sugar and presents a high quantity of oil, varying between 3 and 38%, depending on cultivar, agricultural practices, and maturity. Olive is constituted by the skin (epicarp), the pulp (mesocarp), and the stone wall around the kernel (endocarp) (Charoenprasert and Mitchell 2012). Olive oil and table olives are the main products of olive processing. These are great sources of simple phenolics, such as phenolic acids and phenolic alcohols (hydroxytyrosol and tyrosol), lignans, secoiridoids, and flavonoids (Ghanbari et al. 2012). Olive polyphenols are usually more distributed in the skin and around the seed structure (Charoenprasert and Mitchell 2012). Olive polyphenols are chemically varied, but most of them can present hydrophilicity due to sugar moieties and multiple hydroxylation sites, making them move and remain in by-products as olive pomace (with a high-water content) and olive mill wastewaters (Charoenprasert and Mitchell 2012). Olive oil processing is mainly composed of three sequential steps: crushing or milling, malaxing, and centrifugation. Throughout the process, physical and chemical events lead to modifications on the quantitative and qualitative polyphenols profiles. The crushing step decreases polyphenols' initial amount by 46%, reinforcing crushing as a critical step in all processes. Industrial-scale assays already reported a loss of half of the polyphenols (Klen and Vodopivec 2012). The modifications observed result from the exposure of the pulpous material and from malaxation, the mechanical mixing of the olive paste. Hence, during both processes (crushing and malaxation), chemical, enzymatic, and non-enzymatic hydrolyses and oxidation occurs (Parenti et al. 2008), leading to the compound's differences found in olives and virgin olive oil. Crushing enhances the presence of simple phenols and benzoic acids, whereas lignans are not affected by the milling process. Other compounds decrease or even disappear during this step due to transformation events, and others increase by liberation and formation of new derivatives. The most affected compounds are secoiridoids, such as oleuropein, demethyloleuropein, and ligstroside, converted first into their respective aglycones (oleuropein or ligstroside aglycones) and then to their decarboxymethylated forms (hydroxytyrosol or tyrosol). Hydroxytyrosol and tyrosol increase significantly during this step, mostly due to endogenous esterases cleavage of the ester bond. Also, glucosidases can be responsible for releasing the fruit hydroxytyrosol glucoside and/or verbascoside, and tyrosol could be obtained from nüzhenide and esters. Crushing can impact most polyphenols. However, it is reported that a small fraction of those compounds do not suffer any transformation, as is the case of comselogoside, caffeoyl-6′-secologanoside, and luteolin-3′-O-glucoside, meaning that these compounds present some type of technological resistance. During malaxation, the components present the same quantitative and qualitative behavior observed in the crushing phase, suggesting a balance between the degradation and formation of polyphenols. Therefore, the phase where the losses are more significant is crushing rather than malaxation. Compounds with particular relevance for health, such as hydroxytyrosol, increase during both olive oil processing stages (Klen and Vodopivec 2012). In the Klen and colleague study (2012), only ~0.5% of the olive polyphenols ended up in the olive oil at the end of the olive processing. In this way, it is possible to recognize that along with olive oil, the by-products generated are also a great source of polyphenols.

On the other hand, it is not possible to consume olives as raw fruit due to their astringent flavor attributed to oleuropein, and they should be processed into table olives to be organoleptically acceptable. The most common methods to process table olives are salt curing and alkaline hydrolysis resulting in oleuropein-derived compounds such as hydroxytyrosol (Charoenprasert and Mitchell 2012).

Table olives are highly appreciated and part of the Mediterranean diet. Olive-debittering methods are the primary factor that affects the olives' polyphenols content. The major phenolic found in raw olives is the secoiridoid oleuropein, which confers bitterness to raw olives. The fruits' processing allows the reduction of the oleuropein levels and increases hydroxytyrosol and tyrosol contents (Charoenprasert and Mitchell 2012).

There are three predominant types of olive-processing methods to obtain table olives: California-style black ripe, Spanish-style green, and Greek-style naturally black olives. All methods have a common purpose, debittering olives, but lead to different final amounts of phenolics. Usually, the California-style-processed olives present the lowest amount of polyphenols, especially hydroxytyrosol, compared to the other two methods (Charoenprasert and Mitchell 2012). Also, the profile is distinct. For example, in the Spanish processing method, the major compound identified is hydroxytyrosol, followed by tyrosol, vanillic acid, and oleoside-11-methyl ester. In the Greek-processed olives, it was possible to find hydroxytyrosol, tyrosol, oleoside-11-methyl ester, vanillic acid, oleuropein, and 3,4-dihydroxyphenylglycol (Charoenprasert and Mitchell 2012).

Table olives are considered part of a healthy pattern as the Mediterranean diet contributes with large amounts of phenolics, namely hydroxytyrosol and monounsaturated fatty acids, both protective against chronic diseases.

After olive oil obtention, the olive pomace is transported to other industries, the olive pomace oil extractors, which use organic solvents (*n*-hexane) to remove the remaining oil. The olive pomace oil corresponds to crude oil. To eliminate the compounds responsible for undesirable flavors and colors, the oil is refined, which significantly reduces the content of polyphenols. Then, the refined oil is blended with virgin olive oil, being commercialized as olive pomace oil (Mateos et al. 2020). As it is mixed with virgin olive oil, the polyphenols found are mainly those characteristic of olive oil, which were previously described.

10.2.2 Olive By-Products: Leaves, Pomace, and Olive Mill Wastewaters

The main factors that affect the olive polyphenols content are variety, ripening stage, agricultural practices, and edaphoclimatic conditions. These have an impact on the olive fruit but also on the olive oil and, subsequently, on the by-products (Covas et al. 2009).

The major source of olive leaves is tree pruning. Nevertheless, they are also separated in olive mills from the fruits and represent ~10% of the weight of the delivered products in olive mills. Olive leaves, prepared for consumption as infusion or decoction, have been used for a long time as preventive or the treatment of several diseases by folk medicine (Roselló-Soto et al. 2015; Acar-Tek and Ağagündüz 2020).

The phenolics found in olives are also present in the leaves. Oleuropein is the major compound described. Other reported phenolics are demethyloleuropein, oleuropein diglucoside, verbascoside, ligstroside, hydroxytyrosol glucoside, hydroxytyrosol, tyrosol glucoside, tyrosol, oleoside-11-methyl ester, oleuroside, nuzhenide, caffeic acid, chlorogenic acid, p-coumaric, vanillic acid, and homovanillic. Moreover, the following flavonoids have been also reported: apigenin-7-glucoside, apigenin-7-rutinoside, luteolin-4-glucoside, luteolin-7-rutinoside, luteolin-7-glucoside, luteolin, diosmetin, quercetin, hesperidin, and rutin (Charoenprasert and Mitchell 2012).

The health effects described for leaves are mainly associated with their content in oleuropein. Substantial health-promoting properties have been reported (e.g., antioxidant, hypotensive, cardioprotective, anti-inflammatory, stimulant of the immune system, anti-inflammatory, antiarrhythmic). Also, antihyperglycemic and lipid-regulating effects were reported (Acar-Tek and Ağagündüz 2020).

Most olive oil is currently extracted using a two- or three-phase system. The two-phase system generates a waste called wet olive pomace, or *alperujo*, whereas, in the three-phase system, it generates a pomace with a very low amount of water and olive mill wastewaters (Višnjevec et al. 2021).

Wet olive pomace is a heterogenous biomass composed of olive skin, pulp, stone, and kernel. It contains residual oil and a high-water content that can attain 70%. The pomace is rich in water-soluble (e.g., hydroxytyrosol, tyrosol, and comsegoloside) and liposoluble (e.g., tocopherols and oleic acid) bioactive compounds (Nunes et al. 2018). Other functional compounds have been reported as dietary fiber, sterols and hydrocarbons, β-carotene, and minerals (Difonzo et al. 2021). Nevertheless, polyphenols are the main bioactive compounds present in wet olive pomace. Several studies explored the profile and amount of polyphenols. The main polyphenols in olive pomace identified are hydroxytyrosol, hydroxytyrosol glucoside, hydroxytyrosol diglucoside, hydroxytyrosol rhamnoside, tyrosol, tyrosol glucoside, loganin, loganin glucoside, loganic acid, loganic acid glucoside, 7-deoxyloganic acid, secologanic acid, secologanoside, secologanin, eleanolic acid, oleosid, oleosid glucoside, oleosid diglucoside, oleoside riboside, oleoside-11-methylester, oleoside dimethylester, shikimic acid, phenylalanine, cinnamic acid, ρ-coumaric acid, caffeic acid, protocatechuic acid, vanillic acid, ferulic acid, gallic acid, pinoresinol, hydroxypinoresinol, acetoxypinoresinol, rutin, apigenin, luteolin, apigenin glucoside, luteolin glucoside, taxifolin, diosmetin, quercetin, oleuropein, 10-hydroxy-oleuropein, oleuropein aglycone, and verbascoside and oleuropein derivatives (Peralbo-Molina et al. 2012; Olmo-García et al. 2018).

Different amounts of polyphenols and profiles can be found in pomaces accordingly to the process used (two-phase versus three-phase). These compounds were found in higher levels in the two-phase pomace when compared with the three-phase one. In the latter, a dilution factor must be considered since it is added variable amounts of water in this process. Additionally, differences in the secoiridoid group occur. The pomace from the two-phase process presented a higher amount (~2,000 mg/kg, dry weight), while the three-phase pomace had ~1,300 mg/kg (dry weight). Vanillin followed the same tendency with significant differences between the two- and the three-phase system (43 and 6 mg/kg dry weight, respectively). No differences were found on flavonoid, cinnamic acid, and simple phenolic compound contents. Hence, the two most common and used technological processing methods can also affect the bioactive compounds profile of the by-products (Višnjevec et al. 2021).

The olive mill wastewaters derived from the three-phase system is a mixture of lipids, sugars, pectin minerals, tannins, and polyphenols. It is particularly rich in hydroxytyrosol and potassium. Due to its composition, the olive mill wastewaters are considered phytotoxic and an environmental burden (Bellumori et al. 2018).

The water-saving and ecological two-phase olive-oil-processing system has been progressively replacing the three-phase system (Višnjevec et al. 2021).

10.3 BIOAVAILABILITY OF OLIVE POLYPHENOLS

Health benefits associated with polyphenols are strongly influenced by bioavailability in the gastrointestinal and circulatory systems. The amount of a compound ingested, digested, and absorbed into the systemic circulation is related to bioavailability. Overall, bioavailability refers to the ingested fraction that attains organs and tissues and participates in the essential metabolic processes. Bioaccessibility comprises the digestive biotransformations, the absorption into the intestinal epithelium cells, presystemic intestinal and hepatic metabolism, followed by tissue distribution and bioaction. Absorption and transformation together influence the bioavailability (Nunes et al. 2016; Dima et al. 2020).

Several factors affect the bioaction of polyphenols, such as (1) the structural features of each compound, including the functional groups and degree of polymerization or glycosylation; (2) the interaction with other food matrix components; (3) food processing/cooking; and (4) the individual physiological conditions. Additionally, higher amounts of polyphenols evaluated in in vitro studies do not necessarily mean a positive correlation with those compounds' best bioavailability and bioaccessibility compared with others present in lesser quantity (Shahidi and Peng 2018).

The food matrix is essential in defining the compound release as polyphenols can be found as free, conjugated, and insoluble-bound phenolics. Free phenolics occur as phenolic aglycones, while conjugated phenolics are present in phenolic glycosides form. Most of the phenolic glycosides are rapidly released to the digestive juice by the effect of mechanical and chemical digestions. Usually, the insoluble phenolics are bound to polysaccharides, proteins, and high-polymerized phenolics like lignin and condensed tannins, meaning that considering the total of phenolics ingested in a food matrix, some can be partially or even vaguely released, and few will penetrate the intestinal epithelium and reach the blood system. Other phenolics continue to the colon, where metabolization and release via fermentation can occur (Shahidi and Peng 2018).

Hydroxytyrosol is the major phenolic in olive by-products (e.g., olive pomace) and the most biologically active one. Several research projects and studies have been focusing on the potential of this compound on the human metabolic system and the possibility of its use in other products beyond olive oil (González-Santiago et al. 2010; Robles-Almazan et al. 2018). Because hydroxytyrosol is an amphipathic compound, it can be detected not only in olive oil but mostly in olive pomace, table olives, and olive tree leaves as a result of oleuropein hydrolysis. It can be found in the free form, as acetate or as part of complex compounds like oleuropein, verbascoside, and oleacein, being partially released during digestion (Robles-Almazan et al. 2018; Fabiani et al. 2021).

Hydroxytyrosol is a potent antioxidant, due to its ortho-diphenol moiety, and it has cardio- and neuroprotective properties and antimicrobial, anti-inflammatory, and anticarcinogenic actions. These are dependent on the absorption and metabolization of the compound (Boronat et al. 2019). For example, Vissers et al. (2004) report that, in humans, the absorption of hydroxytyrosol, tyrosol, oleuropein aglycone, and ligstroside aglycone ranges between 55 and 66%; 5% is eliminated in urine as hydroxytyrosol and tyrosol.

Though hydroxytyrosol is associated with the beneficial effects described and reduced attention has been paid to tyrosol due to its low antioxidant activity, preclinical studies identified the bioconversion of tyrosol into hydroxytyrosol via cytochrome P450 isoforms CYP2A6 and CYP2D6 (Boronat et al. 2019). Considering the current data about the endogenous conversion of tyrosol into hydroxytyrosol, both are health-related compounds of interest.

Olive leaves are rich in secoiridoids (oleuropein, ligstroside), flavonoids (luteolin, kaempferol, apigenin), and phenolics (hydroxytyrosol, tyrosol, caffeic acid). Oleuropein is the most abundant phenolic in leaves, but it is found in reduced amounts in olive oil. Due to their richness in such compounds, olive leaves are used in cosmetics, nutraceuticals, and food supplements. Regarding the metabolization and bioavailability of the olive leaf compounds, human studies report that they could be affected by interindividual variations in absorption and metabolism, and the effects are also dose-dependent (51.1 mg oleuropein and 9.7 mg hydroxytyrosol versus 76.6 mg oleuropein and 14.5 mg hydroxytyrosol) (De Bock et al. 2013).

Olive polyphenols resist acidic stomach conditions and are rapidly absorbed. Oleuropein is rapidly absorbed via oral and has a plasma peak two hours after administration. In hydroxytyrosol, the concentration peak in plasma occurs after only five to ten minutes of ingestion. The renal clearance time occurs during the first hour after administration (Piroddi et al. 2017).

After being absorbed in the bowel, polyphenols are subjected to hepatic metabolism. Polyphenols undergo phases 1 and 2 of metabolism, where they are transformed into glucuronide, methylated, and sulfate by-products. In the case of hydroxytyrosol, it can be detected in plasma and urine in conjugated forms (glucuronoconjugates) (98%), whereas only 2% is found in free form (Miro-Casas et al. 2003).

As soon as absorbed, hydroxytyrosol becomes part of the plasmatic high-density lipoproteins acting as an antioxidant. The plasma half-life of this compound is about one to two minutes, and the rapid and optimal distribution in tissues as muscle and liver leads to the recognized health properties of hydroxytyrosol. Moreover, hydroxytyrosol can cross the blood-brain barrier and be present in the brain tissue reinforcing its neuroprotective benefits (Robles-Almazan et al. 2018). The conjugated metabolites are mainly excreted by the kidneys being six hours the time required to complete the human body's elimination (Rodríguez-Morató et al. 2016; Robles-Almazan et al. 2018).

Hydroxytyrosol was already classified as non-mutagenic, non-genotoxic and with no-observed-adverse-effect level (NOAEL), indicating a safety profile and a promising utilization in functional foods and pharmaceutical applications (Rodríguez-Lara et al. 2019; Bertelli et al. 2020).

10.4 EPIGENETIC EFFECTS OF OLIVES AND OLIVE DERIVATIVE POLYPHENOLS

Olive product and by-product polyphenols can impact the outcomes of metabolic syndrome as central obesity, hyperglycemia, hypertension, and dyslipidemia

(Saibandith et al. 2017). Other effects, such as neuroprotective, anti-aging, anti-carcinogenic, and anti-inflammatory properties, have been reported. Three main epigenetic modifications can be responsible for those effects: post-transcriptional gene regulation by non-coding microRNAs (miRNAs), DNA methylation, and histone modifications (acetylation and methylation) (Fabiani et al. 2021).

miRNAs have an important role in regulating gene expression by directly binding to the target mRNAs and inhibiting translation or stability. They are involved in several fundamental physiologic processes and can be biomarkers for dysfunctions such as obesity since associations between circulating miRNA levels and obesity in adults have been reported (Ortega et al. 2013; Scoditti et al. 2019).

The regulation of the epigenome is defined if a gene is expressed or silenced. The disruption of the epigenetic mechanisms has been associated with chronic diseases, namely cancer (Bishop and Ferguson 2015).

The effects of olive compounds are exerted at a genomic level by modulating the expression of key genes related to some disease's onset and progression. Often, the beneficial effects are reported not for a single compound but for a food matrix, such as olive oil that contains polyphenols, fatty acids, squalene and other triterpenes, tocopherols, pigments, and sterols. Like polyphenols, the amount of those minor compounds varies according to the olive's cultivar and ripeness, agricultural practices, and edaphoclimatic conditions. Also, it depends on the olive-oil-processing system (Covas et al. 2009).

The bioactivity of olive compounds, especially polyphenols, have been studied, most especially hydroxytyrosol and oleuropein (Kiritsakis et al. 2020). Figure 10.1 shows the chemical structure of the main olive derivatives polyphenols (hydroxytyrosol, oleuropein, oleocanthal, and tyrosol).

Several health benefits, including immunostimulant and antimicrobial activities, were reported, as well as beneficial effects on several diseases due to their anti-inflammatory and antioxidant properties.

The effects of major olive polyphenols on the expression of genes will be presented considering the major and most representative organic systems dysfunctions (atherosclerotic process, hypertension, dyslipidemia, obesity, T2D, inflammatory bowel diseases, osteoarthritis, Alzheimer's disease, and cancer) that have an impact in the modern society and human well-being. Figure 10.2 is a schematic presentation of some of the olive polyphenols' benefits under the nutrigenomic approach.

10.4.1 Cardiovascular System: Heart and Vessels

Modifiable factors, such as smoking, physical activity, and optimal nutrition can prevent 80% of heart diseases (angina, heart attack, coronary heart disease, congestive heart failure). Despite the increase in diagnostic tests accuracy and the prevention and treatment strategies, the main cardiovascular factors (dyslipidemia, obesity, T2D, smoking, and hypertension) persist. Moreover, 50% of the individuals who normalize the levels of the top five risk factors mentioned continue to have coronary heart disease or myocardial infarction. This is referred to as the coronary heart disease gap since those factors do not explain the currently limited reduction of cardiovascular

Compound

Hydroxytyrosol
IUPAC name:
4-(2-hydroxyethyl)benzene-1,2-diol

Oleuropein
IUPAC name:
methyl (4S,5E,6S)-4-[2-[2-(3,4-dihydroxyphenyl)ethoxy]-2-oxoethyl]-5-ethylidene-6-[(2S,3R,4S,5S,6R)-3,4,5-trihydroxy-6-(hydroxymethyl)oxan-2-yl]oxy-4H-pyran-3-carboxylate

Oleocanthal
IUPAC name:
2-(4-hydroxyphenyl)ethyl (E,3S)-4-formyl-3-(2-oxoethyl)hex-4-enoate

Tyrosol
IUPAC name:
4-(2-hydroxyethyl)phenol

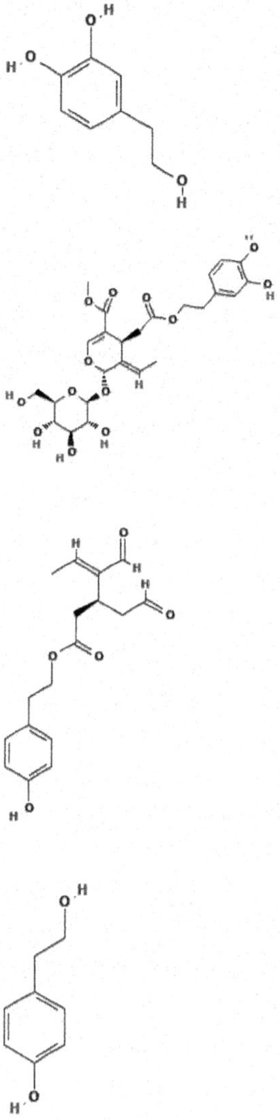

FIGURE 10.1 Chemical structure of the main olive polyphenols (hydroxytyrosol, oleuropein, oleocanthal, and tyrosol). (From the National Center for Biotechnology Information (2021). PubChem Compound Summary for CID 82755, 5281544, 11652416, 10393.)

diseases. The cardiovascular system's response to risk factors involves oxidative stress, vascular immune dysfunction, and inflammation. Therefore, other risk factors and biomarkers can start to be considered for cardiovascular pathogenesis, such as micronutrient testing, genetic evaluation, metabolomics, and nutrigenomics (Houston 2018).

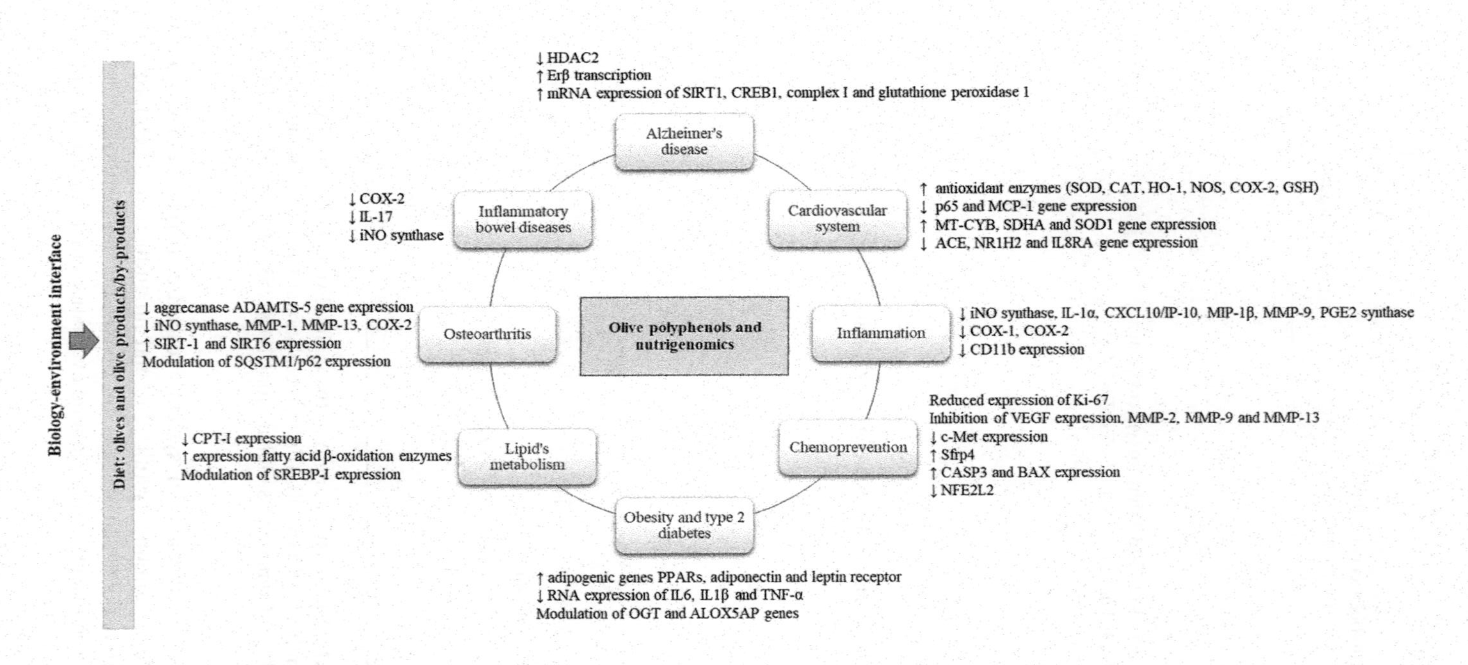

FIGURE 10.2 Olive polyphenols' beneficial effects.

The impact of olive-derived compounds in preventing cardiovascular diseases, mainly in the context of Mediterranean diet or olive oil consumption, has been extensively reviewed (Nocella et al. 2018; Ditano-Vázquez et al. 2019; Marcelino et al. 2019). However, few studies explored the nutrigenomics of those benefits. It is known that oxidative stress is associated with endothelial dysfunction, inflammation, hypertrophy, cell migration, fibrosis, and angiogenesis, which can be a leading factor of atherosclerosis. Atherosclerosis is a vascular disease that causes thickening and inelasticity of arteries. Hence, oxidative stress is also a key factor in hypertension onset and then in cardiovascular disease. The atherosclerotic risk can be reduced by managing a lower ROS production and restoring cellular antioxidant defenses (D'Angelo et al. 2020).

Hydroxytyrosol has the capacity of scavenging oxidant species. Moreover, it can also promote the synthesis and activity of several antioxidant enzymes like glutathione reductase, catalase, superoxide dismutase, glutathione peroxidase, and NO synthase while preserving the cellular high levels of reduced glutathione (D'Angelo et al. 2020). It can induce the synthesis and translocation to the cell nucleus of Nrf2, promoting the transcription of encoding genes of the antioxidant response as phase 2 detoxifying enzymes and DNA-repair proteins (Bertelli et al. 2020).

The inflammatory response is generally fast and self-limited. In these conditions, it is beneficial and protective. However, chronic inflammation is detrimental if endothelial, smooth muscle, and peripheral blood cells are subjected to continuous and high levels of pro-inflammatory cytokines, chemokines, prostaglandins and leukotrienes, and potentially toxic molecules (D'Angelo et al. 2020).

The inflammation process is complex and involves numerous mediators with cells and plasma origins. The development and severity of several chronic diseases are linked to a chronic inflammation state. Hydroxytyrosol can effectively inhibit the pathways that stimulate NO production; the cytokines IL-1α, IL-1β, IL-6, IL-12, and TNF-α; the chemokines CXCL10/IP-10 and CCL2/MPC-1; and the eicosanoid PGE2. Equivalent repression effects occurred in genes, such as the inducible NO synthase, IL-1α, CXCL10/IP-10, MIP-1β, MMP-9, and PGE2 synthase (Piroddi et al. 2017).

The anti-inflammatory effect of hydroxytyrosol and oleuropein was studied using a cell line of murine macrophages and in human granulocytes and monocytes. Nutritionally low relevant doses of hydroxytyrosol, oleuropein, and resveratrol were tested. In concentration-dependent doses (10 μM), the three compounds inhibited the granulocyte oxidative burst and the CD11b expression (resveratrol and hydroxytyrosol). Overall, an anti-inflammatory effect of resveratrol and hydroxytyrosol was shown by the inhibition of the activation of granulocytes and monocytes. Also, the modulation of miR-146a expression and the activation of the transcription factor Nrf2 were observed (Bigagli et al. 2017). Hence, the anti-inflammatory preventive actions of hydroxytyrosol also have a relevant impact on the atherosclerotic process.

In the human umbilical vein, endothelial cells treated with serum obtained from individuals two hours after the intake of olive oil rich in polyphenols decreased the p65 and MCP-1 gene expression and increased MT-CYB, SDHA, and SOD1 gene expression. The same treatment applied after four hours decreased MCP-1 and catalase gene expression and increased MT-CYB gene expression. The genes p65 and MCP-1 are anti-inflammatory, MT-CYB and SDHA are prooxidant enzymes and respiratory chain genes, and SOD1 and catalase are antioxidant enzymes. Olive oil reduced inflammation and increased the expression of oxidative-stress-related genes in the vascular endothelium, reducing the atherosclerotic risk (Meza-Miranda et al. 2016). Therefore, olive oil metabolites, particularly hydroxytyrosol metabolites, can prevent endothelium dysfunction (Catalán et al. 2015; D'Angelo et al. 2020).

Hypertension is a marker for vascular endothelium dysfunction. It can develop silently and can be a severe cause or aggravate cardiovascular diseases or chronic heart failure. The risk of cardiovascular diseases increases progressively as the blood pressure deregulates. The effect of extra-virgin olive oil with high polyphenol content on the expression of the blood-pressure-related genes (ACE, ADRB2, ECE2, IL8RA, MPO, NR1H2, OLR1, and PPARG) involved in the regulation of the renin-angiotensin-aldosterone system (RAAS) was studied. RAAS regulates blood volume and systemic vascular resistance, influencing cardiac output and arterial pressure. Data showed that the daily consumption of virgin olive oil (25 mL) for three weeks decreased the ACE, NR1H2, and IL8RA gene expressions that reflected in a decrease in the systolic blood pressure. In this case, olive oil presented an oleuropein content of 65%, followed by 18% of ligstroside aglycones and 18% hydroxytyrosol (Martín-Peláez et al. 2017). A blood-pressure-lowering effect has been reported to oleuropein, which goes in agreement with the deep-rooted traditional use of olive leaves in decoctions and infusions to treat mild to moderate hypertension. A daily dosage of oleuropein (60 mg) in an animal model resulted in a significant decrease in systolic blood pressure (Khalili et al. 2017) and 30 mg of polyphenol-rich olive oil reduced both systolic and diastolic blood pressures in young women with mild hypertension (Moreno-Luna et al. 2012).

10.4.2 Liver and Biliary Tract: Lipids Metabolism

Liver, biliary tree, and gallbladder structures are considered together due to their anatomic proximity and functions. The liver is exposed to various metabolic, toxic, microbial, circulatory, and neoplastic attacks. This organ acts as a large functional reserve and regulates most chemical levels in the blood. More than 500 vital functions have been identified. Some of the principal and well-known ones are (1) production of cholesterol and proteins to carry fats through the bloodstream, (2) conversion of excess glucose into glycogen and storage, (3) processing of hemoglobin as the liver stores iron, (4) regulation of blood clotting, and (5) clearing the blood of drugs and other toxic substances. Overall, liver functions comprise carbohydrate, protein, and lipid metabolism. The main processes related to lipid metabolism in the liver are lipogenesis, fatty acid oxidation, lipoprotein synthesis, and phospholipid and cholesterol synthesis (Mitra and Metcalf 2012).

High levels of total cholesterol and low-density lipoprotein (LDL) and low levels of high-density lipoproteins (HDL) are associated with the onset of certain diseases such as cardiovascular ones, mainly related to atherosclerotic plaque formation. Therefore, improving the lipid profile and dyslipidemia prevention can have a protective effect (D'Angelo et al. 2020).

The positive impact of extra-virgin olive oil (richer in polyphenols than olive oil) and olive leaf extracts on dyslipidemia is being corroborated and reviewed (Saibandith et al. 2017). As a ROS scavenger, hydroxytyrosol reduces oxidized LDL and platelets aggregation, seeming to be a key mechanism associated with the regulation of dyslipidemia. Hence, potential effects of olive products on lipid metabolism and inflammation arise as linked to metabolic pathways and inflammation-related genes (Correa et al. 2009).

The oxidation of the lipid fraction of LDL results in a modification of the lipoprotein conformation, enabling the atherosclerotic process. Olive polyphenols, mainly hydroxytyrosol, protects LDL from oxidation. Based on this effect, the European Food Safety Authority claimed that daily consumption of 5 mg of hydroxytyrosol and its derivatives protects blood lipids from oxidation (Peyrol et al. 2017). Several other studies, such as the EUROLIVE (Effect of Olive Oils on Oxidative Damage in European Populations), also demonstrate that olive oil with different polyphenol content reduces LDL in a dose-dependent manner. It was observed in rodent and murine models that hydroxytyrosol reduces the accumulation of triglycerides in tissues such as liver and skeletal muscle and low serum cholesterol in high-fat-diet animals (Peyrol et al. 2017).

Molecular targets for hydroxytyrosol, related to its beneficial effects in lipid metabolism, were identified in experimental studies. Recently, López de Las Hazas et al. (2019) reviewed and, afterward, experimentally validated molecular hydroxytyrosol targets. Four miRNAs responded to hydroxytyrosol supplementation (miR-802-5p, miR-423-3p, miR-30a-5p, and miR-146b-5p), and Fgf21 and Rora were newly identified as potential hydroxytyrosol targets in this study. Also, miR-802-5p responded consistently to dietary hydroxytyrosol supplementation in two different tissues (liver and intestine), supporting a miRNA modulating action by hydroxytyrosol (López de Las Hazas et al. 2019).

Nevertheless, most studies performed in humans or animal models have reported a modest or positive effect on circulating lipids and lipid peroxidation (Visioli et al. 2020). Likewise, despite transcriptomics and proteomics greatly contributing to the knowledge of olive compounds' effect on the expression of a vast number of genes related to dyslipidemia, inflammation, endothelial dysfunction, and cardiovascular diseases, the evidence about those mechanisms is far from complete comprehension. The limited number of human studies and the heterogenicity of the doses administered leads to an increasing requirement of transcriptomic and proteomic tools to identify and validate hydroxytyrosol and oleuropein targets (López de Las Hazas et al. 2019).

Non-alcoholic fatty liver disease (NAFLD) is a chronic liver disease that comprises several conditions, from simple steatosis to a severe degree of the diseases characterized by inflammation or non-alcoholic steatohepatitis that can turn into cirrhosis, hepatocarcinoma, and organ failure (Priore et al. 2015). It was reported in rats with NAFLD that olive oil decreased the storage of hepatic triglycerides, increased the secretion of triglycerides (as very-low-density lipoprotein), and decreased the occurring lipolytic flux from the peripheral adipose tissue to the liver. Thus, olive oil can provide protection against liver steatosis (Hussein et al. 2007).

In human studies, olive oil decreased the serum triglycerides by increasing the expression of hepatic fatty acid β-oxidation enzymes through the corresponding genes by the transcription factor peroxisome proliferator-activated receptor-α (Assy et al. 2009; Priore et al. 2015).

10.4.3 Endocrine System: Obesity and Type 2 Diabetes

Adipose tissue was formerly considered a non-dynamic tissue which function was limited to the body energy storage. Currently, it is known that adipose tissue is highly active, with immunological and hormonal regulatory functions (González-Casanova et al. 2020). In obesity, ghrelin, an orexigenic hormone, is increased, and the appetite-suppressing or anorexigenic hormones (insulin, amylin, glucagon-like peptide-1, cholecystokinin, peptide YY, and leptin) are decreased. Hormone regulation is essential to regulate food intake. Hence, appetite and satiety are controlled by a complex communication network comprising adipose tissue, endocrine organs, gastroenteric peptides, and central nervous system (Poddar et al. 2017).

Obesity is a multifactorial and chronic disease. Particularly, the chronic inflammation of adipose tissue contributes largely to cardiometabolic disease. The occurring abnormal adipose tissue expansion in obesity associated with adipocyte hypoxia and death leads to an increased production of ROS and lipid mediators. Also, adipokines like prostaglandins are produced, as well as peptide hormones and cytokines enrolled in the local/systemic chronic inflammation; insulin resistance and vascular dysfunction are also observed. The hypertrophied adipocytes induce the recruitment, infiltration, and pro-inflammatory activation of macrophages and lymphocytes (Scoditti et al. 2019; Wadey et al. 2019). TNFα, a secretory product of those cells, activates the inflammatory signaling, with an abnormal expression and release of pro-inflammatory, pro-atherogenic, pro-thrombotic adipokines and factors associated with the metabolic deregulation, angiogenesis, matrix remodeling, and fibrosis. Overall, the cell products will aggravate systemic inflammation and resistance to insulin (Wadey et al. 2019). The insulin resistance syndrome leads to several other pathologies, such as increased triglyceride levels, blood pressure, and serum glucose, which enhance the severity of T2D and cardiovascular disease. Due to the strong relationship between obesity and diabetes, the combination of the two diseases is often named "diabesity", and they are treated together (Poddar et al. 2017).

miRNAs can regulate the obesity pathophysiological processes by an active regulation of adipokine production, inflammation, and intercellular communication. Along with inflammation, miRNAs can be unregulated. For example, in adipose tissue, miR-34a leads to the pro-inflammatory macrophages activation or miR-155, promoting lipid cell dysfunction and inflammation (Scoditti et al. 2019). Considering the strong hydroxytyrosol anti-inflammatory activity, its application to treat adipocyte inflammation in adipose tissue is appellative. Hydroxytyrosol and oleuropein prevented 3T3-L1 (preadipocytes) differentiation, with the most potent effects in early stages, at 150 and 300 μmol/L, respectively, and without affecting the cell viability. Also, both compounds downregulate the expression of adipogenesis genes (Drira et al. 2011).

Recently, an olive leaf extract with 12% of polyphenols, in which oleuropein represented 10%, reduced the body weight gain in mice and improved the expression of the adipogenic genes PPARs and adiponectin and leptin receptors in adipose tissue. The extracts also ameliorated the anti-inflammatory status in the adipose tissue by reducing the RNA expression of IL-6, IL-1β, and TNFα (Vezza et al. 2019).

Diabetes has two main forms of presentation: immune-mediated β-cell destruction (T1D) and loss and death of β-cell functional mass that leads to the development of T2D. The effect of olive oil's commercial standard polyphenols (10 μM) on β-cell function and survival was studied for each compound for 24 hours showing that hydroxytyrosol, tyrosol, and apigenin preserve β-cells function and survival, meaning that those compounds may ameliorate the insulin secretion and control glycemia (Marrano et al. 2021). In overweight T2D individuals, the daily consumption of olive oil enriched in polyphenols (~580 mg/kg) improved the circulatory inflammatory adipokines (Santangelo et al. 2016), and supplementation with 10 mg hydroxytyrosol/kg (daily) for five weeks improved glucose tolerance and insulin sensitivity in rat models (Pirozzi et al. 2016). Also, after ingestion of 50 mL of olive oil, modest changes were observed in the expression of insulin sensitivity-related genes: after one hour, it was observed downregulation in OGT and ALOX5AP genes; OGT was upregulated at six hours; CD36 was upregulated at one hour; LIAS, PPARBP, ADAM17, and ADRB2 genes were upregulated at six hours (Konstantinidou et al. 2010).

Antidiabetic properties have been attributed to oleuropein, and one of the proposed mechanisms – reduction of serum glucose – seems to be related to its chemical structure. As oleuropein exists in a glycoside form, it can compete with glucose in the intestinal epithelial cells to be absorbed through sodium-dependent glucose transporter 1 (Kerimi et al. 2019). The inhibition of digestive enzymes and the increase of the glucagon-like peptide 1 levels, which attenuate the postprandial glycemia, are other proposed actions (Carnevale et al. 2018).

The studies that address the nutrigenomic effect of hydroxytyrosol or oleuropein in T2D are scarce. These compounds likely have biological properties and mechanisms of action that lead to the positive effects observed, such as inhibition of carbohydrate digestion and glucose absorption, activation of insulin receptors and glucose uptake in the tissues, and effects related to the capacity of modulating the antioxidant and anti-inflammatory status (Alkhatib et al. 2018). Additionally, oxidative stress and inflammation are ameliorated with oleuropein or hydroxytyrosol administration or exposition, indicating that the potential effects of the olive biophenols on T2D occur through metabolic pathways and inflammation-related genes. Most of the studies are performed in cell cultures or animal models, and the studies conducted on humans are still limited.

10.4.4 Gastrointestinal Tract: Inflammatory Bowel Diseases and Microbiota

Ulcerative colitis and Crohn's disease are the two main types of inflammatory bowel disease characterized by an extensive and chronic inflammation process. Usually, they are controlled with massive pharmacological agents. Ulcerative colitis is a colonic mucosal inflammation related to the deregulation of the immune system.

In a mouse model with induced colitis, oleuropein reduced eosinophil, neutrophil, and macrophage in colon tissue and inhibited the expression of COX-2 (Giner et al. 2013). Moreover, oleuropein treatment using the same model reduced the intestinal IL-6, IL-17A, and TNFα concentrations and was able to downregulate the Th17 response, a pro-inflammatory pathway activated in intestinal bowel disease (Giner et al. 2016). In the colonic mucosa from patients with active ulcerative colitis, oleuropein ameliorates the inflammatory state. The expression of COX-2 and IL-17 was lower in the oleuropein-treated samples when compared with those without oleuropein (Larussa et al. 2017). Also, hydroxytyrosol showed an anti-inflammatory effect by suppressing inducible NO synthase and COX-2 in a dose-dependent manner (Zhang et al. 2009).

Hydroxytyrosol acetate supplementation in an animal model also improves histological damage and reduces the COX-2 and inducible NO synthase expression. Due to the presence of an ester group, this has higher solubility in lipophilic phases than free hydroxytyrosol, meaning that hydroxytyrosol acetate can be better absorbed across intestinal epithelial cell monolayers compared to free hydroxytyrosol (Sánchez-Fidalgo et al. 2015). Considering this, the impact of hydroxytyrosol acetate vehiculated by a lipidic format as olive oil or lipid-based nutraceuticals on acute ulcerative colitis can be more significant than free hydroxytyrosol. However, new studies, especially in humans and regarding both compounds, are still necessary. Notwithstanding the promising in vivo results observed for bowel inflammatory diseases treatment, most studies are performed with extra-virgin olive oil since it is the most consumed olive tree product and the base of the Mediterranean diet (Larussa et al. 2019). Moreover, extra-virgin olive oil presents many beneficial compounds that can act synergistically (Piroddi et al. 2017). Hence, more research is needed regarding the interconnection between bowel inflammation, olive compounds, and epigenetics in humans using clinical trials and a higher number of individuals.

The microbes that comprise the gut microbiota play an important role in the human body's physiological maintenance. Dysbiosis, microbiota dysregulation, impairs its beneficial function, modifies intestinal permeability, and triggers inflammation. This process could lead to severe pathological conditions, such as obesity, insulin resistance, and inflammatory status. Therefore, a positive association between gut microbiota and health and its maintenance is required (Marcelino et al. 2019).

Most of the olive polyphenols are rapidly absorbed in the small intestine. Nevertheless, some simple and complex compounds can reach the large intestine and will be metabolized by microbiota. For example, it is known that oleuropein is catabolized in hydroxytyrosol in vitro. *Lactobacillus*, *Bifidobacteria*, and *Enterococcus* hydrolyze oleuropein into hydroxytyrosol (Santos et al. 2012).

The gut microbiota profile is affected by environmental and genetic factors. Diet is the one with the highest dynamic impact. Olive oil (20% of the diet) can increase the microbial diversity in spontaneously hypertensive rats. These authors also suggested that the changes in gut microbiota are linked to a reduction in systolic blood pressure (Hidalgo et al. 2018). Specifically, hydroxytyrosol is shown to modulate the microbiota composition by enhancing the microbiota richness and restraining the pathogenic bacteria (Wang et al. 2019). Moreover, in male mice, it improved obesity and insulin resistance by modifying the microbiota, reduced the release of endotoxins into the bloodstream, and reduced inflammation at a dose of 50 mg/kg/day (eight weeks) (Liu et al. 2019).

To sum up, olive hydroxytyrosol and oleuropein influence the microbiota composition regarding its profile and bacteria content and act as a modulator by controlling pathogenic bacteria's growth and stimulating the proliferation of beneficial ones.

The effects of nutrients on the human body, particularly on gene expression, should be studied under the scope of the microbiome perspective since the axis genome-food-microbiota influence gene expression locally or at a systemic level. Moreover, the mechanisms involved in these processes and the study of isolated compounds are a great research area and essential to complement these recent findings.

10.4.5 Musculoskeletal System: Osteoarthritis

Oleuropein, hydroxytyrosol, and oleocanthal are being pointed out as compounds of interest in the management of osteoarthritis, an inflammatory and degenerative disease. Oleuropein (10, 50, and 100 μM) was able to inhibit the IL-1β-induced production of NO and PGE2, as well as the gene expression of the aggrecanase ADAMTS-5, inducible NO synthase, MMP-1, MMP-13, and COX-2, leading to the degradation of aggrecan (aggregates of proteoglycans and hyaluronic acid) and collagen-II in human primary chondrocytes. The therapeutic effect found was due to the inhibition of NF-Kβ and MAPK signaling pathways (Feng et al. 2017).

In osteoarthritis pathogenesis, autophagy is considered a cellular housekeeping system able to recycle and remove impaired macromolecules and organelles. This is a protective mechanism in normal cartilage. Its aging-related loss is associated with chondrocyte death and the pathogenesis of osteoarthritis. Hydroxytyrosol modulates this homeostatic process by stimulating the induction and flux of the mechanism autophagy. Moreover, when oxidative stress is induced, hydroxytyrosol protects chondrocytes from DNA damage and cell death. SIRT-1, a protein deacetylase that can regulate oxidative stress, inflammation, apoptosis, metabolism, and autophagy, modulates the expression of genes associated with autophagy by deacetylating key transcription factors. Hydroxytyrosol also can enhance the SIRT-1 expression in human chondrocytes, exerting a protective role in cell survival and cartilage homeostasis (Facchini et al. 2014; Cetrullo et al. 2016). Hydroxytyrosol affects several genes expression, such as SQSTM1/p62 (Cetrullo et al. 2016) and miR-9 (D'Adamo et al. 2017). Particularly, miR-9 is overexpressed when chondrocytes are exposed to hydrogen peroxide, one of the major ROS in chondrocytes. Hydroxytyrosol could counteract hydrogen peroxide-induced miR-9 expression, restoring the protein translation of SIRT-1 (D'Adamo et al. 2017).

SIRT6 is also involved in osteoarthritis protection due to its ability to suppress the inflammatory response and chondrocyte senescence. Likewise, in this case, hydroxytyrosol promotes the autophagy flux and inhibits the chondrocytes inflammatory response by increasing the gene expression of SIRT6 (Zhi et al. 2018).

Oleocanthal suppresses the expression of inflammatory cytokines and mediators as TNFα, inducible NO synthase, COX-2, IL-6, and IL-8, among others, as well as the catabolic enzymes MMP13 and ADAMTS-5 (Scotece et al. 2018).

10.4.6 Nervous System and Cognition: Alzheimer's Disease

The normal function of the nervous system is dependent on the maintenance of its structural integrity and metabolic processes. Neurodegenerative diseases comprise a heterogeneous group of diseases that can impair cognitive function. Such examples are Parkinson's and Alzheimer's diseases. Neurodegenerative diseases do not have a cure. However, prevention and treatment in the early stages can manage the symptoms and delay the progression (Agnihotri and Aruoma 2020).

Alzheimer's disease is age-related and gives rise to dementia, causing disability. This disease is characterized by a gradual cognitive decline and memory impairment, and it represents the major form of dementia worldwide. Although it is not entirely understood what causes Alzheimer's directly, two factors are pointed as putative causes: gene mutations in the amyloid precursor protein (APP) and presenilin 1 and 2 genes, which are related to the amyloid-beta (Aβ) peptide synthesis, and processes related to the hyperphosphorylation of the tau protein and its consequent deposition. There is a positive correlation between Alzheimer's disease symptoms and the presence of tau and Aβ protein in their aggregated forms (neurofibrillary tangles and β-amyloid plaques). Nevertheless, a combination of age-related alterations in the brain and genetics, lifestyle, and environmental factors is probably behind this disease's high incidence. Moreover, most of the knowledge about Alzheimer's has been obtained post mortem, and thus, the exact mechanisms of the disease are still poorly understood (Mondragón-Rodríguez et al. 2017; Agnihotri and Aruoma 2020).

Chronic oxidative stress has been demonstrated as detrimental in the pathogenesis of age-related diseases such as Alzheimer's. Oxidative stress can induce several disturbances in mitochondria like DNA mutations, impairment of the mitochondrial respiratory chain and membrane permeability functions, and disturbance in Ca^{2+} homeostasis. Hence, antioxidant therapy has been suggested. Nevertheless, good nutrition is assumed as crucial to prevent or delay the neurodegenerative evolution as it provides, among other nutrients, polyphenols that impair chronic oxidative stress (Agnihotri and Aruoma 2020).

Regarding olive compounds, it was reported that oleocanthal enhances β-amyloid clearance by upregulating major β-amyloid transport proteins in mice brain endothelial cells, more specifically the P-glycoprotein and LDL lipoprotein receptor-related protein-1, and inhibits the tau protein aggregation into neurofibrillary tangles (Monti et al. 2012; Abuznait et al. 2013).

Oleuropein is an epigenetic modulator. Oleuropein aglycone impairs the β-amyloid and tau protein aggregation and neuroinflammation and induces autophagy, decreasing aggregated proteins and reducing cognitive loss. This effect is related to the capacity of oleuropein to activate the gene expression mediated by sirtuins and histone acetylation or EB transcription factor. The gene expression is inhibited by the increase of histone deacetylase 2 (HDAC2). Its overexpression in mice impairs memory. Hence, downregulation or inhibition of HDAC2 is suggested as a therapeutic target for memory-related disturbance. Administration of oleuropein (50 mg/kg; eight weeks) decreased the levels of HDAC2 in mice and synaptic function amelioration (Luccarini et al. 2015; Cordero et al. 2018).

Also, a polyphenol extract obtained from concentrated olive mill wastewater (verbascoside, oleuropein di-aldehyde, hydroxytyrosol, tyrosol) significantly improves the cognitive function of mice. The number and area of Aβ42 and pE-3Aβ (isoform and modified form of Aβ) plaques were significantly reduced in the cortex by oleuropein and in the cortex and hippocampus by the polyphenol extract (Pantano et al. 2017).

An aqueous extract of olive with 40–50% hydroxytyrosol, 5–10% of oleuropein, and 0.3% of tyrosol (Hidrox), administered to rats, promoted a reduction in toxic oxidative stress and neuroinflammation. Moreover, hydroxytyrosol maintained the redox balance and homeostasis by activating the Nrf2 pathway and increasing the expression of phase 2 detoxifying enzymes, reducing neurodegeneration. Also, the treatment improved memory impairment and cognitive dysfunction. This extract decreased the markers associated with Alzheimer's disease as the β-amyloid accumulation and APP and tau overexpression (Cordaro et al. 2021).

It was also reported that hydroxytyrosol acetate improved cognitive function, in animal models, by decreasing inflammatory cytokine levels and improving neuronal apoptosis. The compound was able to induce the transcription of the Erβ receptor (abundant in areas such as hippocampal formation, cerebral cortex, and thalamus), increasing neuronal viability (Qin et al. 2021).

Recently, to investigate the cause and effect of olive leaves, individual compounds (oleocanthal, oleuropein, hydroxytyrosol, oleuroside aglycon, ligstroside, ligustaloside B, ligstroside aglycone, oleuroside, tyrosol, and oleacein) were tested on mitochondrial function in SH-SY5Y-APP695 cells. Then as only oleocanthal and ligstroside were able to enhance the capacity of mitochondrial respiratory chain complexes, their molecular mechanisms on the expression of several genes related to mitochondrial biogenesis, respiration, and antioxidative capacity (PGC-1α, SIRT1, CREB1, NRF1, TFAM, complex I, IV and V, glutathione peroxidase 1, superoxide dismutase 2, and catalase) were explored. It was shown that only ligstroside enhanced the mRNA expression of SIRT1, CREB1, complex I, and glutathione peroxidase 1. On the other hand, just oleocanthal decreased the SH-SY5Y-APP695 cells Aβ 1–40 after 24 hours incubation. Additionally, these authors tested oleocanthal and ligstroside (supplemented diet) in a mouse model of aging for six months. The mice fed with a diet enriched with ligstroside presented an improvement in spatial working memory. Also, in aged mice, ligstroside restored the brain ATP levels and significantly extended lifespan compared to the aged control mice (Grewal et al. 2020).

Because olive derivative compounds such as hydroxytyrosol have been proposed to be included in a food pattern as functional ingredients/products or via dietary supplements, or even included in personalized nutritional models, in the case of neurodegenerative diseases, it is still necessary more studies in other animal models and, if possible, in humans, to evaluate the potential neuroprotective role.

10.4.7 Chemoprevention

Cancer is a multifactor genetic disease. Diet is one of the factors that have been highlighted on cancer's predisposition, development, and prognosis. The knowledge of the effect of bioactive compounds on genome and transcriptome patterns is of great interest to the oncology field since certain compounds specifically activate cancer inhibitory mechanisms, affecting key cancer hallmarks, such as apoptosis or the impairment of angiogenesis (Irimie et al. 2019).

The anticancer effect of many plant-derived polyphenols has been explored over the last years. Polyphenols can interact with other food components or drugs, resulting in additive, synergistic, or antagonistic effects. The combination of polyphenols with chemotherapeutics can enhance the anticancer efficacy, diminish the side effects of chemotherapy, and overcome the radio- or chemo-resistance of cancer cells (Torić et al. 2019). Olive polyphenols can exert chemoprotective and anticancer actions in breast cancer, prostate cancer, melanoma, promyelocytic leukemia, and colon cancer, among others (Torić et al. 2019).

Oleuropein, hydroxytyrosol, oleacein, and oleocanthal as olive derivative compounds show to exert antioxidant and anti-inflammatory effects and also act on the expression of genes that control the proliferation, apoptosis, and differentiation of cancer cells. It is hypothesized that the targets of these anticancer effects could be the genes associated with growth factors (GF) production or growth factor receptors (GFR). The overexpression of GF and GFR in cancer cells results in uncontrolled proliferation and production of signaling molecules that, ultimately, lead to tumor growth. Olive polyphenols can, thus, have an anticancer potential (Torić et al. 2019).

Oleuropein, in vitro, inhibited thyroid cancer cell proliferation by acting on growth-promoting signal pathways (Bulotta et al. 2013) and reduced UVB-radiation-induced tumor volume possibly by the inhibition of the expression of VEGF, MMP-2, MMP-9, and MMP-13 through a reduction in COX-2 levels (Kimura and Sumiyoshi 2009). Several in vitro studies have shown that oleuropein inhibits proliferation and induces apoptosis in different cancer-related cell lines, such as breast, colon, liver, pancreatic, and thyroid cancers, as well as in osteosarcoma, leukemia, neuroblastoma, and mesothelioma cells (Shamshoum et al. 2017).

Despite the promising outputs from the in vitro studies, few animal studies assessed the effects of oleuropein on tumor progression in vivo. In breast cancer, it was found that oleuropein (125 mg/kg) in mice inhibited tumor growth and metastases and prevented the peripulmonary dissemination of the tumor. On the other hand, it was also reported that 0.3 mg/kg of oleuropein in an animal model of glioma did not inhibit tumor growth (Martínez-Martos et al. 2014).

Also, in colon cancer, administration of oleuropein (50 or 100 mg/kg) in mice led to a reduction of the tumor progression, a decrease of inflammation markers, a reduction of the number and dimension of tumors, and impairment of neoplastic cells proliferation. The effects are related to a reduced expression of Ki-67, upregulation of BAX, and inhibition of NF-Kβ phosphorylation, Wnt/b-catenin, Akt, and STAT-3 (Giner et al. 2016).

In skin cancer, effects related to the inhibition of VEGF expression, MMP-2, MMP-9, and MMP-13 were found. In this case, the treatment with oleuropein (male mice) (10 and 25 mg/kg; 30 weeks; twice daily) reduced the tumor incidence and volume. The positive results observed were dose-related. Overall, it was shown that the olive leaf extract administered (300 and 1,000 mg/kg; 30 weeks; twice daily), and oleuropein inhibited the increase of skin thickness and reduction in skin elasticity, skin carcinogenesis, and tumor growth in UVB irradiated mice (three times/week; 30 weeks) (Kimura et al. 2009).

Data also showed that oleuropein could have a preventive effect on tongue cancer. The administration of an oleuropein extract (3 mg/kg; 31 weeks) in a rat model of 4-NQO-induced tongue cancer led to a reduced tumor incidence and volume due to a decrease of c-Met and Ki67 expression. C-Met is an oncogene able to induce cell proliferation and survival, whereas Ki-67 is a protein required through the cell cycle and its expression inhibits cell proliferation (Grawish et al. 2011).

Likewise, studies with hydroxytyrosol are promising. As hydroxytyrosol is a metabolite of oleuropein, some of the results reported to oleuropein could be effectively due to metabolized hydroxytyrosol (Shamshoum et al. 2017). The administration of 10 mg/kg of hydroxytyrosol for 14 days (female mice) reduced tumor size, vessel lumina, and blood perfusion to the tumor in colon cancer cells. These effects resulted from the downregulation of HIF-1α, VEGF, and mPGEs-1 (Terzuoli et al. 2010). Also, mammary tumor growth was inhibited when hydroxytyrosol was administered (0.5 mg/kg; six weeks). It was shown that hydroxytyrosol modifies genes related to cell proliferation, apoptosis, and the Wnt signaling pathway, promoting a high expression of Sfrp4, a major isoform able to chemo-sensitize tumor cells to chemotherapeutics (Granados-Principal et al. 2011).

Using a human cell line, it was also shown that cholangiocarcinoma, a digestive tumor with a high rate of mortality, growth was reduced by hydroxytyrosol administration (500 mg/kg; daily; three weeks). Moreover, in vivo assays revealed that, after hydroxytyrosol treatment, tumor growth was significantly suppressed (Li et al. 2014).

The anticancer actions of hydroxytyrosol may be due to its capacity to suppress cell survival and/or to activate pro-apoptotic mechanisms. Another proposed action of hydroxytyrosol is the induction of ubiquitination followed by lysosomal degradation of EGFR, which reduced expression is associated with the decrease of cell proliferation in colon cancer cells (Emma et al. 2021). Recently, in a human colorectal cancer cell line, it was demonstrated that hydroxytyrosol increased the expression of CASP3 and BAX, both proapoptotic genes, and downregulated the expression of the NFE2L2 gene (Hormozi et al. 2020).

In breast cancer, cell treatment with hydroxytyrosol and oleuropein reversed 3-MA-dependent suppression of autophagic flux (3-MA is an inhibitor of autophagy), increasing LC3II/LC3I and reducing p62 expression. In this way, it was observed the reduction of tumor cell migration and invasion by activated autophagy (Lu et al. 2019).

Data obtained from in vivo animal and in vitro studies regarding the effect of oleuropein and hydroxytyrosol on carcinogenesis in several cell lines is already extensive and suggests that both compounds can inhibit cancer initiation and metastasis. However, the results should be ascertained in human studies (Shamshoum et al. 2017; Torić et al. 2019). Different conditions (isolated compounds versus extracts) and, mainly, different concentrations have led to the opposite and even controversial effects (Emma et al. 2021).

10.5 CONCLUSION

Nutrition is a multidisciplinary field aligned with physiology and food technology but increasingly includes environmental, socioeconomic, and political sciences.

Also, sustainable agro-food policies and practices have focused on nutrition to base its practices on food security (Raubenheimer and Simpson 2016). The nutrition-environment-gene axis should not be overlooked since, increasingly, other products beyond the traditionally consumed ones start to be part of dietary patterns and consumed as functional foods.

Most of the nutrigenomic studies are focused on olive oil or olive leaves rather than on their individual compounds, namely polyphenols. The emerging R&D of new products using the olive by-products and claiming health benefits based on individual compounds should be validated. Moreover, extraction and bioactive compound processing change the way they naturally exist and take the food composition out of balance, turning the investigation on the bioavailability a challenge.

New food presentations using olive polyphenols will arise on the market. Olive leaves are an example. Olive leaves have been traditionally used mainly to prepare infusions but, nowadays, have also been increasingly used to produce food additives, dietary supplements, and nutraceuticals. Thus, epigenetic effects regarding by-products as foodstuff models could also contribute to the development of the nutrigenomics field.

Overall, eco-nutrition principles promote ethical and sustainable food consumption, considering the environmental and agricultural resources, but above all, they support healthy dietary patterns (Bisht 2021). These bounding lines emerge and should be considered by the food industry and research institutions in a joint effort to contribute to nutrigenomics by investigating if a specific olive compound, incorporated or not in a food matrix, prevents the onset of disorders or diseases.

An integrated approach between genomics and nutrition supports personalized diets, a key factor to prevent diseases and, above all, to maintain optimal global health status. Olive compounds will be one of the future contributors to functional food products, and their impact in genomics ought to be explored.

This chapter presents the main phenolics present in olive products and by-products and their impact on gene regulation and subsequent consequences. Hydroxytyrosol and oleuropein are the compounds most described and bioactive. Although tyrosol, oleocanthal, and ligstroside are present in minor amounts, significant beneficial effects have been reported. The nutrigenomic study associated with cancer and cardiovascular diseases is in great advancement, but lipids metabolism or inflammatory bowel diseases fields are now exciting and promising areas for nutrigenomic research.

ACKNOWLEDGMENTS

The authors acknowledge projects UIDB/50006/2020 (Fundação Para a Ciência e Tecnologia/Ministério da Ciência, Tecnologia e Ensino Superior, Portugal) and AgriFood XXI I&D&I (NORTE-01–0145-FEDER-000041), co-financed by European Regional Development Fund, through the NORTE 2020 (Programa Operacional Regional do Norte 2014/2020), Maria Antónia da Mota Nunes (SFRH/BD/130131/2017), and Rita Carneiro Alves (CEECIND/01120/2017). Thanks to Fundação Para a Ciência e Tecnologia (Portugal).

REFERENCES

Abuznait, A. H., Qosa, H., Busnena, B. A., El Sayed, K. A., and Kaddoumi, A. 2013. Olive-oil-derived oleocanthal enhances β-amyloid clearance as a potential neuroprotective mechanism against Alzheimer's disease: *In vitro* and *in vivo* studies. *ACS Chemical Neuroscience* 4(6):973–82. https://doi.org/10.1021/cn400024q

Acar-Tek, N., and Ağagündüz, D. 2020. Olive leaf (*Olea europaea* L. *folium*): Potential effects on glycemia and lipidemia. *Annals of Nutrition and Metabolism* 76(1):10–15. https://doi.org/10.1159/000505508

Agnihotri, A., and Aruoma, O. I. 2020. Alzheimer's disease and Parkinson's disease: A nutritional toxicology perspective of the impact of oxidative stress, mitochondrial dysfunction, nutrigenomics and environmental chemicals. *Journal of the American College of Nutrition* 39(1):16–27. https://doi.org/10.1080/07315724.2019.1683379

Alkhatib, A., Tsang, C., and Tuomilehto, J. 2018. Olive oil nutraceuticals in the prevention and management of diabetes: From molecules to lifestyle. *International Journal of Molecular Sciences* 19(7):2024. www.mdpi.com/1422-0067/19/7/2024

Assy, N., Nassar, F., Nasser, G., and Grosovski, M. 2009. Olive oil consumption and non-alcoholic fatty liver disease. *World Journal of Gastroenterology* 15(15):1809–15. https://doi.org/10.3748/wjg.15.1809

Bellumori, M., Cecchi, L., Romani, A., Mulinacci, N., and Innocenti, M. 2018. Recovery and stability over time of phenolic fractions by an industrial filtration system of olive mill wastewaters: A three-year study. *Journal of the Science of Food and Agriculture* 98(7):2761–9. https://doi.org/10.1002/jsfa.8772

Bertelli, M., Kiani, A. K., Paolacci, S., et al. 2020. Hydroxytyrosol: A natural compound with promising pharmacological activities. *Journal of Biotechnology* 309:29–33. https://doi.org/10.1016/j.jbiotec.2019.12.016

Bigagli, E., Cinci, L., Paccosi, S., Parenti, A., D'Ambrosio, M., and Luceri, C. 2017. Nutritionally relevant concentrations of resveratrol and hydroxytyrosol mitigate oxidative burst of human granulocytes and monocytes and the production of pro-inflammatory mediators in LPS-stimulated RAW264.7 macrophages. *International Immunopharmacology* 43:147–55. https://doi.org/10.1016/j.intimp.2016.12.012

Bishop, K. S., and Ferguson, L. R. 2015. The interaction between epigenetics, nutrition and the development of cancer. *Nutrients* 7(2):922–47. https://doi.org/10.3390/nu7020922.

Bisht, I. S. 2021. Agri-food system dynamics of small-holder hill farming communities of Uttarakhand in north-western India: Socio-economic and policy considerations for sustainable development. *Agroecology and Sustainable Food Systems* 45(3):417–49.

Bora, P., Chauhan, P., Pardeshi, K. A., and Chakrapani, H. 2018. Small molecule generators of biologically reactive sulfur species. *RSC Advances* 8(48):27359–74. https://doi.org/10.1039/C8RA03658F

Boronat, A., Mateus, J., Soldevila-Domenech, N., et al. 2019. Cardiovascular benefits of tyrosol and its endogenous conversion into hydroxytyrosol in humans. A randomized, controlled trial. *Free Radical Biology and Medicine* 143:471–81. https://doi.org/10.1016/j.freeradbiomed.2019.08.032

Bulotta, S., Corradino, R., Celano, M., et al. 2013. Antioxidant and antigrowth action of peracetylated oleuropein in thyroid cancer cells. *Journal of Molecular Endocrinology* 51(1):181–9. https://doi.org/10.1530/jme-12-0241

Carnevale, R., Silvestri, R., Loffredo, L., et al. 2018. Oleuropein, a component of extra virgin olive oil, lowers postprandial glycaemia in healthy subjects. *British Journal of Clinical Pharmacology* 84(7):1566–74. https://doi.org/10.1111/bcp.13589

Catalán, Ú., López de Las Hazas, M.-C., Rubió, L., et al. 2015. Protective effect of hydroxytyrosol and its predominant plasmatic human metabolites against endothelial dysfunction in human aortic endothelial cells. *Molecular Nutrition and Food Research* 59(12):2523–36. https://doi.org/10.1002/mnfr.201500361

Cetrullo, S., D'Adamo, S., Guidotti, S., Borzì, R. M., and Flamigni, F. 2016. Hydroxytyrosol prevents chondrocyte death under oxidative stress by inducing autophagy through sirtuin 1-dependent and -independent mechanisms. *Biochimica et Biophysica Acta (BBA) – General Subjects* 1860(6):1181–91. https://doi.org/10.1016/j.bbagen.2016.03.002

Charoenprasert, S., and Mitchell, A. 2012. Factors influencing phenolic compounds in table olives (*Olea europaea*). *Journal of Agricultural and Food Chemistry* 60(29):7081–95. https://doi.org/10.1021/jf3017699

Cordaro, M., Salinaro, A. T., Siracusa, R., et al. 2021. Hidrox® roles in neuroprotection: Biochemical links between traumatic brain injury and Alzheimer's disease. *Antioxidants* 10(5):818. https://doi.org/10.3390/antiox10050818

Cordero, J. G., García-Escudero, R., Avila, J., Gargini, R., and García-Escudero, V. 2018. Benefit of oleuropein aglycone for Alzheimer's disease by promoting autophagy. *Oxidative Medicine and Cellular Longevity* 2018:5010741. https://doi.org/10.1155/2018/5010741

Correa, J. A., López-Villodres, J. A., Asensi, R., Espartero, J. L., Rodríguez-Gutiérez, G., and De La Cruz, J. P. 2009. Virgin olive oil polyphenol hydroxytyrosol acetate inhibits *in vitro* platelet aggregation in human whole blood: Comparison with hydroxytyrosol and acetylsalicylic acid. *British Journal of Nutrition* 101(8):1157–64. https://doi.org/10.1017/s0007114508061539

Covas, M. I., Konstantinidou, V., and Fitó, M. 2009. Olive oil and cardiovascular health. *Journal of Cardiovascular Pharmacology* 54(6):477–82. https://doi.org/10.1097/FJC.0b013e3181c5e7fd

D'Adamo, S., Cetrullo, S., Guidotti, S., Borzì, R. M., and Flamigni, F. 2017. Hydroxytyrosol modulates the levels of microRNA-9 and its target sirtuin-1 thereby counteracting oxidative stress-induced chondrocyte death. *Osteoarthritis and Cartilage* 25(4):600–10. https://doi.org/10.1016/j.joca.2016.11.014

D'Angelo, C., Franceschelli, S., Quiles, J. L., and Speranza, L. 2020. Wide biological role of hydroxytyrosol: Possible therapeutic and preventive properties in cardiovascular diseases. *Cells* 9(9):1932. www.mdpi.com/2073-4409/9/9/1932

de Bock, M., Thorstensen, E. B., Derraik, J. G., Henderson, H. V., Hofman, P. L., and Cutfield, W. S. 2013. Human absorption and metabolism of oleuropein and hydroxytyrosol ingested as olive (*Olea europaea* L.) leaf extract. *Molecular Nutrition and Food Research* 57(11):2079–85. https://doi.org/10.1002/mnfr.201200795

Difonzo, G., Troilo, M., Squeo, G., Pasqualone, A., and Caponio, F. 2021. Functional compounds from olive pomace to obtain high-added value foods – a review. *Journal of the Science of Food and Agriculture* 101(1):15–26. https://doi.org/10.1002/jsfa.10478

Dima, C., Assadpour, E., Dima, S., and Jafari, S. M. 2020. Bioavailability and bioaccessibility of food bioactive compounds; overview and assessment by *in vitro* methods. *Comprehensive Reviews in Food Science and Food Safety* 19(6):2862–84. https://doi.org/10.1111/1541-4337.12623

Ditano-Vázquez, P., Torres-Peña, J. D., Galeano-Valle, F., et al. 2019. The fluid aspect of the Mediterranean diet in the prevention and management of cardiovascular disease and diabetes: The role of polyphenol content in moderate consumption of wine and olive oil. *Nutrients* 11(11):2833.

Drira, R., Chen, S., and Sakamoto, K. 2011. Oleuropein and hydroxytyrosol inhibit adipocyte differentiation in 3 T3-L1 cells. *Life Sciences* 89(19):708–16. https://doi.org/10.1016/j.lfs.2011.08.012

Durazzo, A., Lucarini, M., Souto, E. B., et al. 2019. Polyphenols: A concise overview on the chemistry, occurrence, and human health. *Phytotherapy Research* 33(9):2221–43. https://doi.org/10.1002/ptr.6419

Emma, M. R., Augello, G., Di Stefano, V., et al. 2021. Potential uses of olive oil secoiridoids for the prevention and treatment of cancer: A narrative review of preclinical studies. *International Journal of Molecular Sciences* 22(3):1–22. https://doi.org/10.3390/ijms22031234

Fabiani, R., Vella, N., and Rosignoli, P. 2021. Epigenetic modifications induced by olive oil and its phenolic compounds: A systematic review. *Molecules* 26(2):273. https://doi.org/10.3390/molecules26020273

Facchini, A., Cetrullo, S., D'Adamo, S., et al. 2014. Hydroxytyrosol prevents increase of osteoarthritis markers in human chondrocytes treated with hydrogen peroxide or growth-related oncogene α. *PLoS One* 9(10):e109724. https://doi.org/10.1371/journal.pone.0109724

Feng, Z., Li, X., Lin, J., et al. 2017. Oleuropein inhibits the IL-1β-induced expression of inflammatory mediators by suppressing the activation of NF-κB and MAPKs in human osteoarthritis chondrocytes. *Food and Function* 8(10):3737–44. https://doi.org/10.1039/c7fo00823f

Ferguson, J. F., Allayee, H., Gerszten, R. E., et al. 2016. Nutrigenomics, the microbiome, and gene-environment interactions: New directions in cardiovascular disease research, prevention, and treatment: A scientific statement from the American heart association. *Circulation: Genomic and Precision Medicine* 9(3):291–313. https://doi.org/10.1161/hcg.0000000000000030

Fraga, C. G., Galleano, M., Verstraeten, S. V., and Oteiza, P. I. 2010. Basic biochemical mechanisms behind the health benefits of polyphenols. *Molecular Aspects of Medicine* 31(6):435–45. https://doi.org/10.1016/j.mam.2010.09.006

Ghanbari, R., Anwar, F., Alkharfy, K. M., Gilani, A.-H. and Saari, N. 2012. Valuable nutrients and functional bioactives in different parts of olive (*Olea europaea* L.) – a review. *International Journal of Molecular Sciences* 13(3):3291–340. www.mdpi.com/1422-0067/13/3/3291

Giner, E., Recio, M. C., Ríos, J. L., Cerdá-Nicolás, J. M., and Giner, R. M. 2016. Chemopreventive effect of oleuropein in colitis-associated colorectal cancer in c57bl/6 mice. *Molecular Nutrition and Food Research* 60(2):242–55. https://doi.org/10.1002/mnfr.201500605

Giner, E., Recio, M.-C., Ríos, J.-L. and Giner, R.-M. 2013. Oleuropein protects against dextran sodium sulfate-induced chronic colitis in mice. *Journal of Natural Products* 76(6):1113–20. https://doi.org/10.1021/np400175b

González-Casanova, J. E., Pertuz-Cruz, S. L., Caicedo-Ortega, N. H., and Rojas-Gomez, D. M. 2020. Adipogenesis regulation and endocrine disruptors: Emerging insights in obesity. *BioMed Research International* 2020:7453786. https://doi.org/10.1155/2020/7453786

González-Santiago, M., Fonollá, J., and Lopez-Huertas, E. 2010. Human absorption of a supplement containing purified hydroxytyrosol, a natural antioxidant from olive oil, and evidence for its transient association with low-density lipoproteins. *Pharmacological Research* 61(4):364–70. https://doi.org/10.1016/j.phrs.2009.12.016

Gorzynik-Debicka, M., Przychodzen, P., Cappello, F., et al. 2018. Potential health benefits of olive oil and plant polyphenols. *International Journal of Molecular Sciences* 19(3):686. www.mdpi.com/1422-0067/19/3/686

Granados-Principal, S., Quiles, J. L., Ramirez-Tortosa, C., et al. 2011. Hydroxytyrosol inhibits growth and cell proliferation and promotes high expression of sfrp4 in rat mammary tumours. *Molecular Nutrition and Food Research* 55(S1):S117–S26. https://doi.org/10.1002/mnfr.201000220

Grawish, M. E., Zyada, M. M., and Zaher, A. R. 2011. Inhibition of 4-NQO-induced F433 rat tongue carcinogenesis by oleuropein-rich extract. *Medical Oncology* 28(4):1163–68. https://doi.org/10.1007/s12032-010-9612-2

Grewal, R., Reutzel, M., Dilberger, B., et al. 2020. Purified oleocanthal and ligstroside protect against mitochondrial dysfunction in models of early Alzheimer's disease and brain ageing. *Experimental Neurology* 328:113248. https://doi.org/10.1016/j.expneurol.2020.113248

Hidalgo, M., Prieto, I., Abriouel, H., et al. 2018. Changes in gut microbiota linked to a reduction in systolic blood pressure in spontaneously hypertensive rats fed an extra virgin olive oil-enriched diet. *Plant Foods for Human Nutrition* 73(1):1–6. https://doi.org/10.1007/s11130-017-0650-1

Hormozi, M., Salehi Marzijerani, A., and Baharvand, P. 2020. Effects of hydroxytyrosol on expression of apoptotic genes and activity of antioxidant enzymes in LS180 cells. *Cancer Management and Research* 12:7913–19. https://doi.org/10.2147/CMAR.S253591

Houston, M. 2018. The role of noninvasive cardiovascular testing, applied clinical nutrition and nutritional supplements in the prevention and treatment of coronary heart disease. *Therapeutic Advances in Cardiovascular Disease* 12(3):85–108. https://doi.org/10.1177/1753944717743920. https://doi.org/10.1080/21683565.2020.1825585. https://doi.org/10.3390/nu11112833

Hussein, O., Grosovski, M., Lasri, E., Svalb, S., Ravid, U., and Assy, N. 2007. Monounsaturated fat decreases hepatic lipid content in non-alcoholic fatty liver disease in rats. *World Journal of Gastroenterology* 13(3):361–8. https://doi.org/10.3748/wjg.v13.i3.361

Irimie, A. I., Braicu, C., Pasca, S., et al. 2019. Role of key micronutrients from nutrigenetic and nutrigenomic perspectives in cancer prevention. *Medicina* 55(6):283. https://doi.org/10.3390/medicina55060283

Ji, M., Gong, X., Li, X., Wang, C., and Li, M. 2020. Advanced research on the antioxidant activity and mechanism of polyphenols from *Hippophae* species – A review. *Molecules* 25(4):917. https://doi.org/10.3390/molecules25040917

Kerimi, A., Nyambe-Silavwe, H., Pyner, A., et al. 2019. Nutritional implications of olives and sugar: Attenuation of post-prandial glucose spikes in healthy volunteers by inhibition of sucrose hydrolysis and glucose transport by oleuropein. *European Journal of Nutrition* 58(3):1315–30. https://doi.org/10.1007/s00394-018-1662-1669

Khalili, A., Nekooeian, A. A., and Khosravi, M. B. 2017. Oleuropein improves glucose tolerance and lipid profile in rats with simultaneous renovascular hypertension and type 2 diabetes. *Journal of Asian Natural Products Research* 19(10):1011–21. https://doi.org/10.1080/10286020.2017.1307834

Kimura, Y., and Sumiyoshi, M. 2009. Olive leaf extract and its main component oleuropein prevent chronic ultraviolet B radiation-induced skin damage and carcinogenesis in hairless mice. *Journal of Nutrition* 139(11):2079–86. https://doi.org/10.3945/jn.109.104992

Kiritsakis, A. K., Kiritsakis, K. A., and Tsitsipas, C. K. 2020. A review of the evolution in the research of antioxidants in olives and olive oil during the last four decades. *Journal of Food Bioactives* 11:31–56. https://doi.org/10.31665/JFB.2020.11236

Klen, T. J., and Vodopivec, B. M. 2012. The fate of olive fruit phenols during commercial olive oil processing: Traditional press versus continuous two- and three-phase centrifuge. *LWT – Food Science and Technology* 49(2):267–74. https://doi.org/10.1016/j.lwt.2012.03.029

Klen, T. J., Wondra, A. G., Vrhovšek, U., Sivilotti, P., and Vodopivec, B. M. 2015. Olive fruit phenols transfer, transformation, and partition trail during laboratory-scale olive oil processing. *Journal of Agricultural and Food Chemistry* 63(18):4570–79. https://doi.org/10.1021/jf506353z

Kolluru, G. K., Shen, X., and Kevil, C. G. 2020. Reactive sulfur species. *Arteriosclerosis, Thrombosis, and Vascular Biology* 40(4):874–84. https://doi.org/10.1161/ATVBAHA.120.314084

Konstantinidou, V., Covas, M.-I., Muñoz-Aguayo, D., et al. 2010. *In vivo* nutrigenomic effects of virgin olive oil polyphenols within the frame of the Mediterranean diet: A randomized controlled trial. *FASEB Journal* 24(7):2546–57. https://doi.org/10.1096/fj.09-148452

Larussa, T., Imeneo, M., and Luzza, F. 2019. Olive tree biophenols in inflammatory bowel disease: When bitter is better. *International Journal of Molecular Sciences* 20(6):1390. https://doi.org/10.3390/ijms20061390

Larussa, T., Oliverio, M., Suraci, E., et al. 2017. Oleuropein decreases cyclooxygenase-2 and interleukin-17 expression and attenuates inflammatory damage in colonic samples from ulcerative colitis patients. *Nutrients* 9(4):391. https://doi.org/10.3390/nu9040391

Li, S., Han, Z., Ma, Y., et al. 2014. Hydroxytyrosol inhibits cholangiocarcinoma tumor growth: An *in vivo* and *in vitro* study. *Oncology Reports* 31(1):145–52. https://doi.org/10.3892/or.2013.2853

Liu, Z., Wang, N., Ma, Y., and Wen, D. 2019. Hydroxytyrosol improves obesity and insulin resistance by modulating gut microbiota in high-fat diet-induced obese mice. *Frontiers in Microbiology* 10(390):1–12. https://doi.org/10.3389/fmicb.2019.00390

López de Las Hazas, M.-C., Martin-Hernández, R., Crespo, M.-C., et al. 2019. Identification and validation of common molecular targets of hydroxytyrosol. *Food and Function* 10(8):4897–910. https://doi.org/10.1039/C9FO01159E

Lu, H. Y., Zhu, J. S., Zhang, Z., et al. 2019. Hydroxytyrosol and oleuropein inhibit migration and invasion of MDA-MB-231 triple-negative breast cancer cell via induction of autophagy. *Anti-Cancer Agents in Medicinal Chemistry* 19(16):1983–90. https://doi.org/10.2174/1871520619666190722101207

Luccarini, I., Grossi, C., Rigacci, S., et al. 2015. Oleuropein aglycone protects against pyroglutamylated-3 amyloid-ß toxicity: Biochemical, epigenetic and functional correlates. *Neurobiology of Aging* 36(2):648–63. https://doi.org/10.1016/j.neurobiolaging.2014.08.029

Marcelino, G., Hiane, P. A., Freitas, K. C., et al. 2019. Effects of olive oil and its minor components on cardiovascular diseases, inflammation, and gut microbiota. *Nutrients* 11(8):1826. www.mdpi.com/2072-6643/11/8/1826

Marrano, N., Spagnuolo, R., Biondi, G., et al. 2021. Effects of extra virgin olive oil polyphenols on beta-cell function and survival. *Plants* 10(2):286. https://doi.org/10.3390/plants10020286

Martínez-Martos, J. M., Mayas, M. D., Carrera, P., et al. 2014. Phenolic compounds oleuropein and hydroxytyrosol exert differential effects on glioma development via antioxidant defense systems. *Journal of Functional Foods* 11:221–34. https://doi.org/10.1016/j.jff.2014.09.006

Martín-Peláez, S., Castañer, O., Konstantinidou, V., et al. 2017. Effect of olive oil phenolic compounds on the expression of blood pressure-related genes in healthy individuals. *European Journal of Nutrition* 56(2):663–70. https://doi.org/10.1007/s00394-015-1110-z

Mateos, R., Sarria, B., and Bravo, L. 2020. Nutritional and other health properties of olive pomace oil. *Critical Reviews in Food Science and Nutrition* 60(20):3506–21. https://doi.org/10.1080/10408398.2019.1698005

Meza-Miranda, E. R., Rangel-Zúñiga, O. A., Marín, C., et al. 2016. Virgin olive oil rich in phenolic compounds modulates the expression of atherosclerosis-related genes in vascular endothelium. *European Journal of Nutrition* 55(2):519–27. https://doi.org/10.1007/s00394-015-0868-3

Milenkovic, D., Jude, B., and Morand, C. 2013. miRNA as molecular target of polyphenols underlying their biological effects. *Free Radical Biology and Medicine* 64:40–51. https://doi.org/10.1016/j.freeradbiomed.2013.05.046

Miro-Casas, E., Covas, M. I., Farre, M., et al. 2003. Hydroxytyrosol disposition in humans. *Clinical Chemistry* 49(6):945–52. https://doi.org/10.1373/49.6.945

Mitra, V., and Metcalf, J. 2012. Metabolic functions of the liver. *Anaesthesia and Intensive Care Medicine* 13(2):54–5. https://doi.org/10.1016/j.mpaic.2011.11.006

Mondragón-Rodríguez, S., Perry, G., and Peña-Ortega, F. 2017. Tau proteins. In: *Drug Discovery Approaches for the Treatment of Neurodegenerative Disorders*, ed. A. Adejare, 145–60. Academic Press, Amsterdam Holland.

Monti, M. C., Margarucci, L., Riccio, R., and Casapullo, A. 2012. Modulation of tau protein fibrillization by oleocanthal. *Journal of Natural Products* 75(9):1584–8. https://doi.org/10.1021/np300384h

Moreno-Luna, R., Muñoz-Hernandez, R., Miranda, M., et al. 2012. Olive oil polyphenols decrease blood pressure and improve endothelial function in young women with mild hypertension. *American Journal of Hypertension* 25(12):1299–304. https://doi.org/10.1038/ajh.2012.128

Nishida, M., Kumagai, Y., Ihara, H., Fujii, S., Motohashi, H., and Akaike, T. 2016. Redox signaling regulated by electrophiles and reactive sulfur species. *Journal of Clinical Biochemistry and Nutrition* 58(2):91–8. https://doi.org/10.3164/jcbn.15-111

Nocella, C., Cammisotto, V., Fianchini, L., et al. 2018. Extra virgin olive oil and cardiovascular diseases: Benefits for human health. *Endocrine, Metabolic and Immune Disorders* 18(1):4–13. https://doi.org/10.2174/1871530317666171114121533

Nunes, M. A., Costa, A. S. G., Bessada, S., et al. 2018. Olive pomace as a valuable source of bioactive compounds: A study regarding its lipid- and water-soluble components. *Science of the Total Environment* 644:229–36. https://doi.org/10.1016/j.scitotenv.2018.06.350

Nunes, M. A., Pimentel, F., Costa, A. S. G., Alves, R. C., and Oliveira, M. B. P. P. 2016. Cardioprotective properties of grape seed proanthocyanidins: An update. *Trends in Food Science and Technology* 57:31–9. https://doi.org/10.1016/j.tifs.2016.08.017

Olmo-García, L., Kessler, N., Neuweger, H., et al. 2018. Unravelling the distribution of secondary metabolites in *Olea europaea* L.: Exhaustive characterization of eight olive-tree derived matrices by complementary platforms (LC-ESI/APCI-MS and GC-APCI-MS). *Molecules* 23(10):2419. https://doi.org/10.3390/molecules23102419

Olson, K. R. 2020. Reactive oxygen species or reactive sulfur species: Why we should consider the latter. *The Journal of Experimental Biology* 223(4):jeb196352. https://doi.org/10.1242/jeb.196352

Ortega, F. J., Mercader, J. M., Catalán, V., et al. 2013. Targeting the circulating microRNA signature of obesity. *Clinical Chemistry* 59(5):781–92. https://doi.org/10.1373/clinchem.2012.195776

Pantano, D., Luccarini, I., Nardiello, P., Servili, M., Stefani, M., and Casamenti, F. 2017. Oleuropein aglycone and polyphenols from olive mill waste water ameliorate cognitive deficits and neuropathology. *British Journal of Clinical Pharmacology* 83(1):54–62. https://doi.org/10.1111/bcp.12993

Parenti, A., Spugnoli, P., Masella, P., and Calamai, L. 2008. The effect of malaxation temperature on the virgin olive oil phenolic profile under laboratory-scale conditions. *European Journal of Lipid Science and Technology* 110(8):735–41. https://doi.org/10.1002/ejlt.200700307

Peña-Romero, A. C., Navas-Carrillo, D., Marín, F., and Orenes-Piñero, E. 2018. The future of nutrition: Nutrigenomics and nutrigenetics in obesity and cardiovascular diseases. *Critical Reviews in Food Science and Nutrition* 58(17):3030–41. https://doi.org/10.1080/10408398.2017.1349731

Peralbo-Molina, Á., Priego-Capote, F., and Luque de Castro, M. D. 2012. Tentative identification of phenolic compounds in olive pomace extracts using liquid chromatography – tandem mass spectrometry with a quadrupole – quadrupole-time-of-flight mass

detector. *Journal of Agricultural and Food Chemistry* 60(46):11542–50. https://doi.org/10.1021/jf302896m
Peyrol, J., Riva, C., and Amiot, M. J. 2017. Hydroxytyrosol in the prevention of the metabolic syndrome and related disorders. *Nutrients* 9(3):306. https://doi.org/10.3390/nu9030306
Piroddi, M., Albini, A., Fabiani, R., et al. 2017. Nutrigenomics of extra-virgin olive oil: A review. *Biofactors* 43(1):17–41. https://doi.org/10.1002/biof.1318
Pirozzi, C., Lama, A., Simeoli, R., et al. 2016. Hydroxytyrosol prevents metabolic impairment reducing hepatic inflammation and restoring duodenal integrity in a rat model of NAFLD. *Journal of Nutritional Biochemistry* 30:108–15. https://doi.org/10.1016/j.jnutbio.2015.12.004
Poddar, M., Chetty, Y., and Chetty, V. T. 2017. How does obesity affect the endocrine system? A narrative review. *Clinical Obesity* 7(3):136–44. https://doi.org/10.1111/cob.12184
Priore, P., Cavallo, A., Gnoni, A., Damiano, F., Gnoni, G. V., and Siculella, L. 2015. Modulation of hepatic lipid metabolism by olive oil and its phenols in nonalcoholic fatty liver disease. *IUBMB Life* 67(1):9–17. https://doi.org/10.1002/iub.1340
Qin, C., Hu, S., Zhang, S., et al. 2021. Hydroxytyrosol acetate improves the cognitive function of APP/PS1 transgenic mice in ERβ-dependent manner. *Molecular Nutrition and Food Research* 65(3):e2000797. https://doi.org/10.1002/mnfr.202000797
Raubenheimer, D., and Simpson, S. J. 2016. Nutritional ecology and human health. *Annual Review of Nutrition* 36:603–26. https://doi.org/10.1146/annurev-nutr-071715-051118
Robles-Almazan, M., Pulido-Moran, M., Moreno-Fernandez, J., et al. 2018. Hydroxytyrosol: Bioavailability, toxicity, and clinical applications. *Food Research International* 105:654–67. https://doi.org/10.1016/j.foodres.2017.11.053
Rodis, P. S., Karathanos, V. T., and Mantzavinou, A. 2002. Partitioning of olive oil antioxidants between oil and water phases. *Journal of Agricultural and Food Chemistry* 50(3):596–601. https://doi.org/10.1021/jf010864j
Rodríguez-Lara, A., Mesa, M. D., Aragón-Vela, J., et al. 2019. Acute/subacute and sub-chronic oral toxicity of a hidroxytyrosol-rich virgin olive oil extract. *Nutrients* 11(9):2133. https://doi.org/10.3390/nu11092133
Rodríguez-López, P., Lozano-Sanchez, J., Borrás-Linares, I., Emanuelli, T., Menéndez, J. A., and Segura-Carretero, A. 2020. Structure – biological activity relationships of extra-virgin olive oil phenolic compounds: Health properties and bioavailability. *Antioxidants* 9(8):685. www.mdpi.com/2076-3921/9/8/685
Rodríguez-Morató, J., Boronat, A., Kotronoulas, A., et al. 2016. Metabolic disposition and biological significance of simple phenols of dietary origin: Hydroxytyrosol and tyrosol. *Drug Metabolism Reviews* 48(2):218–36. https://doi.org/10.1080/03602532.2016.1179754
Roselló-Soto, E., Koubaa, M., Moubarik, A., et al. 2015. Emerging opportunities for the effective valorization of wastes and by-products generated during olive oil production process: Non-conventional methods for the recovery of high-added value compounds. *Trends in Food Science and Technology* 45(2):296–310. https://doi.org/10.1016/j.tifs.2015.07.003
Saibandith, B., Spencer, J. P. E., Rowland, I. R., and Commane, D. M. 2017. Olive polyphenols and the metabolic syndrome. *Molecules* 22(7):1082. www.mdpi.com/1420-3049/22/7/1082
Sánchez-Fidalgo, S., Villegas, I., Aparicio-Soto, M., et al. 2015. Effects of dietary virgin olive oil polyphenols: Hydroxytyrosyl acetate and 3, 4-dihydroxyphenylglycol on DSS-induced acute colitis in mice. *Journal of Nutritional Biochemistry* 26(5):513–20. https://doi.org/10.1016/j.jnutbio.2014.12.001
Santangelo, C., Filesi, C., Varì, R., et al. 2016. Consumption of extra-virgin olive oil rich in phenolic compounds improves metabolic control in patients with type 2 diabetes mellitus: A possible involvement of reduced levels of circulating visfatin.

Journal of Endocrinological Investigation 39(11):1295–301. https://doi.org/10.1007/s40618-016-0506-9

Santos, M. M., Piccirillo, C., Castro, P. M. L., Kalogerakis, N., and Pintado, M. E. 2012. Bioconversion of oleuropein to hydroxytyrosol by lactic acid bacteria. *World Journal of Microbiology and Biotechnology* 28(6):2435–40. https://doi.org/10.1007/s11274-012-1036-z

Santos-Sánchez, N. F., Salas-Coronado, R., Villanueva-Cañongo, C., and Hernández-Carlos, B. 2019. Antioxidant compounds and their antioxidant mechanism. In: *Antioxidants*, ed. E. Shalaby, 1–28. IntechOpen, London. https://10.5772/intechopen.85270

Scoditti, E., Carpi, S., Massaro, M., et al. 2019. Hydroxytyrosol modulates adipocyte gene and miRNA expression under inflammatory condition. *Nutrients* 11(10):2493. Available from: www.mdpi.com/2072-6643/11/10/2493

Scotece, M., Conde, J., Abella, V., et al. 2018. Oleocanthal inhibits catabolic and inflammatory mediators in LPS-activated human primary osteoarthritis (OA) chondrocytes through MAPKs/NF-κB pathways. *Cellular Physiology and Biochemistry* 49(6):2414–26. https://doi.org/10.1159/000493840

Shahidi, F., and Peng, H. 2018. Bioaccessibility and bioavailability of phenolic compounds. *Journal of Food Bioactives* 4:11–68. https://doi.org/10.31665/JFB.2018.4162

Shamshoum, H., Vlavcheski, F., and Tsiani, E. 2017. Anticancer effects of oleuropein. *Biofactors* 43(4):517–28. https://doi.org/10.1002/biof.1366

Terzuoli, E., Donnini, S., Giachetti, A., et al. 2010. Inhibition of hypoxia inducible factor-1alpha by dihydroxyphenylethanol, a product from olive oil, blocks microsomal prostaglandin-E synthase-1/vascular endothelial growth factor expression and reduces tumor angiogenesis. *Clinical Cancer Research* 16(16):4207–16. https://doi.org/10.1158/1078-0432.Ccr-10-0156

Torić, J., Marković, A. K., Brala, C. J., and Barbarić, M. 2019. Anticancer effects of olive oil polyphenols and their combinations with anticancer drugs. *Acta Pharmaceutica* 69(4):461–82. https://doi.org/10.2478/acph-2019-0052

Vezza, T., Rodríguez-Nogales, A., Algieri, F., et al. 2019. The metabolic and vascular protective effects of olive (*Olea europaea* L.) leaf extract in diet-induced obesity in mice are related to the amelioration of gut microbiota dysbiosis and to its immunomodulatory properties. *Pharmacological Research* 150:104487. https://doi.org/10.1016/j.phrs.2019.104487

Visioli, F., Davalos, A., López de Las Hazas, M.-C., Crespo, M. C., and Tomé-Carneiro, J. 2020. An overview of the pharmacology of olive oil and its active ingredients. *British Journal of Pharmacology* 177(6):1316–1330. https://doi.org/10.1111/bph.14782

Višnjevec, A. M., Baker, P., Charlton, A., et al. 2021. Developing an olive biorefinery in Slovenia: Analysis of phenolic compounds found in olive mill pomace and wastewater. *Molecules* 26(1):7. www.mdpi.com/1420-3049/26/1/7

Vissers, M. N., Zock, P. L., and Katan, M. B. 2004. Bioavailability and antioxidant effects of olive oil phenols in humans: A review. *European Journal of Clinical Nutrition* 58(6):955–65. https://doi.org/10.1038/sj.ejcn.1601917

Wadey, R. M., Connolly, K. D., Mathew, D., Walters, G., Rees, D. A., and James, P. E. 2019. Inflammatory adipocyte-derived extracellular vesicles promote leukocyte attachment to vascular endothelial cells. *Atherosclerosis* 283:19–27. https://doi.org/10.1016/j.atherosclerosis.2019.01.013

Wang, N., Ma, Y., Liu, Z., et al. 2019. Hydroxytyrosol prevents PM2.5-induced adiposity and insulin resistance by restraining oxidative stress related NF-κB pathway and modulation of gut microbiota in a murine model. *Free Radical Biology and Medicine* 141:393–407. https://doi.org/10.1016/j.freeradbiomed.2019.07.002

Winterbourn, C. C. 2020. Biological chemistry of superoxide radicals. *ChemTexts* 6(1):7. https://doi.org/10.1007/s40828-019-0101-8

Zhang, X., Cao, J., and Zhong, L. 2009. Hydroxytyrosol inhibits pro-inflammatory cytokines, iNOS, and COX-2 expression in human monocytic cells. *Naunyn-Schmiedeberg's Archives of Pharmacology* 379(6):581–6. https://doi.org/10.1007/s00210-009-0399-7

Zhi, L. Q., Yao, S. X., Liu, H. L., Li, M., Duan, N., and Ma, J. B. 2018. Hydroxytyrosol inhibits the inflammatory response of osteoarthritis chondrocytes via SIRT6-mediated autophagy. *Molecular Medicine Reports* 17(3):4035–42. https://doi.org/10.3892/mmr.2017.8353

11 Metabolomic Approach

Specific Markers for Authenticity, Nutritional Safety, and Quality of Milk and Milk Products

*Richa Singh**, *Ravali Parvartam, and Sumit Arora*

CONTENTS

11.1 INTRODUCTION

Global livestock production accounts for 40% of total agricultural gross domestic product (GDP) in developed countries and 20% of total agricultural GDP in developing countries and supports the livelihood of at least 1.3 billion people. The global demand for livestock products (milk and meat) is expected to increase by 70% around the year 2050 since the world's population is expected to reach 9.6 billion people (Food and Agriculture Organization 2021). Milk, a liquid product produced by mammary glands, is rich in lactose, proteins, lipids, vitamins, minerals, and bio-functional molecules (e.g., peptides, oligosaccharides, and immunoglobulins) (Sundekilde et al. 2013). Milk is a livestock product, which is primarily consumed by all age groups. The nutrients in milk vary with breed, feed, stage of lactation, season, health of the animal, and processing of milk (Walker et al. 2004; Elgersma et al. 2006; Garnsworthy et al. 2006). These factors may have remarkable quantitative effects on milk nutrients, as well as on the physical and technological properties (heat

* Corresponding author email: richasingh.ndri@gmail.com

DOI: 10.1201/9781003142195-11

stability, coagulation properties, and fermentation quality) of the milk. Therefore, information regarding the chemical composition of milk and milk products is important for understanding their nutritional and technological properties.

Metabolites are low molecular biomolecules (50–1,500 Da) (Fiehn 2002) that are the intermediates and end products of cellular metabolism (Lu and Thompson 2012). In milk, metabolites often reflect metabolic activity in the mammary glands, where several pathways and mechanisms are in place to transport compounds across the cell membrane for the synthesis of milk components. Major metabolic pathways in the mammary gland are gluconeogenesis, lipogenesis, pyruvate metabolism, urea, and tricarboxylic acid (TCA) cycle (Silanikove et al. 2014). In special cases like disease, stress paracellular pathways are also open that may change the metabolic profile markedly (McManaman and Neville 2003). Around 75% of the metabolites are shared between the mammary gland and milk, and not all the compounds in milk are metabolites as some do not originate from cellular metabolism (Sundekilde et al. 2011). Some metabolites may also be secreted by microorganisms present in raw milk, from somatic cells, or some may be originating from enzymatic reactions occurring in milk (Hettinga et al. 2009).

Metabolomics is an analytical profiling method used for measuring and comparing large numbers of metabolites found in biological samples. Metabolomics provides an insight in the metabolic pathways as high-throughput analytical chemistry techniques (LC-MS/MS, NMR, GC-MS) are combined with multivariate data processing. The term "metabolic profiling" was first used during the analysis of human urine sample (Horning and Horning 1971), and the word "metabolome" was first coined in 1998 (Oliver et al. 1998). Metabolomics is majorly used as a technology to understand the metabolism and physiology of living systems (microorganisms, plants, animals, and humans) and in biomedical research (for biomarker discovery and disease mechanism research), crop characterization in agriculture science (where metabolomics is commonly used in crop trait selection), pesticide monitoring, crop breeding, and crop evaluation (Simó et al. 2014; Sumner et al. 2015). However, the technique also has a potential for application in food systems; it allows for the assessment of the quality of food resources (affected by environment and genetic factors), is useful in determining authenticity and traceability (depending upon geographical origin), and investigates changes caused by climatic and seasonal factors that otherwise are difficult to ascertain by using conventional analytical techniques unless a major change has occurred (Bernillon et al. 2013; Li et al. 2017). Metabolite analysis offers an advantage over conventional methods as it has the ability to detect metabolites, each belonging to a different class simultaneously, which offers an opportunity to derive different interpretations per requirement. Milk contains approximately 223 metabolites (Boudonck et al. 2009) belonging to chemically diverse compounds such as lipids, organic acids, carbohydrates, amino acids, nitrogenous compounds, etc. These metabolites depend on the species, breed of animal, conditions, stage of lactation, and feeding practices and also on the processing of milk and milk products (Sundekilde et al. 2013). The variability among metabolites can help in monitoring the technological and nutritional quality of milk and milk products and also identify specific markers for predicting its authenticity and nutritional quality. It can also be used to study the metabolic characteristics of food resources in relation to

TABLE 11.1
General Applications of Metabolomics

Area	Application	References
Genomics	To map genotypic changes in terms of quantifiable metabolic outputs	Fernie et al. 2004
Personalized medicine	To classify hundreds of metabolites, allowing for disease detection at an early stage	Lindon et al. 2006; Vinayavekhin and Saghatelian 2010; Wishart 2016
Physiology	To assess the physiological effects of metabolites on health	Blow 2008; Kim et al. 2016; Carneiro et al. 2019
Biomarker	To distinguish between two groups of samples and also identify and quantify metabolites associated with disease and its symptoms	Lindon et al. 2006; Lewis et al. 2008; Carneiro et al. 2019
Agriculture	To study complex biochemistry at various stages of plant growth	Saito et al. 2006; Nadella et al. 2012; Tian et al. 2016
Animal science	To diagnose disease and animal health, heat stress, maintenance, and regulation of lactation	Tian et al. 2016; Blakebrough-Hall et al. 2020; Stella et al. 2021
Food science	To identify geographical origin, discriminate growth-promoter-treated and genetically modified food, and monitor food processing, food safety, and food packaging	Martínez-Hernández et al. 2016; Creydt et al. 2018; Cubero-Leon et al. 2018

environmental and genetic factors, thus allowing the evaluation of food quality. The study of metabolites appears to be a very fascinating, but the major challenge arises due to the complexity of metabolome; however, recent developments in analytical chemistry and metabolite data analysis methods have opened up metabolomics to a broader range of research disciplines (Table 11.1).

11.2 DIFFERENT ANALYTICAL TOOLS TO ANALYZE METABOLITES

The diverse application of metabolites, good experimental design, and methods are essential to achieve high-quality results. Metabolomic studies involve a large number of samples, necessitating high-throughput analytical methods that are fast, repeatable, and stable over time. Analytical techniques such as NMR spectroscopy, liquid chromatography–mass spectrometry (LC-MS), gas chromatography–mass spectrometry (GC-MS), and ultra-performance liquid chromatography – quadrupole time-of-flight mass spectrometry (UPLC-QTOFMS) have already proven to be effective in ensuring food quality and protection (Sundekilde et al. 2013). NMR is the most powerful and non-destructive technique used in identifying milk metabolites with minimal sample preparation, but the sensitivity is lower than MS-based metabolomic techniques. The MS-based metabolomic techniques (LC-MS and GC-MS) offer advantages of high speed and sensitivity (Emwas 2015) but also suffer from disadvantages, like lack of well-established and standardized methods, problems encountered in identifying metabolites due to their complexity and chemical diversity, variation in detection of trace-level metabolites, and limitations of available software in processing huge data of metabolomics with unknown compositions (Sampson et al. 2013). Furthermore, the polarity of metabolites also plays a role in their identification by LC-MS or GC-MS. GC-MS is mostly used for hydrophilic, apolar and volatile metabolites. Derivatization is an important prerequisite in analyzing polar compounds using GC-MS. LC-MS is gaining popularity as it can process both apolar and polar compounds with minimal sample preparation; however, for small and highly polar compounds, specific columns are required (Courant et al. 2014).

Targeted (selective) and untargeted metabolomic approaches can both be used in milk metabolite profiling. The untargeted approach is used to detect as many metabolites as possible without prejudice from a variety of biological samples. This method is globally used when no specific metabolites are targeted in the biological sample. In this approach, metabolite detection is highly dependent upon the method of data acquisition. However, in the targeted approach quantification of a particular collection of metabolites is carried out to address a specific biochemical query. This can be a particular metabolite, an individual metabolic pathway or even a collection of pathways. Unlike the untargeted approach, absolute recovery and quantification accuracy are of great importance in this approach. Extraction and acquisition methods may be altered in order to preferentially detect certain metabolites and remove interference from less-important metabolites. Since it is focused, generally fewer replicates of samples are required than for the untargeted approach (Shulaev 2006).

Raw data processing in metabolomics is perhaps the most complex and time-consuming stage in data analysis. Noise reduction, spectrum deconvolution, peak detection, integration, chromatogram alignment, and compound recognition and quantification are all standard steps in the processing of a collection of raw chromatograms (Shulaev 2006). Without the right statistical and visualization methods, metabolomics generates complex data tables that are difficult to summarize and interpret (Wiklund et al. 2008). Principal component analysis (PCA), partial least-squares (PLS), and orthogonal PLS (OPLS) are important chemometric tools since they provide effective and robust methods for the modeling, analysis, and interpretation of complex chemical and biological data (Sundekilde et al. 2013).

11.3 OVERVIEW OF METABOLOMIC RESEARCH IN DAIRY

The technique of recognizing metabolites in biofluids has a long history. Sweet-tasting urine was discovered to be an indicator of disease in ancient China, later known as diabetes. Roger Williams proposed in the late 1940s that each person has a "metabolic activity" that is expressed in their body fluids. There has been a revolution in techniques and approaches used in molecular biology over the past decade. Progress in technology and resources has led to simultaneous measurement of a number of metabolites, each belonging to a different class. This has enabled metabolomics to elucidate different metabolic pathways aimed at answering different questions (Smith et al. 2020). The definition and techniques of metabolomics were first used in the field of cancer research (Spratlin et al. 2009), where they proved to be extremely useful in identifying biomarkers of specific carcinogenic pathways. These have been investigated and incorporated into diagnostic and therapeutic processes. Metabolomic studies have recently become increasingly popular in the fields of nutrition sciences, food matrices, and dairy cattle research since food systems have a direct impact on human nutrition and health. Analysis of metabolomics can help in obtaining the metabolic fingerprint of individual animals and identify functionally important metabolites that serve as biomarker candidates (Sun et al. 2017). Milk metabolomes represent the metabolism of cows and offer new animal health predictors (Melzer et al. 2013). It may be possible to apply new management or breeding techniques to dairy farming if specific milk metabolites essential to cow or human health can be established and further delineated as to how and why they are present in milk. Metabolomics also helps in correlating milk metabolites with microbiome, which may result in the detection and prevention of diseases so as to increase the production, quality and safety of milk products (Tong et al. 2019).

Understanding the relation between milk metabolites and technological properties can also lead to the manufacture of milk products with better shelf life. Sundekilde et al. (2011) reported the association of milk metabolites with coagulation properties in bovine milk and showed that choline (positively), carnitine, citrate, and lactose (negatively) were associated with coagulation properties of milk.

Lu et al. (2013) used metabolomics and proteomics to gain a deeper understanding of the mammary physiology of cows in negative energy balance (NEB). Dairy cows enter and stay in a negative energy balance throughout the early lactation period as their feed intake cannot sustain the energy required for body maintenance and sudden demands for milk production, a condition that is linked to a variety of metabolic diseases. Cows recover positive energy balance when their feed consumption can once again meet their energy needs (Sundekilde et al. 2011). Hence, milk's metabolic profiles can potentially be of interest as indicators for energy balance in lactating dairy cows and also reveal variation in metabolite profile in milk during early and late lactation.

Furthermore, metabolomics can be used in conjunction with genomics to identify complex animal characteristics and to investigate the metabolite profile of milk with genetic variability. While genomics and transcriptomics recognize genes and pathways essential in specific processes, proteomics integrates knowledge of protein function and structure (Burtis and Bruns 2014). Understanding milk synthesis and its relationship with the metabolic status of the animal is a complex concept; hence, metabolomics can provide the missing link. Unlike other omics techniques, metabolomics directly represents the physiological status, biochemical activity, and condition of cells or tissues; thus, it can be a strong and effective method for studying the metabolism and physiology of living organisms stimulated by environmental changes (Tian et al. 2015; Nie et al. 2016). Metabolomics can be used to classify disease biomarkers, investigate unknown metabolic pathways and stress tolerance mechanisms, and grow microbial strains in a variety of living systems (Zhang et al. 2012; Fontanesi 2016). This unique aspect of metabolomics among the omics technologies can measure metabolites providing a retrospective and wide-ranging account of the biological processes that have occurred within an individual and may be relevant to health and disease status. As a consequence, metabolome has been regarded as the best descriptor of physiological phenomena (Blow 2008). A metabolomic technique can be a powerful tool for elucidating changes in phenotype induced by any perturbations, such as gene alteration, environmental influences, and physical stress (Fiehn et al. 2015). However, there are different challenges associated with metabolomic analysis. One of the major challenges is to interpret MS data since it is difficult to discriminate metabolites with similar chemical characteristics. After identification, further correlation of metabolites with a specific pathway is difficult as many metabolites are the products or substrates of a variety of activities and thus take part in multiple pathways. Therefore, pinpointing a metabolite to a specific pathway is tricky. Another challenge after the identification of a metabolite is to establish reproducible quantification (Lindon et al. 2006). It is evident from the literature that blood, urine, and milk can be used as a start material to analyze the metabolic profile. Among all, milk can be considered to be the most appropriate biological fluid for the analysis of metabolites due to its easy and regular collection. The most challenging part of metabolomic analysis of milk and milk products is to prevent variation in the samples. As milk is perishable, collection, preparation, and storing of samples play a vital role in the analysis as any mishandling may lead to changes in the metabolite profile of milk. Table 11.2 summarizes a few of the applications of metabolomics in dairy research.

TABLE 11.2
Applications of Metabolomics in Dairy Research

Application	Details	References
Energy balance	To identify metabolites that help in estimating energy balance	Klein et al. 2012; Lu et al. 2013; Xu et al. 2018, 2020
Health of animal	To enhance the detection and prevention of diseases	Melzer et al. 2013; Sundekilde et al. 2013; Tong et al. 2019
Technological properties	To associate milk metabolites with coagulation properties	Sundekilde et al. 2011, 2013, 2014; Caboni et al. 2019
Authentication	To indentify milk adulteration, maintain quality control, and trace and control geographical origin	Boudonck et al. 2009; Scano et al. 2014; Pisano et al. 2016; Sun et al. 2017; Salzano et al. 2020
Composition of milk	To study the correlation between characteristics and metabolites in milk	Melzer et al. 2013

11.4 METABOLOMIC APPROACH FOR AUTHENTICITY OF MILK AND MILK PRODUCTS

The quality, authenticity, and traceability of food products have become important for the protection of global food systems, especially to those foods that have a high price and demand among consumers (Danezis et al. 2016; Pustjens et al. 2016). The high price of these foods makes them susceptible to substitution with falsely labeled, non-authentic foods (De La Fuente et al. 2005). Milk, being a perishable product with high price and demand, is usually susceptible to adulteration. The market value of milk and dairy products is associated with the origin, species, and composition of the milk used (Brescia et al. 2005). Milk produced from cows, buffalo, goats, sheep, and other species is processed into various dairy products of different qualities and commercial values.

Different breeds of animals have biochemical heterogeneity, which may result into different biochemical and metabolic profiles. This can be used to authenticate the source of milk based on the identification of possible markers for a specific type of milk. However, identifying the specific marker based on the difference in species is difficult as the difference in metabolites may also differ due to the difference in age, stage of lactation, feeding practices, and processing of milk (McJarrow and van Amelsfort-Schoonbeek 2004; Elgersma et al. 2006; Arnould and Soyeurt 2009; Åkerstedt et al. 2011; Sundekilde et al. 2011). Metabolomics can also be used to detect milk adulteration (Santos et al. 2013). A few metabolomic studies have established markers for distinguishing milk types, milk origin, and farming methods (Sundekilde et al. 2013).

Boudonck et al. (2009) observed biochemical variability of bovine milk obtained after conventional (grain-based fodder containing cereal, maize, and protein supplements) and organic (fed on a diet consisting of fresh grass and clover) feeding. They further reported that different metabolites (e.g., tyrosine, isoleucine, mannose, glycerate, ribose, carnitine, butyrylcarnitine, and hippurate) were present in higher a concentration in the milk of animals fed on an organic diet; however, proline, 4-hydroxyproline, glucose-1-phosphate, ribose-5-phosphate, glycerol-3-phosphate, and glycerol-2-phosphate were present in a lower concentration.

Mazzei and Piccolo (2012) reported NMR-based metabolomics to assess the authenticity of Italian mozzarella cheese prepared with buffalo milk. The trademark Mozzarella di Buffalo Campana (MBC) is used for cheese made in the Campana region of Italy from buffalo milk and is known for its typical organoleptic properties. NMR coupled with PCA analysis has been successfully applied to assess the authenticity of MBC based on the presence of four metabolites β-galactose, β-lactose, acetic acid, and glycerol.

Scano et al. (2014) characterized the metabolic profile of caprine (goat) and bovine milk using GC-MS and reported that valine and glycine metabolites were found to be specific to goat milk and talose and malic acid metabolites were specific to cow milk.

Sun et al. (2015) performed GC-MS-based metabolomics to elucidate the impact of forage quality on milk production with a special focus on milk protein yield and found eight different metabolites in animals fed with alfalfa hay (AH) and corn stover (CS). These metabolites were involved in glycine, serine, and threonine metabolism, tyrosine metabolism, and phenylalanine metabolism. It was shown that AH-fed animals have higher amino-acid metabolism than CS-fed animals.

Yang et al. (2016) characterized the metabolite profile of dairy animals (Holstein, Jersey cow, buffalo, goat, and camel milk) by using NMR and LC-MS/MS. They reported that choline and citrate metabolites could differentiate milk from Holstein and Jersey cow; choline was higher in Holstein milk, and citrate was relatively higher in Jersey milk. Metabolites like leucine, valine, and pyruvate were higher in Holstein milk than Jersey, buffalo, and goat milk. These metabolites are responsible for milk protein synthesis. They further reported that oleic, linoleic, and α-linolenic acid were higher in camel milk than cow, buffalo, and goat milk, which may be associated with biohydrogenation of fat in ruminants.

Li et al. (2017) used NMR-based metabolomics for differentiating intermixing of bovine, goat, and soy milk. They reported ten different metabolites – carnitine, N-acetyl carbohydrate, acetate, choline, ethanolamine, citrate, creatine, lecithin, lactose, and sucrose – that can be used to detect intermixing of different types of milk. The limit of quantification was reported to be 2% for adulteration of soy milk in bovine milk, 2% soy milk in goat milk, and 5% bovine milk in goat milk.

Salzano et al. (2020) compared metabolomics of unprocessed buffalo milk and mozzarella cheese made from the same buffalo milk in PDO (European Union protected designation of origin, which has geographical indication) and non-PDO origin in Italy using GC-MS. They reported that unprocessed buffalo milk from PDO origin has a lower concentration of galactopyranoside, hydroxybutyric acid, allose, citric acid metabolites, and buffalo milk from non-PDO origin has a lower concentration of talopyranose, pantothenic acid, and mannobiose. The mozzarella cheese made from PDO origin milk samples had a higher concentration of metabolites, like talopyranose, 2,3-dihydroxypropyl icosanoate, and so on, while non-PDO samples had a higher concentration of tagatose, lactic acid dimer, ribitol. Figure 11.1 represents the major metabolites found in milk and cheese of PDO and non-PDO origin.

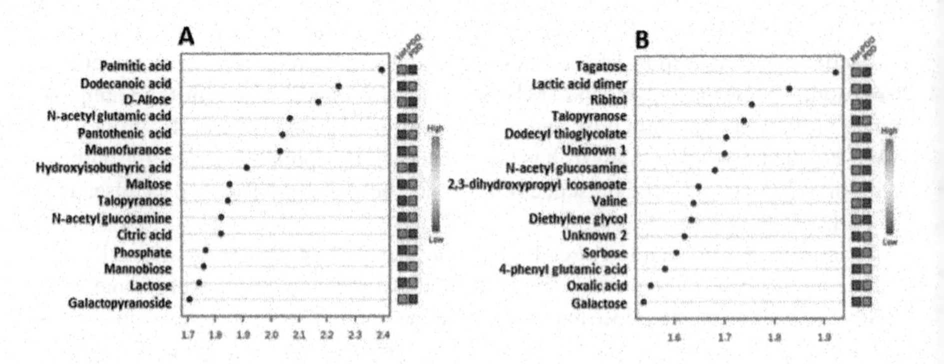

FIGURE 11.1 Major metabolites found in milk (A) and mozzarella cheese (B) samples of PDO and non-PDO origin. The shaded boxes on the right indicate the relative amount of the corresponding metabolite. (Adapted from Salzano et al. 2020.)

The difference in metabolite profile of milk from breeds of different geographical origin arise due to difference in breed, environment, and feeding practices followed, which will contribute toward authentication of milk and milk products. In metabolite profiling, a specific biomarker or an indicator in the product is determined to identify the origin. The metabolite profile may also help in understanding the technological properties of milk from different breeds of animals so that milk from specific breeds with desirable characteristics can be chosen for the production of particular dairy products.

Metabolomics can thus work as a useful and important tool to characterize and verify the authenticity of food items since a variety of metabolites can be detected and quantified (Cevallos-Cevallos et al. 2009; Marincola et al. 2012; Piras et al. 2013; Scano et al. 2014). Although there are strict guidelines and regulatory requirements for product classification, the metabolite profile is not always realistic ways to judge product authenticity. However, metabolite profiling can be used in conjunction with conventional methods to avoid food adulteration (Pinu 2016) and to assess the ability to distinguish between genuine and adulterated foods (Hou et al. 2015). Metabolomics can also recognize a molecular fingerprint that reliably describes the food product in all of its aspects and can also differentiate between genuine and fake varieties (Lindon et al. 2011).

11.5 METABOLOMIC APPROACH FOR NUTRITIONAL SAFETY AND QUALITY OF MILK AND MILK PRODUCTS

As already mentioned, milk composition is influenced by a range of different factors (genetic and processing factors), and these factors may have remarkable effects on the quality and nutritional safety of milk and milk products. The variability in metabolite profiles of processed milk occurs as it is subjected to various heat treatments and processing operations, such as cooling, heating, homogenization, separation, clarification, and packaging, all of which affect its commercial value and quality. Further, milk is converted into different products, and all these treatments may alter the overall metabolite composition of milk (Sundekilde et al. 2013). The microbial susceptibility also affects the metabolite profile.

Coagulation properties, such as rennet coagulation or curd syneresis, heat stability of milk, and milk fermentation consistency, are critical for the dairy industry in manufacturing different products (e.g., cheese, yogurt, ice cream, evaporated and powdered milk). Milk proteins, especially caseins, have a significant impact on the coagulation properties of curd. Sundekilde et al. (2011) reported that choline, carnitine, citrate, and lactose are essential metabolites that influence the coagulation properties of milk. Therefore, the identification of metabolites in milk can be correlated with different technological properties, which can further be used as biomarkers for detecting the quality and nutritional safety of milk and milk products.

Sundekilde et al. (2011) conducted the NMR metabolic profiling of milk from two different bovine breeds and investigated its relationship with coagulation properties. They further reported that carnitine and lactose are metabolites that are responsible for the difference in two breeds, whereas metabolites responsible for the difference in coagulation properties are citrate, choline, carnitine, and lactose.

Harzia et al. (2012) correlated the coagulation property of milk and milk metabolites measured through LC-MS/MS. Several marker ions responsible for differential coagulation were found, and the most significant differences were found for carnitine and oligosaccharides.

Melzer et al. (2013) analyzed milk metabolites of Holstein cows to characterize the relationship between metabolites with somatic cell count, quantity, the energy content of milk, and its composition (fat, saturated and unsaturated fatty acids, protein, casein, urea, lactose, pH, etc.). The somatic cell counts were predicted with the highest (78%) mean value of predicted precision followed by casein and protein (60%). Mean prediction precision was observed between 17 and 41% for others traits (quantity, energy content, abovementioned compositional parameters, except casein and protein). The most important metabolites identified with important compositional parameters of milk are listed in Table 11.3.

Xi et al. (2017) investigated metabolites in the milk of healthy cows and subclinical and clinical mastitis cows and found a significant difference in some metabolites. In the milk of cows with clinical mastitis, there was a lower concentration of glucose, d-glycerol-1-phosphate, 4-hydroxyphenyllactate, l-carnitine, sn-glycero-3-phosphocholine, citrate, and hippurate, and in the milk of cows of subclinical mastitis, a lower concentration of d-glycerol-1-phosphate, benzoic acid, l-carnitine, and cis-aconitate was found in comparison to milk from healthy animals. The concentration

TABLE 11.3
Important Metabolites Identified Related to Compositional Parameters of Milk

Compositional parameter	Metabolites
Protein	myo-inositol-1-phosphate; phosphoenolpyruvic acid; pyroglutamic acid; spermidine; thiazole, 4-methyl-5-hydroxyethyl-thiazole
Casein	2-piperidinecarboxylic acid; adipic acid, 2-amino-; alanine; arabitol; asparagine; aspartic acid; butanoic acid, 2-amino-; cinnamic acid, 3,4,5-trimethoxy-, trans-; glycerol-3-phosphate; myo-inositol-1-phosphate; phosphoenolpyruvic acid; pyroglutamic acid; spermidine; 4-methyl-5-hydroxyethyl-thiazole
Fat	1,3-dihydroxyaceton; arabitol; aspartic acid; galactitol; glucaric acid-1,4-lactone; myo-inositol-1-phosphate; pyroglutamic acid
Short-chain fatty acid	1,3-dihydroxyacetone; glycerol
Unsaturated fatty acids	galactitol; serine
Lactose	1,3-dihydroxyacetone; glucaric acid-1,4-lactone; leucine; methionine; phenylalanine; tyrosine

Source: Melzer et al. 2013.

of arginine and leucine was found to increase in the milk of both clinical and subclinical mastitis groups.

Zhang et al. (2018) differentiated milk on the basis of heat processing (raw, pasteurized, and UHT) using LC-MS-based metabolomics and identified biomarkers as 9-hydroxydecanoic acid, 12-hydroxydodecanoic acid, 2-hydroxymyristic acid, 3-hydroxytetradecanoic acid, 5-hydroxyeicosatetraenoic acid, 3-hydroxyhexadecanoic acid, 10-hydroxyoctadecanoic acid, and lysophosphatidylethanolamine.

Caboni et al. (2019) used GC-MS-based metabolomics to differentiate the quality of cheese made from raw and thermized ovine milk. The macro-compositional parameters of cheese and free fatty acids were not able to provide evidence regarding the effect of thermization due to the predominant effect of milk seasonality and ripening of cheese. However, cheese produced from raw and the thermized milk has shown great differences at the metabolite level, particularly with regard to free amino acids and saccharides.

One specific challenge these days is to monitor the labeling claims on high-quality dairy products. The NMR-spectroscopy-based metabolomics has been used to measure lactose content in different milks to verify labeling in relation to milk nutrition and composition (Monakhova et al. 2012).

Somatic cell count (SCC) is another parameter related to milk quality and can indicate mastitis inflammation, both subclinical and clinical. As different bacteria have been shown to increase unique milk metabolites, somatic cells present in milk have an effect on the metabolome, as different somatic cell types can release different metabolites into the milk. Udder health and physiology, milk production and its efficiency, and dairy sustainability are all affected by changes in bacterial diversity and abundance (Firkins and Yu 2006; Mansor et al. 2013; Yang et al. 2016). Tong et al. (2019) studied the relation between the microbiota associated with bovine mammary glands and their health. They reported a relationship between milk quality and the presence of spoilage bacteria. The study of these bacteria could reveal how variations in milk synthesis between healthy cows and those with subclinical mastitis are related to changes in milk metabolomic profiles.

Sundekilde et al. (2013) reported that β-hydroxybutyric acid (BHBA), butyrate, and isoleucine were found in higher concentrations in milk with higher SCC, while fumarate and hippurate were found in lower concentrations in milk with higher SCC. Rollin et al. (2015) identified acetate, lactose, and lactate metabolites as biomarkers of elevated SCC, which further can be correlated with mastitis.

Sundekilde et al. (2014) analyzed the correlation between milk metabolites and its rennet coagulation ability. They reported that lactate, acetate, glutamate, creatinine, choline, carnitine, galactose 1-phosphate, and glycerophosphocholine were significantly different in non-coagulating milk and well-coagulating milk.

Chemical contaminants and foodborne pathogens have also been identified using metabolomics in dairy products (Tengstrand et al. 2013; Layne et al. 2014). Foodborne pathogens, such as *E. coli* O157:H7, *Salmonella typhimurium*, *Salmonella muenchen*, *Salmonella hartford*, and *Listeria* in milk and milk products must be detected quickly and reliably to prevent foodborne outbreaks and product recalls (Cevallos-Cevallos et al. 2009; Beale et al. 2014; Jadhav et al. 2015).

Aside from technical and microbial properties, there have been breeding programs in place to actively enhance milk production. Currently, breeding programs are focused on enhancing total fat and protein content in milk, with a strong incentive to increase milk quality through selective breeding. Thus, utilizing metabolomics to study the chemical variability of milk is important for defining new alternative breeding targets. Only a few large-scale metabolomic studies regarding metabolite profiles of milk from individual cows have been performed to date. Investigations of milk metabolites combined with genetic analyses could pave the way for a better understanding of new quality parameters that can be improved by breeding strategies. Biofilm formation is another big issue in the dairy industry since it has been linked to several foodborne outbreaks. Metabolomics can be used to evaluate and understand the metabolic processes in bacterial biofilms, as well as to prevent the development of bacterial biofilms linked to foodborne outbreaks. This may also help to develop new drugs and therapies for biofilm-related diseases.

From the above discussion, it is evident that in recent years, significant research has been carried out in milk metabolomics for its application as a tool for assessing milk quality and authenticity. Different techniques like NMR, GC-MS, and LC-MS are used for determining metabolites in milk and milk products. Table 11.4 describes the application of different techniques used in milk metabolomics.

TABLE 11.4
Application of Different Techniques in Milk Metabolomics and Their Significant Findings

Analytical techniques used in metabolomics	Findings	Reference
Ultra-fast LC-triple TOF-MS and ^{1}H-NMR with PCA, and OPLS-DA	Effect of heat stress on milk metabolites	Tian et al. 2016
GC-MS with PCA, PLS-DA, and OPLS-DA	Metabolomic differences between buffalo and cow mozzarella cheese	Pisano et al. 2016
UHPLC-QTOF-MS with PCA, PLS-DA	Amino-acid metabolite difference between commercially available and traditional cheese	Pan et al. 2018
^{1}H NMR	Effect of feeding on unsaturated lipid and phospholipid content	Mazzei and Piccolo 2012
^{1}H-NMR with PLS-DA	Effect of feeding on milk metabolites	O'Callaghan et al. 2018
^{1}H-NMR with PCA and PLS	Relation of milk metabolites with seasonal variations and feeding	Tenori et al. 2018
UHPLC-QTOF-MS with PCA and OPLS-DA	Discrimination between PDO and non-PDO Grana Padano cheeses	Rocchetti et al. 2018
^{1}H-NMR with PCA and PLS-DA	Difference in metabolites with change in feeding and ripening stage	Boiani et al. 2019

TABLE 11.4 (CONTINUED)

Analytical techniques used in metabolomics	Findings	Reference
LC-QTRAP-MS/MS with PLS-DA	Effect of bovine diet on the metabolomic profile of skim milk and whey protein ingredients	Magan et al. 2019
^{1}H-NMR with PLS-DA	Difference in milk metabolites of Friesian and indigenous breeds of northern Italy	Tomassini et al. 2019
LC-MS and ^{1}H NMR with Pearson's correlations	Energy balance of a cow is corelated with the yield of fat, choline, ethanolamine, fucose, etc., in milk	Xu et al. 2020
UHPLC-QTOF-MS with PCA	Changes in metabolites of milk and yogurt samples as a result of processing	Gauglitz et al. 2020
UHPLC-QTOF-MS with OPLS-DA	Effect of feeding on milk metabolites	Rocchetti et al. 2020
GC-MS with PCA and OPLS-DA	Effect of feeding on ovine milk metabolites	Scano et al. 2020
^{1}H-NMR with PLS-DA	Difference in metabolites of milk and colostrum	O'Callaghan et al. 2021

11.6 CONCLUSION AND FUTURE PERSPECTIVES

Metabolomics has proven to be an important tool for the advancement in food-science-related areas, such as compliance to regulations, processing, quality, safety, and microbiology. Milk is a popular food commodity liked by all age groups. The difference in milk compositions originates from different factors (e.g., species, breeds, lactation, environmental conditions, animal management, and production systems). In recent years, consumers are laying greater emphasis on the authenticity and origin of some food products, especially cheese varieties from PDO and non-PDO origin and organic milk and milk products that are free from contaminants (antibiotics, pesticides, etc.), and are often willing to pay a premium price for such products. Therefore, it is pertinent to establish methods that can evaluate the quality and also authenticate milk and milk products. The characterization of the milk metabolome using advanced analytical techniques (LC-MS/MS, GC-MS, NMR, etc.) is a promising approach in establishing quality and authenticity. In this chapter, it has been shown that milk metabolomics can be used as an effective tool for screening health status and stress conditions in milk animals. This will ensure the quality and safety of milk and milk products during production and processing by analyzing variations in milk metabolites. Significant progress has been made in characterizing the various metabolites found in milk, but further research is needed to learn more about the factors, which influence their relative concentrations in milk. Moreover, the effects of certain metabolites on the processability and nutritional value of milk and on the quality of final products need further elucidation. In addition, potential validation of functional biomarker compounds in milk and the methods for their rapid, reliable detection and measurement will be critical.

REFERENCES

Åkerstedt, M., Forsbäck, L., Larsen, T., and Svennersten-Sjaunja, K. 2011. Natural variation in biomarkers indicating mastitis in healthy cows. *Journal of Dairy Research* 78(1):88–9.

Arnould, V. R., and Soyeurt, H. 2009. Genetic variability of milk fatty acids. *Journal of Applied Genetics* 50(1):29–11.

Beale, D. J., Morrison, P. D., and Palombo, E. A. 2014. Detection of *Listeria* in milk using non-targeted metabolic profiling of *Listeria monocytogenes*: A proof-of-concept application. *Food Control* 42:343–4.

Bernillon, S., Biais, B., Deborde, C., et al. 2013. Metabolomic and elemental profiling of melon fruit quality as affected by genotype and environment. *Metabolomics* 9(1):57–21.

Blakebrough-Hall, C., Dona, A., D'occhio, M. J., McMeniman, J., and González, L. A. 2020. Diagnosis of bovine respiratory disease in feedlot cattle using blood ^{1}H NMR metabolomics. *Scientific Reports* 10(1):1–12.

Blow, N. 2008. Biochemistry's new look. *Nature* 455(7213):697–701.

Boiani, M., Sundekilde, U., Bateman, L. M., et al. 2019. Integration of high and low field ^{1}H NMR to analyse the effects of bovine dietary regime on milk metabolomics and protein-bound moisture characterisation of the resulting mozzarella cheeses during ripening. *International Dairy Journal* 91:155–9.

Boudonck, K. J., Mitchell, M. W., Wulff, J., and Ryals, J. A. 2009. Characterization of the biochemical variability of bovine milk using metabolomics. *Metabolomics* 5(4):375–411.

Brescia, M. A., Monfreda, M., Buccolieri, A., and Carrino, C. 2005. Characterisation of the geographical origin of buffalo milk and mozzarella cheese by means of analytical and spectroscopic determinations. *Food Chemistry* 89(1):139–48.

Burtis, C. A., and Bruns, D. E. 2014. *Tietz Fundamentals of Clinical Chemistry and Molecular Diagnostics*. Elsevier Saunders, Amsterdam Holland.

Caboni, P., Maxia, D., Scano, P., et al. 2019. A gas chromatography-mass spectrometry untargeted metabolomics approach to discriminate Fiore Sardo cheese produced from raw or thermized ovine milk. *Journal of Dairy Science* 102(6):5005–13.

Carneiro, G., Radcenco, A. L., Evaristo, J., and Monnerat, G. 2019. Novel strategies for clinical investigation and biomarker discovery: A guide to applied metabolomics. *Hormone Molecular Biology and Clinical Investigation* 38(3):20180045.

Cevallos-Cevallos, J. M., Reyes-De-Corcuera, J. I., Etxeberria, E., Danyluk, M. D., and Rodrick, G. E. 2009. Metabolomic analysis in food science: A review. *Trends in Food Science and Technology* 20(11–12):557–9.

Courant, F., Antignac, J. P., Dervilly-Pinel, G., and Le Bizec, B. 2014. Basics of mass spectrometry-based metabolomics. *Proteomics* 14(21–22):2369–79.

Creydt, M., Hudzik, D., Rurik, M., Kohlbacher, O., and Fischer, M. 2018. Food authentication: Small-molecule profiling as a tool for the geographic discrimination of German white asparagus. *Journal of Agricultural and Food Chemistry* 66(50):13328–411.

Cubero-Leon, E., De Rudder, O., and Maquet, A. 2018. Metabolomics for organic food authentication: Results from a long-term field study in carrots. *Food Chemistry* 239:760–810.

Danezis, G. P., Tsagkaris, A. S., Camin, F., Brusic, V., and Georgiou, C. A. 2016. Food authentication: Techniques, trends and emerging approaches. *Trends in Analytical Chemistry* 85:123–211.

De La Fuente, M. A., and Juárez, M. 2005. Authenticity assessment of dairy products. *Critical Reviews in Food Science and Nutrition* 45(7–8):563–622.

Elgersma, A., Tamminga, S., and Ellen, G. 2006. Modifying milk composition through forage. *Animal Feed Science and Technology* 131(3–4):207–18.

Emwas, A. H. M. 2015. The strengths and weaknesses of NMR spectroscopy and mass spectrometry with particular focus on metabolomics research. In: *Metabonomics*, ed. J. Bjerrum, 161–232. Humana Press, New York.

Fernie, A. R., Trethewey, R. N., Krotzky, A. J., and Willmitzer, L. 2004. Metabolite profiling: From diagnostics to systems biology. *Nature Reviews Molecular Cell Biology* 5(9):763–7.

Fiehn, O. 2002. Metabolomics – the link between genotypes and phenotypes. *Plant Molecular Biology* 48(1–2):155–71.

Fiehn, O., Putri, S. P., Saito, K., Salek, R. M., and Creek, D. J. 2015. Metabolomics continues to expand: Highlights from the 2015 metabolomics conference. *Metabolomics* 11(5):1036–44.

Firkins, J. L., and Yu, Z. 2006. Characterisation and quantification of the microbial populations of the rumen. In: *Ruminant physiology, digestion, metabolism and impact of nutrition on gene expression, immunology and stress*, eds. K. Sejrsen, T. Hvelplund, and M. O. Nielsen, 19–35. Wageningen Academic Publishers, Netherland.

Fontanesi, L. 2016. Metabolomics and livestock genomics: Insights into a phenotyping frontier and its applications in animal breeding. *Animal Frontiers* 6(1):73–6.

Food and Agriculture Organization. 2021. Animal production. Available from: www.fao.org/animal-production

Garnsworthy, P. C., Masson, L. L., Lock, A. L., and Mottram, T. T. 2006. Variation of milk citrate with stage of lactation and de novo fatty acid synthesis in dairy cows. *Journal of Dairy Science* 89(5):1604–8.

Gauglitz, J. M., Aceves, C. M., Aksenov, A. A., et al. 2020. Untargeted mass spectrometry-based metabolomics approach unveils molecular changes in raw and processed foods and beverages. *Food Chemistry* 302:125290.

Harzia, H., Kilk, K., Jõudu, I., Henno, M., Kärt, O., and Soomets, U. 2012. Comparison of the metabolic profiles of noncoagulating and coagulating bovine milk. *Journal of Dairy Science* 95(2):533–47.

Hettinga, K. A., van Valenberg, H. J. F., Lam, T. J. G. M., and van Hooijdonk, A. C. M. 2009. The origin of the volatile metabolites found in mastitis milk. *Veterinary Microbiology* 137(3–4):384–94.

Horning, E. C., and Horning, M. G. 1971. Human metabolic profiles obtained by GC and GC/MS. *Journal of Chromatographic Science* 9(3):129–211.

Hou, B., Meng, X., Zhang, L., Guo, J., Li, S., and Jin, H. (2015). Development of a sensitive and specific multiplex PCR method for the simultaneous detection of chicken, duck and goose DNA in meat products. *Meat science* 101:90–4.

Jadhav, S., Gulati, V., Fox, E. M., et al. 2015. Rapid identification and source-tracking of *Listeria monocytogenes* using MALDI-TOF mass spectrometry. *International Journal of Food Microbiology* 202:1–9.

Kim, S., Kim, J., Yun, E. J., and Kim, K. H. 2016. Food metabolomics: From farm to human. *Current Opinion in Biotechnology* 37:16–7.

Klein, M. S., Buttchereit, N., Miemczyk, S. P., et al. 2012. NMR metabolomic analysis of dairy cows reveals milk glycerophosphocholine to phosphocholine ratio as prognostic biomarker for risk of ketosis. *Journal of Proteome Research* 11(2):1373–8.

Layne, J., Lomas, S., and Misa, A. 2014. LC method development considerations for food contaminants analysis. *American Laboratory* 46(3):29–33.

Lewis, G. D., Asnani, A., and Gerszten, R. E. 2008. Application of metabolomics to cardiovascular biomarker and pathway discovery. *Journal of the American College of Cardiology* 52(2):117–26.

Li, Q., Yu, Z., Zhu, D., et al. 2017. The application of NMR-based milk metabolite analysis in milk authenticity identification. *Journal of the Science of Food and Agriculture* 97(9):2875–7.

Lindon, J. C., Holmes, E., and Nicholson, J. K. 2006. Metabonomics techniques and applications to pharmaceutical research and development. *Pharmaceutical Research* 23(6):1075–83.

Lindon, J. C., Nicholson, J. K., and Holmes, E. 2011. *The Handbook of Metabonomics and Metabolomics*, 557. Elsevier, Netherlands.

Lu, C., and Thompson, C. B. 2012. Metabolic regulation of epigenetics. *Cell Metabolism* 16(1):9–8.

Lu, J., Antunes Fernandes, E., Páez Cano, A. E., et al. 2013. Changes in milk proteome and metabolome associated with dry period length, energy balance, and lactation stage in postparturient dairy cows. *Journal of Proteome Research* 12(7):3288–98.

Magan, J. B., O'Callaghan, T. F., Zheng, J., et al. 2019. Impact of bovine diet on metabolomic profile of skim milk and whey protein ingredients. *Metabolites* 9(12):305–13.

Mansor, R., Mullen, W., Albalat, A., et al. 2013. A peptidomic approach to biomarker discovery for bovine mastitis. *Journal of Proteomics* 85:89–99.

Marincola, F. C., Noto, A., Caboni, P., et al. 2012. A metabolomic study of preterm human and formula milk by high resolution NMR and GC/MS analysis: Preliminary results. *The Journal of Maternal-Fetal and Neonatal Medicine* 25(5):62–5.

Martínez-Hernández, G. B., Boluda-Aguilar, M., Taboada-Rodríguez, A., Soto-Jover, S., Marín-Iniesta, F., and López-Gómez, A. 2016. Processing, packaging, and storage of tomato products: Influence on the lycopene content. *Food Engineering Reviews* 8(1):52–63.

Mazzei, P., and Piccolo, A. 2012. ^{1}H HRMAS-NMR metabolomic to assess quality and traceability of mozzarella cheese from Campania buffalo milk. *Food Chemistry* 132(3):1620–7.

McJarrow, P., and van Amelsfort-Schoonbeek, J. 2004. Bovine sialyl oligosaccharides: Seasonal variations in their concentrations in milk, and a comparison of the colostrums of Jersey and Friesian cows. *International Dairy Journal* 14(7):571–8.

McManaman, J. L., and Neville, M. C. 2003. Mammary physiology and milk secretion. *Advanced Drug Delivery Reviews* 55(5):629–32.

Melzer, N., Wittenburg, D., Hartwig, S., et al. 2013. Investigating associations between milk metabolite profiles and milk traits of Holstein cows. *Journal of Dairy Science* 96(3):1521.

Monakhova, Y. B., Kuballa, T., Leitz, J., Andlauer, C., and Lachenmeier, D. W. 2012. NMR spectroscopy as a screening tool to validate nutrition labeling of milk, lactose-free milk, and milk substitutes based on soy and grains. *Dairy Science and Technology* 92(2):109–11.

Nadella, K. D., Marla, S. S., and Kumar, P. A. 2012. Metabolomics in agriculture. *Omics: A Journal of Integrative Biology* 16(4):149–210.

Nie, W., Yan, L., Lee, Y. H., Guha, C., Kurland, I. J., and Lu, H. 2016. Advanced mass spectrometry-based multi-omics technologies for exploring the pathogenesis of hepatocellular carcinoma. *Mass Spectrometry Reviews* 35(3):331–418.

O'Callaghan, T. F., O'Donovan, M., Murphy, J. P., et al. 2021. The bovine colostrum and milk metabolome at the onset of lactation as determined by ^{1}H-NMR. *International Dairy Journal* 113:104881.

O'Callaghan, T. F., Vázquez-Fresno, R., Serra-Cayuela, A., et al. 2018. Pasture feeding changes the bovine rumen and milk metabolome. *Metabolites* 8(2):27–33.

Oliver, S. G., Winson, M. K., Kell, D. B., and Baganz, F. 1998. Systematic functional analysis of the yeast genome. *Trends in Biotechnology* 16(9):373–5.

Pan, L., Yu, J., Mi, Z., et al. 2018. A metabolomics approach uncovers differences between traditional and commercial dairy products in Buryatia (Russian Federation). *Molecules* 23(4):735–814.

Pinu, F. R. 2016. Metabolomics: Applications to food safety and quality research. In: *Microbial Metabolomics*, eds. D. Beale, K. Kouremenos, and E. Palombo, 225–34. Springer, Cham, Switzerland.

Piras, C., Marincola, F. C., Savorani, F., et al. 2013. A NMR metabolomics study of the ripening process of the Fiore Sardo cheese produced with autochthonous adjunct cultures. *Food Chemistry* 141(3):2137.

Pisano, M. B., Scano, P., Murgia, A., Cosentino, S., and Caboni, P. 2016. Metabolomics and microbiological profile of Italian mozzarella cheese produced with buffalo and cow milk. *Food Chemistry* 192:618–26.

Pustjens, A. M., Muilwijk, M., Weesepoel, Y., and van Ruth, S. M. 2016. Advances in authenticity testing of geographical origin of food products. In: *Advances in Food Authenticity Testing*, ed G. Downey, 339–428. Woodhead Publishing, The Netherlands.

Rocchetti, G., Gallo, A., Nocetti, M., Lucini, L., and Masoero, F. 2020. Milk metabolomics based on ultra-high-performance liquid chromatography coupled with quadrupole time-of-flight mass spectrometry to discriminate different cows feeding regimens. *Food Research International* 134:109279.

Rocchetti, G., Lucini, L., Gallo, A., Masoero, F., Trevisan, M., and Giuberti, G. 2018. Untargeted metabolomics reveals differences in chemical fingerprints between PDO and non-PDO Grana Padano cheeses. *Food Research International* 113:407–16.

Rollin, E., Dhuyvetter, K. C., and Overton, M. W. 2015. The cost of clinical mastitis in the first 30 days of lactation: An economic modeling tool. *Preventive Veterinary Medicine* 122(3):257–67.

Saito, K., Dixon, R. A., and Willmitzer, L. 2006. *Plant Metabolomics*, Vol. 57, 348. Springer Verlag, Germany.

Salzano, A., Manganiello, G., Neglia, G., et al. 2020. A preliminary study on metabolome profiles of buffalo milk and corresponding mozzarella cheese: Safeguarding the authenticity and traceability of protected status buffalo dairy products. *Molecules* 25(2):304–10.

Sampson, J. N., Boca, S. M., Shu, X. O., et al. 2013. Metabolomics in epidemiology: Sources of variability in metabolite measurements and implications. *Cancer Epidemiology and Prevention Biomarkers* 22(4):631–9.

Santos, P. M., Pereira-Filho, E. R., and Rodriguez-Saona, L. E. 2013. Rapid detection and quantification of milk adulteration using infrared microspectroscopy and chemometrics analysis. *Food Chemistry* 138(1):19–25.

Scano, P., Carta, P., Ibba, I., Manis, C., and Caboni, P. 2020. An untargeted metabolomic comparison of milk composition from sheep kept under different grazing systems. *Dairy* 1(1):30–41.

Scano, P., Murgia, A., Pirisi, F. M., and Caboni, P. 2014. A gas chromatography-mass spectrometry-based metabolomic approach for the characterization of goat milk compared with cow milk. *Journal of Dairy Science* 97(10):6057–9.

Shulaev, V. 2006. Metabolomics technology and bioinformatics. *Briefings in Bioinformatics* 7(2):128.

Silanikove, N., Merin, U., Shapiro, F., and Leitner, G. 2014. Milk metabolites as indicators of mammary gland functions and milk quality. *The Journal of Dairy Research* 81(3):358–65.

Simó, C., Ibáez, C., Valdés, A., Cifuentes, A., and García-Cañas, V. 2014. Metabolomics of genetically modified crops. *International Journal of Molecular Sciences* 15(10):18941.

Smith, A. M., Natowicz, M. R., Braas, D., et al. 2020. A metabolomics approach to screening for autism risk in the children's autism metabolome project. *Autism Research* 13(8):1270–85.

Spratlin, J., Serkova, N. J and Eckhardt, S. G. 2009. Clinical applications of metabolomics in oncology: A review. *Clinical Cancer Research* 15(2):431–39.

Stella, R., Bovo, D., Mastrorilli, E., et al. 2021. A novel tool to screen for treatments with clenbuterol in bovine: Identification of two hepatic markers by metabolomics investigation. *Food Chemistry* 353:129366.

Sumner, L. W., Lei, Z., Nikolau, B. J., and Saito, K. 2015. Modern plant metabolomics: Advanced natural product gene discoveries, improved technologies, and future prospects. *Natural Product Reports* 32(2):212–7.

Sun, H. Z., Shi, K., Wu, X. H., et al. 2017. Lactation-related metabolic mechanism investigated based on mammary gland metabolomics and 4 biofluids' metabolomics relationships in dairy cows. *BMC Genomics* 18(1):1–14.

Sun, H. Z., Wang, D. M., Wang, B., et al. 2015. Metabolomics of four biofluids from dairy cows: Potential biomarkers for milk production and quality. *Journal of Proteome Research* 14(2):1287.

Sundekilde, U. K., Frederiksen, P. D., Clausen, M. R., Larsen, L. B., and Bertram, H. C. 2011. Relationship between the metabolite profile and technological properties of bovine milk from two dairy breeds elucidated by NMR-based metabolomics. *Journal of Agricultural and Food Chemistry* 59(13):7360–7.

Sundekilde, U. K., Gustavsson, F., Poulsen, N. A., et al. 2014. Association between the bovine milk metabolome and rennet-induced coagulation properties of milk. *Journal of Dairy Science* 97(10):6076–8.

Sundekilde, U. K., Poulsen, N. A., Larsen, L. B., and Bertram, H. C. 2013. Nuclear magnetic resonance metabonomics reveals strong association between milk metabolites and somatic cell count in bovine milk. *Journal of Dairy Science* 96(1):290–9.

Tengstrand, E., Rosén, J., Hellenäs, K. E., and Åberg, K. M. 2013. A concept study on non-targeted screening for chemical contaminants in food using liquid chromatography – mass spectrometry in combination with a metabolomics approach. *Analytical and Bioanalytical Chemistry* 405(4):1237–46.

Tenori, L., Santucci, C., Meoni, G., Morrocchi, V., Matteucci, G., and Luchinat, C. 2018. NMR metabolomic fingerprinting distinguishes milk from different farms. *Food Research International* 113:131–8.

Tian, H., Zheng, N., Wang, W., et al. 2016. Integrated metabolomics study of the milk of heat-stressed lactating dairy cows. *Scientific Reports* 6(1):1–10.

Tian, Y., Nie, X., Xu, S., et al. 2015. Integrative metabonomics as potential method for diagnosis of thyroid malignancy. *Scientific Reports* 5(1):1–12.

Tomassini, A., Curone, G., Solè, M., et al. 2019. NMR-based metabolomics to evaluate the milk composition from Friesian and autochthonous cows of Northern Italy at different lactation times. *Natural Product Research* 33(8):1085–6.

Tong, J., Zhang, H., Zhang, Y., Xiong, B., and Jiang, L. 2019. Microbiome and metabolome analyses of milk from dairy cows with subclinical *Streptococcus agalactiae* mastitis – Potential biomarkers. *Frontiers in Microbiology* 10:2547.

Vinayavekhin, N., and Saghatelian, A. 2010. Untargeted metabolomics. *Current Protocols in Molecular Biology* 90(1):30–41.

Walker, G. P., Dunshea, F. R., and Doyle, P. T. 2004. Effects of nutrition and management on the production and composition of milk fat and protein: A review. *Australian Journal of Agricultural Research* 55(10):1009–19.

Wiklund, S., Johansson, E., Sjöström, L., et al. 2008. Visualization of GC/TOF-MS-based metabolomics data for identification of biochemically interesting compounds using OPLS class models. *Analytical Chemistry* 80(1):115–7.

Wishart, D. S. 2016. Emerging applications of metabolomics in drug discovery and precision medicine. *Nature Reviews Drug Discovery* 15(7):473–511.

Xi, X., Kwok, L. Y., Wang, Y., Ma, C., Mi, Z., and Zhang, H. 2017. Ultra-performance liquid chromatography-quadrupole-time of flight mass spectrometry MSE-based untargeted milk metabolomics in dairy cows with subclinical or clinical mastitis. *Journal of Dairy Science* 100(6):4884–912.

Xu, W., Vervoort, J., Saccenti, E., Kemp, B., van Hoeij, R. J., and van Knegsel, A. T. 2020. Relationship between energy balance and metabolic profiles in plasma and milk of dairy cows in early lactation. *Journal of Dairy Science* 103(5):4795–810.

Xu, W., Vervoort, J., Saccenti, E., van Hoeij, R., Kemp, B., and van Knegsel, A. 2018. Milk metabolomics data reveal the energy balance of individual dairy cows in early lactation. *Scientific Reports* 8(1):1–11.

Yang, Y., Zheng, N., Zhao, X., et al. 2016. Metabolomic biomarkers identify differences in milk produced by Holstein cows and other minor dairy animals. *Journal of Proteomics* 136:174–8.

Zhang, A., Sun, H., Wang, P., Han, Y., and Wang, X. 2012. Modern analytical techniques in metabolomics analysis. *Analyst* 137(2):293–7.

Zhang, Y. D., Li, P., Zheng, N., et al. 2018. A metabolomics approach to characterize raw, pasteurized, and ultra-high temperature milk using ultra-performance liquid chromatography – quadrupole time-of-flight mass spectrometry and multivariate data analysis. *Journal of Dairy Science* 101(11):9630–6.

12 Application of Metabolomic Tools to Survey the Phenolic Composition of Food, Medicinal Plants, and Agro-Industrial Residues

*Ticiane Carvalho Farias, Carolina Thomaz dos Santos D'Almeida, Thaiza Serrano de Souza, Talita Pimenta do Nascimento, Fernanda de Sousa Bezerra, Roberta Nogueira Pereira da Silva, Mariana Simões Larraz Ferreira, Andrea Furtado Macedo, and Maria Gabriela Bello Koblitz**

CONTENTS

* Corresponding author email: maria.koblitz@unirio.br

DOI: 10.1201/9781003142195-12

12.1 INTRODUCTION

Polyphenols are a class of compounds present in plants, especially plant-based crops (fruits, vegetables, and grains), that are often concentrated in their by-products (peels, seeds, stems, and roots). Food by-products are derivatives from food processing and represent an enormous quantity of waste that is rich in bioactive compounds. The recovery of these by-products can solve economic and environmental problems of agro-waste, whereas food-related phenolic compounds are valuable bioactive compounds (Duba and Fiori 2015; Fernández et al. 2018). In the vegetable oil industry, for instance, up to 30% of the total raw material becomes by-product or waste, from which phenolic compounds may be recovered by applying organic solvents and/or natural solvents associated with modern extraction techniques such as ultrasound, microwave, and hydrostatic pressure, among others (Bezerra et al. 2020). Medicinal plants are also considered a rich source of bioactive compounds related to their use over conventional drugs, enabled by their potentially high bioactivity. These herbs are known to have negligible side effects and toxicity and an enormous therapeutic potential to treat several diseases (Rajput and Kumar 2020).

Phenolic compounds are secondary plant metabolites, considered non-essential for the general survival of the organism but are important components for overall plant adaptation and protection against biotic and abiotic stress conditions (Aires 2017; Gálvez-Ranilla 2020). These compounds are a diversified group derived from the amino acids phenylalanine and tyrosine and comprise simple phenols, hydroxybenzoic acids, and cinnamic acid derivatives, flavonoids, coumarins, stilbenes, and tannins, among others (Aires 2017). Many phenolic compounds may also be found in conjunction with carbohydrates and proteins in soluble and insoluble forms. The most used nomenclature to designate the two groups is free (soluble, conjugated or not) and bound (insoluble) phenolic compounds (Santos et al. 2019).

Epidemiological studies have linked a plant-based diet to the reduced hazard of several chronic degenerative diseases (obesity, cardiovascular disease, and diabetes, among others). This suggests that long-term consumption of fruits, vegetables, and grains may exert a protective effect on the body and should be considered as part of a general strategy against non-communicable diseases (NCDs), which are responsible for up to 70% of all deaths worldwide, according to the WHO reports. Since 2003, WHO and FAO recommend the daily consumption of at least 400 g of fruits and vegetables for the control of NCDs, which was translated in different countries as five-a-day campaigns, where people are urged to include at least five portions of fruits and vegetables in their daily diet (WHO 2020). The benefits related to the ingestion of fruits and vegetables are linked to their composition, rich in bioactive compounds, such as polyphenols and carotenoids (Aune et al. 2017). According to Bhuyan and Basu (2017), due to their antioxidant potential, phenolic compounds may help prevent different oxidative-stress-related NCDs, such as various forms of cancer and neurodegenerative diseases (Vuong 2017). The frequency of consumption, the chemical nature, the bioavailability, and the metabolic pathways involved may also influence this bioactivity. Excessive consumption, however, is inadvisable, as polyphenols may exert anti-nutritional or pro-oxidant activities, and studies are still being carried out to find a recommended dose (Aune et al. 2017; Luna-Guevara et al. 2018; Adebo and Medina-Meza 2020).

The great chemical diversity of these plant metabolites, such as phenolic compounds, requires the use of techniques that enable a comprehensive metabolomic analysis. Metabolomics can be defined as the comprehensive, qualitative, and quantitative analysis of metabolites and aims to identify and quantify all small molecules (1,000–1,500 Da) present in a biosystem (Gong and Pegg 2017; Valdés et al. 2017). As such, the use of metabolomic tools is a reliable approach to elucidate the phenolic composition in different plant matrices and has been widely used for the detailed characterization of secondary metabolites in fruits, cereals, medicinal plants, and agro-industrial residues (Table 12.1).

The steps for a metabolomic analysis should be adapted to the objective of the study, the type of sample, and the analytical platform and generally include the extraction of metabolites, the sample preparation, the analytical step, the post-processing of spectra data, statistical analysis, and identification/quantification of metabolites with the application of bioinformatics and chemometric tools. The annotation of the metabolites of interest, either with the use of patterns or structural information via NMR or MS, is the usual final step in metabolomic analyses (Valdés et al. 2017). MS has shown vast potential as a useful tool for metabolomic study, such as high sensitivity and resolution, as well as comprehensive investigation on all metabolites. As with any chemical analysis, however, the results depend on the very initial steps that involve sample collection and extraction (Mushtaq et al. 2014).

The genetic diversity but also external factors, such as location and growing conditions, may strongly impact phenolic composition and content in plants. Several metabolomic studies have focused on understanding the complex biochemical mechanisms

TABLE 12.1
Phenolic Diversity of Some Food, Medicinal Plants, and Agro-Industrial Residues Surveyed by Metabolomic Tools

Food/Medicinal plant/By-product	Most abundant phenolic compounds	Metabolomic approach	Reference
Brewer spent grain	Trans-ferulic acid ρ-Coumaric acid Ferulic acid Caffeic acid Protocatechuic acid 3,7-Dimethylquercetin	UPLC-ESI-QTOF-MS^{E}[1]	Maia et al. 2020
Pineapple crown flour	ρ-Coumaric acid Ferulic acid Daidzein 3,7-Dimethylquercetin 5-Caffeoylquinic acid	UPLC-ESI-QTOF-MS^{E}[1]	Brito et al. 2021
Cabbage stalk flour	4-ρ-Coumaroylquinic acid Quercetin 3-O-Glucuronide Sinapic acid Caffeic acid	UPLC-ESI-QTOF-MS^{E}[1]	Brito et al. 2021
Red and black rice bran	Ferulic acid Dihydroxybenzoic acid Feruloylquinic acid Quercetin ρ-Coumaric	HPLC-DAD[3] UPLC-ESI-QTOF-MS^{E} 1	Santos et al. 2021
Fruit and vegetable residues	Kaempferol Quercetin Epicatechin Ferulic acid Gallic acid	UPLC-ESI-QTOF-MS[1]	Gonçalves et al. 2018
Apple press cake, seeds, skin, flesh, stems	Catechin Epicatechin Caffeic acid-*O*-glucoside Chlorogenic acid	LC-DAD-ESI-MS/MS[2]	Radenkovs et al. 2020
Olive pomace	Caffeic acid Luteolin Ruthin Tyrosol Trans-ferulic acid 3-hydroxytyrosol	HPLC-DAD[3]	Fernández et al. 2018

TABLE 12.1 (CONTINUED)

Food/Medicinal plant/By-product	Most abundant phenolic compounds	Metabolomic approach	Reference
Cunila menthoides seeds	Rosmarinic acid Vertinone Savianolic acid Cinnamic/Hydroxycinnamic acid Isoswertisin 2-rhamnoside hesperetin 7-*O*-glucoside sesartemin	UPLC-Qq-oaTOF-MS[4]	Oliveira, Hakimi et al. 2018; Oliveira, Koblitz et al. 2018
Rosaceae, Asteraceae, and *Lamiceae* leaves	Syringic acid Vanillic acid Chlorogenic acid Ferulic acid ρ-Anisic acid	HPLC-DAD[3]	Sytar et al. 2018
Traditional Chinese medicinal plants	Caffeic acid Ferulic acid Gallic acid Catechin Quercetin	HPLC-DAD[3]	Cai et al. 2006
Wild medicinal plant flowers	Chrysin derivative Quercetin-3-*O*-rutinaside 5-*O*-caffeoylquinic acid	HPLC-DAD-ESI/MS[5]	Barros et al. 2012
P. tortuosus; R. raetam; E. alata; Z. lotus; C. spinoza; C. comosum	Quinic acid Catechin Gallic acid Epicatechin Ruthin ρ-Coumaric acid	LC-ESI-MS[6]	Benabderrahim et al. 2019
Clematis cirrhosa	Gallic acid Chlorogenic acid Catechin Benzoic acid	HPLC-DAD[3]	Chohra et al. 2020
Sorghum grains	Protocatechuic acid B,3,4-Trihydroxy benzenepropanoic acid Catechin hexoside Caffeic acid hexose Catechin	HPLC-MS[7]	Kang et al. 2016

TABLE 12.1 (CONTINUED)
Phenolic Diversity of Some Food, Medicinal Plants, and Agro-Industrial Residues Surveyed by Metabolomic Tools

Food/Medicinal plant/By-product	Most abundant phenolic compounds	Metabolomic approach	Reference
Mango fruit	Gallic acid Protocatechuic acid Chlorogenic acid Vanillic acid	HPLC – ESI-MS[8]	Palafox-Carlos et al. 2012
Eggplant	Dihydrocoumaroyl glucoside amide N-Caffeoylputrescine Homovanillic acid hexose Dicaffeoylquinic acid	HPLC-DAD-QTOF-MS[9]	García-Salas, P., Gómez-Caravaca, A. M., Morales-Soto, A., Segura-Carretero, A. and Fernández-Gutiérrez, A.
Psidium cattleianum Sabine	3-*O*-Caffeoyl-shikimic acid *p*-Coumaroyl-feruloyl glycerol Aconitic acid Gallic acid 3-*O*-Feruloylquinic acid	LC-DAD-ESI-MS/MS[2]	Mallmann et al. 2020
Crataegus pinnatifida	Gallic acid Protocatechuic acid Chlorogenic acid Caffeic acid Vanillic acid Syringic acid	HPLC-ESI-MS/MS[8]	Lou et al. 2020

[1] Ultra-high-performance liquid chromatography electrospray ionization-quadrupole time-of-flight with multiplex tandem mass spectrometry. [2] Liquid chromatography diode array detector electrospray ionization–mass spectrometry. [3] High-performance liquid chromatography diode array detector–mass spectrometry. [4] Ultra-performance liquid chromatography–hybrid quadrupole orthogonal time-of-flight with multiplex tandem mass spectrometry. [5] High-performance liquid chromatography diode array detector electrospray ionization–mass spectrometry. [6] Liquid chromatography electrospray ionization–mass spectrometry. [7] High-performance liquid chromatography–mass spectrometry. [8] High-performance liquid chromatography electrospray ionization–mass spectrometry. [9] High-performance liquid chromatography electrospray ionization-quadrupole time-of-flight tandem mass spectrometry.

involved in response to environmentally directed biotic and abiotic stress factors in plants. During the grain growth and maturation, biochemical changes occur, such as the accumulation of dry mass (starch and proteins) and a reduction in the redox potential of cells. The content of phenolic compounds decreases progressively, as well as the antioxidant activity. Immature wheat grains from different genotypes showed a more complex composition and higher abundance of phenolic than mature grains (Santos et al. 2019).

Metabolomics-based methods have also been successfully applied to study plants' capacity to stress adaptation at the molecular level, helping to understand the dynamics of secondary metabolism of these plants (Oliveira, Hakimi et al. 2018; Oliveira, Koblitz et al. 2018).

Metabolomics is also becoming an important tool for phenotyping. The metabolic phenotype provides a link between gene sequence and visible phenotypes that is, metabolites can be used as relevant biomarkers for trait prediction in crop genetic improvement (Harrigan et al. 2016; Gálvez-Ranilla 2020). In this chapter, the application of metabolomic tools for the analysis of the phenolic composition of food, medicinal plants, and agro-industrial residues is presented. To that end, the sample preparation for analysis and data acquisition in LC-MS/MS metabolomic, bioinformatic, and chemometric tools will be further discussed.

12.2 PREPARATION OF FOOD, HERBS, AND RESIDUE SAMPLES FOR METABOLOMIC ANALYSIS

12.2.1 Sample Preparation

For metabolomic analysis of biological samples, those should be collected, extracted, measured, and the resulting data characterized and evaluated, as shown in the flowchart of Figure 12.1. Sample preparation is a fundamental step for the extraction process and closely linked to the analysis step, which must be considered from the beginning of the experiment. From the raw material studied, it is possible to define the best way to use and identify the compounds in question. Samples must be prepared as similar as possible, with no difference between the repetitions, increasing the reliability and precision of the method. In metabolomics, there are two paths: (1) target analysis, when studies focus on the identification and precise quantification of a defined set of metabolites, and (2) untargeted analysis, which is used to measure and compare the widest possible set of compounds between two or more groups; in this case, chemical standards are not necessary, and the detected signals can be transformed into metabolite IDs using specific databases (Gong et al. 2017; Bingol 2018; Dudzik et al. 2018). Regardless of the approach, every metabolomic strategy can include the identification and quantitation of metabolites; the latter can be absolute or relative.

In general, for the preparation of plant extracts for metabolomic analysis, the steps of harvesting/collecting, drying, extracting plant material, and preparing the sample are performed (Kim and Verpoorte 2009). In this section, the extraction focuses on obtaining phenolic compounds, so the preliminary steps will only be mentioned briefly. The main way to preserve the compounds for future analysis is drying, thus decreasing the moisture content of the sample and inhibiting enzymatic and microbial activities, and as a result, there is an increase in the conservation of the samples, allowing them to be used for an extended period. This can be achieved by air-circulating drying, by oven-drying, preferentially under vacuum using low temperatures

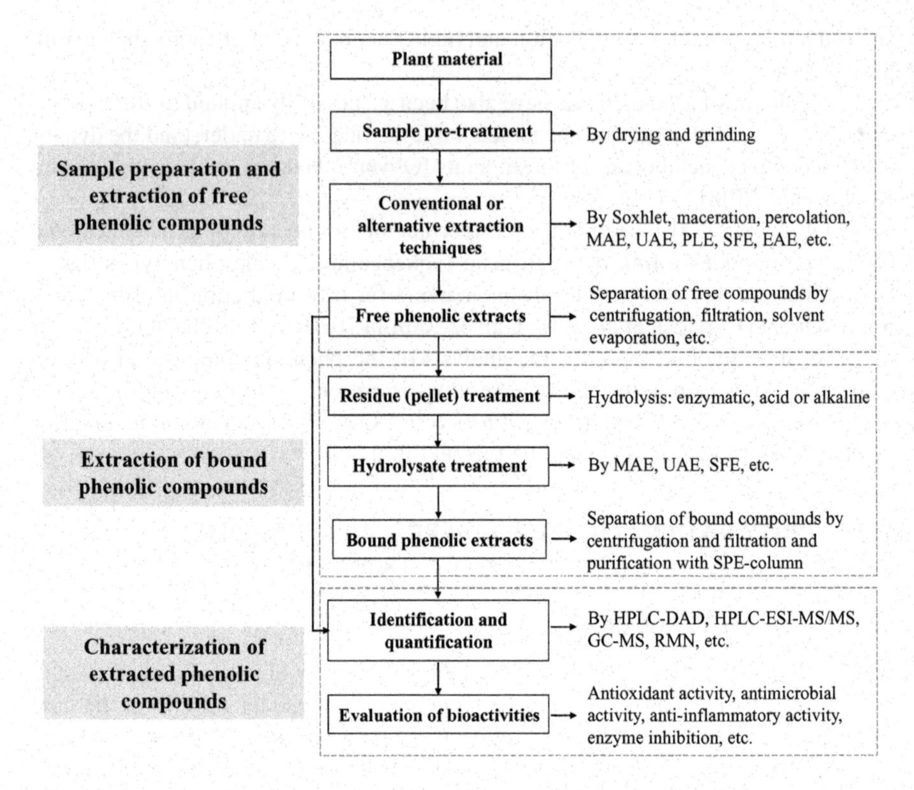

FIGURE 12.1 Flowchart of the steps involved in sample extraction of free and bound phenolic compounds and their characterization. (Adapted from Domínguez-Rodríguez et al. 2017; Dzah et al. 2020). Abbreviations: MAE (microwave-assisted extraction), UAE (ultrasound-assisted), PLE (pressurized liquid extraction), SFE (supercritical fluid extraction), EAE (enzyme-assisted extraction), SPE (solid-phase extraction).

or using specific equipment. The most used method is freeze-drying since it tends to eliminate water without altering the components to be extracted; hence, it is suitable for thermolabile compounds or unstable in aqueous solutions for prolonged storage periods, but that are stable in their dry state (Santos et al. 2019; Filho et al. 2019; Aires and Carvalho 2020; Hazarika and Gosztola 2020).

For the sample preparation, several methodologies can be used to enhance the extraction, such as fermentation to improve and efficiently release bound phenolics from complex food matrices, such as cereal by-products (Maia et al. 2020), thermo-mechanical processes (cooking by extrusion), and hydrolysis (e.g., enzymatic, alkaline, and acid) are also described for increasing the release of bound phenolics (Acosta-Estrada et al. 2014). The most applied forms of sample preparation will be discussed in more detail throughout this chapter.

After preparation, phenolics are generally extracted by pure water, organic solvents, such as alkyl alcohols, acetone, diethyl ether, and ethyl acetate or mixtures thereof, or by using modern alternative extraction techniques. The most common solvents used are ethanol and methanol, as identified in the recent literature on foods, herbs, and food residue (Santos et al. 2019; Nascimento et al. 2019; Aires and Carvalho 2020; Brito et al. 2021). More recently, another class of solvents, called deep eutectic solvents (DES), has been applied and presents a very promising extraction capacity, sometimes even better than traditional solvents, and shows a more natural and biodegradable composition (Bezerra et al. 2020).

12.2.2 Solvent Extraction

The most suitable solvents for the extraction of phenolic compounds, from an environmental, food-safety, and ease-of-handling point of view, are pure water and mixtures of ethanol and acetone with water (Chew et al. 2011; Dorta et al. 2012). According to Nascimento et al. (2019), water was the best extractor of phenolic compounds when compared with mixtures of methanol and acetone to extract phenolics from breadfruit. Alcântara et al. (2018) reported the combinations water-acetone and water-ethanol-acetone as the most efficient for the phenolic extraction in chia seeds. The combination of water and organic solvents leads to the creation of a moderate polar environment suitable for phenolic extraction since extremely polar phenolic acids, such as benzoic and cinnamic acids, would not be effectively extracted with pure organic solvents (Acosta-Estrada et al. 2014). The mixture of equal parts of ethanol and water was also reinforced in the optimization of the phenolic extraction from the medicinal plant *Orthosiphon stamineus*, where most parts of the phenolic compounds were found in the extracts and showed a moderately polar characteristic (Chew et al. 2011).

The use of DES has been widely proposed as a promising strategy to improve the yield extraction of phenolic compounds from food residues. Chanioti and Tzia (2018) investigated the extraction of phenolics from the olive pomace, using mixtures of natural solvents compared to the conventional mixture of ethanol-water (70–30%) and pure water in different types of preparation, and the best results were obtained by the extraction with choline chloride/citric acid (DES-CA) and choline chloride/lactic acid (DES-LA). One of the advantages of DES extraction is the strong solubilization capacity associated with the possibility, depending on its composition, to provide enriched extracts with high phytochemical concentration and diversity (Ramon et al. 2017). However, to resolve the complexity of DES extracts, the application of high-throughput techniques, such as the metabolomic approach, is required to elucidate the chemical complexity. The use of this novel green class of solvents in metabolomic studies is something very new. Santos et al. (2021) compared conventional ethanol mixtures and DES for phenolic extraction in pigmented rice bran and showed that although the phenolic profile is highly dependent on the extraction solvent, specific phenolic compounds with interesting radical scavenging activity can be only extracted using the acidic DES.

12.2.3 Extraction Aids

Extraction is an important and critical step in metabolomics. Its primary aim is to acquire a high number of metabolites from the sample. To achieve this goal, different extraction methods have been used (Mushtaq et al. 2014). The extraction of plant-derived polyphenols can be performed by conventional techniques, such as maceration, percolation, and Soxhlet, or by modern alternative extraction techniques like microwave-assisted extraction (MAE), ultrasound-assisted extraction (UAE), pressurized liquid extraction (PLE), supercritical fluid extraction (SFE), and enzyme-assisted extraction (EAE) (Ameer et al. 2017).

Traditional solvent extraction methods, such as maceration, percolation, and Soxhlet, are based on solid-liquid extraction, where a powdered sample is homogenized and mixed with a solvent, usually under constant agitation; thus, the extraction is based on diffusion and mass-transfer phenomena (Rocchetti et al. 2019; Sut et al. 2019). In addition, those methods require a recovery step followed by the evaporation of the solvents used to concentrate the extract. Those techniques are considered low-cost and simple; however, as disadvantages, they may present low efficiency, are very time-consuming, and require the use of a high volume of organic solvents, generating pollution and environmental concerns (Aires 2017). To overcome the limitations of the traditional methods, novel and more environmentally friendly methods have been tested, as they present rapid processing of samples and higher reproducibility, demand low quantities of solvents, lead to higher extraction yields, and are less destructive to extracted compounds (Sut et al. 2019; Zengin et al. 2019). In Table 12.2, the advantages and disadvantages of alternative extraction techniques are presented.

12.2.3.1 Microwave-Assisted Extraction (MAE)

In MAE, non-ionizing electromagnetic waves penetrate a material, interact with polar compounds, and transform electromagnetic energy into heat (Bordoloi and Goosen 2020). Two phenomena occur with the absorption of the waves by the sample: dipole rotation (through reversals of dipoles) and ionic conduction (through the displacement of ions present in the solute and the solvent), which usually occur simultaneously (Ibrahim and Zaini 2018). Both phenomena are directly related to the temperature, where the dipole rotation is reduced as the sample temperature rises, while the ion conduction increases at a higher temperature. Hence, heating is initially governed by dipole rotation, and as the temperature rises, ionic conduction becomes predominant (Vinatoru et al. 2017).

In MAE, the sample stays in direct contact with the solvents, which are heated by the microwave energy (2.45 GHz) (Mushtaq et al. 2014), and the heat produced enhances the diffusivity of the solvent onto the powdered sample, enabling the dissolution of the components into the liquid matrices by extracting and diffusing the phytochemicals out of the matrix (Aires 2017). To improve the mass transfer and microwave penetration, agitation has been applied, as it accelerates the equilibrium between aqueous and vapor phases (Ibrahim and Zaini 2018). When choosing a solvent for MAE, the interaction of the solvent with the sample, the solubility of the target analyte, and the microwave absorption ability of the solvent should be considered. The absorption ability depends on the solvent dielectric constant (K), where, in theory, the higher the K, the higher the ability to absorb energy and generate heat (Mushtaq et al. 2014). For example, hexane ($K = 1.89$) is not heated up by microwaves, whereas water ($K = 78.5$), methanol ($K = 32.6$), and ethanol ($K = 24.6$) present good absorption ability (Aires 2017). MAE is mostly used to extract monomeric polyphenols, like phenolic acids and flavonoids, and less used in polymeric

TABLE 12.2
Pros and Cons of Alternative Extraction Techniques

Technique	Advantages	Disadvantages	Reference
MAE	Rapid extraction; uses a lesser amount of solvent, affords higher extraction yields, and shows the better quality of the extracts in lower times of extraction when compared with the traditional extraction techniques	The recovery of non-polar compounds and the modification of the chemical structure of target compounds, leading to altered bioactivities	Gil-Chávez et al. 2013; Sonar and Rathod 2020
UAE	Simple technique; increases extraction yields; shows rapid extraction rate of thermolabile components at mild/low-temperature ranges; less time-consuming when compared to traditional techniques and presents a minimum degree of interaction between ultrasonic waves and extracted materials during the process	May degrade active principles from plant matrices due to oxidative pyrolysis during cavitation phenomenon, and high-ultrasound waves can lead to undesirable changes in the extracted components through deleterious effects on active constituents in plants by the formation of free radicals	Ameer et al. 2017
PLE	Rapid extraction and requires a lower quantity of solvents when compared with the classical extraction approach; water can be used as a solvent; generates a cleaner extract compared to classical, MAE, and UAE extractions, reducing background noise during the subsequent analytical quantification	Low selectivity toward the analytes; interferents may be extracted during the extraction process; an excessive dilution of the analytes; high cost; not suitable for thermolabile compounds as high temperature can have deleterious effects on their structure and functional activity	Gil-Chávez et al. 2013; Aires 2017
SFE	Easy remotion of the solvent from the extracted material by simple expansion; ease manipulation of solvation characteristics by slight changes in gas and temperature of the supercritical fluid, which allows the control of their physicochemical properties; high selectivity; short times of extraction; increased pollution prevention; the use of non-toxic organic solvents	High power consumption; high operating pressure; expensive setup; laborious sample processing	Gil-Chávez et al. 2013; Mushtaq et al. 2014; Bordoloi and Goosen 2020

polyphenols extraction, such as tannins and anthocyanins, as they may be degraded by the extraction conditions applied (Aires 2017). In metabolomics, this technique is more often applied in plants than in animal studies, due to their high diversity of metabolites, leading to the need for a more complex extraction protocol (Mushtaq et al. 2014). Sonar and Rathod (2020) evaluated the content of total phenolics, flavonoids, and marmelosin from *Aegle marmelos* using MAE, Soxhlet, and batch extraction techniques. MAE requires just 30 seconds to obtain the highest yield of marmelosin, while the other techniques demanded up to seven hours with a comparatively lower yield.

12.2.3.2 Ultrasound-Assisted Extraction (UAE)

The UAE is based on the mechanical effect caused by the propagation of high-frequency sound waves (>20 kHz) through the medium by compression and rarefaction cycles, which results in the formation of cavitation bubbles (Bordoloi and Goosen 2020). Compression induces positive pressure, leading to the approximation of molecules, and rarefaction causes negative pressure resulting in separate molecules (Nazir and Azad 2019). This effect leads to the implosion of micro-sized bubbles, which induces a fast tissue disruption, enabling the release of compounds into the solvent. UAE is usually used to isolate target compounds from the plant material and its different parts, such as leaves, stems, stalks, fruits, and seeds (Aires 2017). Li et al. (2016) optimized UAE to evaluate the extraction of total phenolic compounds, antioxidants, and rosmarinic acid from *Perilla frutescens* leaves. The results indicated that optimized UAE used less solvent, lower temperature, and shorter extraction time and also extracted polyphenols, which may be of interest for the pharmaceutical and food industries. Zengin et al. (2019) studied the phytochemical composition of *Salvia viridis* L. ethanolic root extracts obtained by different extraction methods – MAE, SFE, UAE, maceration, and Soxhlet. It was observed that the extraction technique influenced compound extractability, where the extract produced by UAE presented the highest total phenolic and flavonoid contents and the highest antioxidant activities. Besides that, HPLC-MS/MS screening indicated a total of 76 compounds in the extracts obtained by Soxhlet, UAE, and maceration, 73 compounds for MAE, and only 24 compounds for SFE.

12.2.3.3 Pressurized Liquid Extraction (PLE)

The PLE, also known as accelerated solvent extraction (ASE), uses organic solvents at high temperature (50 to 200°C) and pressure (1,450 to 2,175 psi), which ensures a fast extraction rate of compounds (Gil-Chávez et al. 2013). The combination of high temperature and pressure enhances the solubility and desorption of molecules, leading to a lower solvent viscosity and better penetration into the matrix, which improves the yield of the polyphenols extracted (Bijttebier et al. 2016; Aires 2017). The most used solvents in PLE are water (called subcritical water extraction [SWE]), ethanol, methanol, or ethyl acetate and their mixtures (Gallego et al. 2019). The SWE is possible when using elevated temperature, as the dielectric water properties are changed, and the water behaves like an organic solvent (Aires 2017). For example, under ambient conditions, water's K is close to 80, although this value is decreased to around 30 at 250°C, showing a K similar to that of ethanol and methanol (Gil-Chávez et al. 2013). Even presenting lower K, water has greater diffusivity in subcritical conditions, which facilities the diffusion in the plant matrix and the release of moderately polar and non-polar compounds from the solid phase into the liquid phase (Zhang et al. 2018). Effective binary solvents, like methanol-water or ethanol-water, have been used in PLE and, as each solvent has different polarities, this method is able to extract a broad range of compounds, from very polar components (e.g., sugars and proteins) to mid-/non-polar compounds (e.g., phenolic compounds, carotenoids, and glycerides) (Ameer et al. 2017; Gallego et al. 2019). PLE has been used in several plants and its different anatomical parts, including seeds, grains, herbs, rhizomes, and agro-industrial by-products, to extract metabolites such as polyphenols and carotenoids (Bijttebier et al. 2016). Gonçalves et al. (2018) evaluated the phenolic profile of fruit and vegetable residues, using PLE as extraction technique and ethanol and water as solvents. It was observed that the highest phenolic acid content was achieved with high temperature while lower temperatures were more efficient in extracting flavonoids. The extracts were characterized by UPLCESI-Q-TOF-MS and 28 phenolic acids, 32 flavonoids, and 28 other polyphenols were identified.

12.2.3.4 Supercritical Fluid Extraction (SFE)

In the SFE, the target compounds are separated from others through the use of a supercritical fluid (SF) (Mushtaq et al. 2014). SF is defined as a liquid that is above its critical temperature and pressure, which carries characteristics of both liquids (dissolves substances like liquids) and gases (diffuses into a solid like a gas) (Mushtaq et al. 2014; Ameer et al. 2017). As an SF combines properties of two individual phases – liquid and gas – simultaneously, it is considered as a solvent of choice, which improves the mass transfer rate during extraction (Ameer et al. 2017). Different substances can be used as SF, such as ethylene, methane, nitrogen, xenon, or fluorocarbons; however, the most used is carbon dioxide (CO_2) due to its low cost and safety, as it is non-toxic, non-flammable, and attainable with a high degree of purity (Gil-Chávez et al. 2013; Aires 2017). Besides that, CO_2 is gaseous at room temperature and pressure, which leads to easy compound recovery, produces solvent-free extracts, and is almost inert in the standard operating conditions (31°C and 7.37 MPa), which makes it suitable to extract heat-labile and non-polar compounds. Despite that, the main disadvantage of CO_2 is its non-polar nature; therefore, it is less effective in extracting highly polar compounds. This limitation, however, may be overcome with the addition of modifiers or co-solvents (Gil-Chávez et al. 2013; Mushtaq et al. 2014). SFE is mostly used to extract non-polar or mid-polar compounds, such as lipids, essential oils, and carotenoids (Gallego et al. 2019). Supercritical fluid extraction–CO_2 (SC-CO_2) has been employed to extract bioactive compounds, like phenols and sesquiterpenes by using pure CO_2 or CO_2 with methanol as a modifier (Mushtaq et al. 2014). Pinto et al. (2020) optimized the SC-CO_2 extraction using ethanol as a co-solvent to recover bioactive compounds with antioxidant properties from *Castanea sativa* shells. As a result, they found the presence of ellagic acid, epigallocatechin, catechin/epicatechin, and caffeic acid derivative as the phenolic composition of the optimal extract, which indicated that SC-CO_2 with ethanol might be an interesting technique to obtain phenolic-compound-enriched extracts in agro-residues with possible application in the nutraceutical industry.

12.2.3.5 Hydrolysis-Assisted Extraction

The enzyme-assisted extraction (EAE) is based on the capacity of the enzymes to degrade cell wall components under mild conditions (Bordoloi and Goosen 2020). Phenolic compounds may be bound to cell walls by either hydrogen bonds or by hydrophobic interactions (Casas and González 2017). In traditional solvent extraction, only the most accessible polyphenols, which are the free compounds (soluble or soluble-conjugated esterified with low-mass compounds), may be extracted (Casas and González 2017; Brito et al. 2021). To release bound phenolic compounds, enzymes may be applied, as they increase extraction via hydrolytic degradation of the cell wall polysaccharides or by breaking glycosidic linkages and hydrogen bonding interactions (Casas and González 2017). Enzymes, such as cellulases, hemicellulases, pectinases, amylases, and glycanases, have been used to hydrolyse cell wall components, and proteases have been used to degrade protein bounds, enabling efficient extraction of phenolic compounds, by facilitating the release of linked compounds (Acosta-Estrada et al. 2014; Aires 2017; Dzah et al. 2020).

Non-extractible polyphenols (NEPs) are largely found in plant residues, such as peels, brans, husks, and skins (Dzah et al. 2020). Those parts usually are discarded as waste; however, these by-products are low-cost and a source of bioactive compounds, including a variety of phenolic compounds, which could be a rich source of antioxidants and other bioactive substances (Casas and González 2017; Dzah et al. 2020). EAE is considered an effective extraction of bioactive compounds from foods and agro-industrial by-products and has been used to improve the extraction efficiency of antioxidants, including phenolics, flavonoids, anthocyanins, and carotenoids (Aires 2017; Xu et al. 2017). Meini et al. (2019) optimized the extraction of phenolics from red grape pomace by EAE by using the enzymes tannase and cellulase. They observed that the extraction was improved by up to 66% and the antioxidant capacity recovery by up to 80% by optimizing the simultaneous enzymatic treatment. The phenolic content was analyzed by HPLC-DAD, and it was found that tannase raised the antioxidant capacity of the extract by the liberation of gallic acid, while cellulase favored the liberation of ρ-coumaric acid and malvidin-3-O-glucoside.

Besides enzymatic hydrolysis, acid and alkaline hydrolysis have also been used to hydrolyze plant materials and release NEPs bound to sugars, fibers, and proteins (Dzah et al. 2020). Acid and alkaline hydrolysis are the most frequently used methods to release bound polyphenols. In the acid treatment, glycosidic bonds are broken, and sugars are solubilized, while ester bonds usually remain intact (Acosta-Estrada et al. 2014). In the alkaline treatment, the ether and ester bonds linking phenolic acids to the cell wall are effectively broken, which makes it especially efficient in the release of polyphenols from polysaccharides (Zhang et al. 2020). In Table 12.3, some advantages and disadvantages of the main hydrolytic methods used to improve the release of NEPs are presented. For acid hydrolysis, 1–5% hydrochloric acid in water/methanol is generally used to hydrolyze insoluble-bound phenolics (Shahidi and Yeo 2016). For alkaline hydrolysis, 1–4 M of sodium hydroxide, room temperature, and different extraction times (15 minutes up to overnight) have been used to release bound phenolics (Acosta-Estrada et al. 2014). Alkaline treatments are mostly used to extract NEPs and other related compounds from cereal grains, legumes, and other seeds (Zhang et al. 2020). Tang et al. (2016) evaluated the phenolic compounds from the meal of quinoa seeds by acid, alkaline, and enzymatic hydrolyses. They identified at least 19 bound phenolic compounds, predominantly phenolic acids and flavonoids. The concentration of bound phenolics, by spectrophotometric assay or by HPLC, was highest in black quinoa, followed by the red and white varieties, regardless of the hydrolysis method used. It was also observed that the alkaline, acidic, and enzymatic (by pectinase, xylanase, and feruloyl esterase) hydrolysis effectively released bound phenolics; however, not all hydrolysis methods released the same phenolic profile. In Table 12.3, the advantages and disadvantages of the use of different hydrolysis techniques are presented, while Table 12.4 presents an overview of the alternative methods used to improve the extraction yield of polyphenols in different matrices, and Table 12.5 summarizes the use of hydrolysis methods to assist the extraction of insoluble-bound phenolics from different plant matrices, herbs, and by-products.

TABLE 12.3
Pros and Cons of Different Hydrolysis Methods Used to Release Bonded Polyphenols

Technique	Advantages	Disadvantages	Reference
EAE	It is a highly specific and efficient method; it is considered an ecofriendly method due to the use of water as a solvent instead of toxic organic chemicals; it shows specificity in targeting desired end products and reduced processing time; it uses lower temperatures that do not induce polyphenol degradation.	In some cases, EAE introduces metabolite artifacts as the used enzyme may induce side reaction; enzymes are high-cost; the activity of enzymes vary with the environmental factors.	Ameer et al. 2017; Xu et al. 2017; Bordoloi and Goosen 2020; Dzah et al. 2020; Zhang et al. 2020
Acid hydrolysis	This method presents simple steps and allows the direct injection of the extracted bound phenolics into a chromatographic system after neutralization and filtration.	At acidic pH and high temperature, this method might cause degradation of some phenolic compounds; it is considered an aggressive treatment; it is non-specific and might change the conformation of NEPs being difficult to know the real structure.	Acosta-Estrada et al. 2014; Shahidi and Yeo 2016; Domínguez-Rodríguez et al. 2017; Zhang et al. 2020
Alkaline hydrolysis	This method leads to a lower rate of loss of phenolics during the process than the acid hydrolysis method as it is conducted at room temperature.	It is a complex procedure, which requires a pretreatment process where the reaction needs to be conducted in darkness under an inert gas atmosphere, and the presence of EDTA is usually necessary to prevent the oxidation of the NEPs; it requires long extraction times; it is non-specific and might change the conformation of NEPs being difficult to know the real structure.	Domínguez-Rodríguez et al. 2017; Wang et al. 2020

TABLE 12.4
Use of Alternative Techniques to Extract Polyphenols from Various Plant Matrices, Herbs, and By-Products

Sample evaluated	Target compound	Extraction technique, extraction condition, and method	Application	References
Walnut leaves (*Juglans regia* L.)	Polyphenols	MAE: 3 min, 107.5°C, and 67.9% ethanol; ME: 112.5 min, 61.3°C, and 50.4% of ethanol; quantification by HPLC-DAD	Walnut leaves as are valorized as a source of quercetin to be used as ingredients for the development of functional foods.	Vieira et al. 2017
Sesame bran	Antioxidants	MAE combined with EAE: 98 min, 49°C, and 1.94 AU/100 g enzyme concentration; identification by LC/Q-TOF/MS	It is a potential source to produce antioxidant-rich protein isolate.	Görgüç et al. 2019
Berberis species (*B. jaeschkeana* and *B. asiatica*)	Alkaloids and polyphenols	MAE: 2 min, 100% methanol, pH 2.0, 598 W of power; quantification by HPLC-DAD	It has the potential, in extract preparation, to harness its nutraceutical and pharmaceutical properties.	Belwal et al. 2020
Salvia viridis L. roots	Bioactive compounds	MAE: 30 min, 96% (w/w) ethanol (1:20 ratio), 600 W; ME: 24 h, 100% methanol; SFE: 50°C, 350 bar; SE: 6 h, 96% (w/w) ethanol; UAE: 60 min, 30°C, 96% (w/w) ethanol; identification by HPLC-MS/MS	It has a possible therapeutic application for the management of chronic complications, such as Alzheimer's disease, diabetes, and skin hyperpigmentation disorders.	Zengin et al. 2019
Grapevine leaves (*Vitis vinifera* L.)	Polyphenols and antioxidants	CSE: 30.96 min, 37.5°C; 29% ethanol (v/v), 72:1 (LSR – mg/g); MAE: 47 s, 34% ethanol (v/v), 40:1 (LSR – mg/g); identification by HPLC – DAD-IT-MS and UPLC-QqQ-MS/MS	It is a possible source of phytochemical constituents for the food industry and/or pharmaceutical applications.	Djemaa-Landri et al. 2020

TABLE 12.4 (CONTINUED)

Sample evaluated	Target compound	Extraction technique, extraction condition, and method	Application	References
Chia (*Salvia hispanica* L.)	Polyphenols and antioxidants	UAE: 40 min, 25°C, methanol/water (60:40), 20 kHz of frequency, 50% power with continuous stirring; identification and quantification by GC-MS	The studied fractions with the highest levels of compounds with nutraceutical value have potential interest for the food and feed industries.	de Falco et al. 2018
Propolis	Polyphenols and antioxidants	UAE: 17 min, frequency of 20 kHz, 140 W of power, 80% ethanol; PE: 6 h shaken and stood for 18 h, 80% ethanol; SFE: 6.5 h, CO_2, 95% ethanol, 317 bars, 45°C, gas flow rate of 2 L/min; identification by UPLC-ESI-QTOF-MS/MS	UAE showed more phenolic types, the highest total phenolic content, and high antioxidant activity, among the techniques used, so it might be considered to be used to extract bioactive compounds from propolis.	Yuan et al. 2019
Seaweed (*S. compressa*)	Polyphenols	UAE: 30 min, 50°C, 3.8 W of power, 32.22% ethanol; identification and quantification by HPLC-DAD and HPLC-MS-TOF	UAE increases the phlorotannin yield extraction, leading to a natural product of high commercial value that might be used in the pharmaceutical, food, and cosmetic industries.	Vázquez-Rodríguez et al. 2020
Sesame	Antioxidants	UAE: 65 min, 50°C, 410 W of power, 75% ethanol, 20:1 (LSR – mL/g); identification by HPLC-MS /MS	It may be suitable for the development of functional products.	Wang et al. 2019

(Continued)

TABLE 12.4 (CONTINUED)

Sample evaluated	Target compound	Extraction technique, extraction condition, and method	Application	References
Extra-virgin olive oil (*Apulian coratina*)	Polyphenols	UAE combined with SHE: a range of 20–25°C, 23 kHz of frequency, 100 W of power; identification by NMR spectroscopy	NMR can provide useful information to develop new extraction strategies for plant optimization and to increase the healthy bioactive product components in extra-virgin olive oil products.	Del Coco et al. 2021
Seaweed (*Fucus vesiculosus*)	Polyphenols, antioxidants, bioactive compounds	PLE: 40°C, 1500 psi pressure, preliminary water extraction step (10 min static cycle), followed by subsequent extractions with 100% methanol and 100% dichloromethane (5 min static cycle for both solvents); identification by UPLC-QTOF-MS/MS	Among the compounds identified (phlorotannins, carotenoids, chlorophylls, betaine lipids, phospholipids, and tocopherols), phlorotannin showed the greatest radical scavenging and apoptotic activities against pancreas cancer cells.	Heavisides et al. 2018
Grape skin	Polyphenols and antioxidants	ASE: 14.82 min, 50.79°C, 48.8% ethanol, 10.1 MPa pressure; CSE: 5 h, 50°C, 49% ethanol; identification by HPLC and UPLC	The phenolic with significant antioxidant potential can be used as an excellent natural antioxidant agent for industrial application.	Li J et al. 2019

TABLE 12.4 (CONTINUED)

Sample evaluated	Target compound	Extraction technique, extraction condition, and method	Application	References
Black pepper (*Piper nigrum*)	Bioactive compounds	ASE: 10 min, 70°C, solvent di-chloromethane, 100 atm pressure; quantification by UHPLC-DAD	The combination of ASE-UHPLC-DAD produced a fast and sensitive method to quantify the active drug Piperine in commercial food samples as a marker for the determination of adulteration.	Ahmad et al. 2019
Ginseng roots (*Panax ginseng* C. A. Mey)	Bioactive compounds	SWE: 20 min, 200°C, 6.0 MPa pressure; CSE: 3 h, pure water or 70% (v/v) ethanol, at 100°C and 60°C respectively; identification and quantification by UFLC-MS/MS	SWE was more feasible and efficient than the conventional solid-liquid heating extraction method for the extraction of sugars, antioxidant TP, proteins, and ginsenoside Rg2.	Zhang et al. 2018
Stems, leaves, and berries of *Aronia melanocarpa*	Bioactive compounds	SWE: 20 min, 130°C, 35 bar pressure; identification and quantification by HPLC-DAD	All three aronia parts demonstrated biological potential to develop newly designed functional products.	Cvetanović et al. 2018
Camelina sativa seed	Bioactive compounds	SC-CO_2: 20 min, 70°C, 45 MPa pressure, 10% (w/w) ethanol as co-solvent; identification and quantification by HPLC	The method enriched the oil in terms of phenolic compounds, which can protect omega-3 oils against oxidation.	Belayneh et al. 2017
Hibiscus sabdariff	Polyphenols, antioxidants, bioactive compounds	SC-CO_2: 90 min, 50°C, 250 bar pressure, 16.7% ethanol as co-solvent; quantification by HPLC-ESI-TOF-MS	SC-CO_2 demonstrated to be a suitable and selective technique to maximize the extraction of several phytochemical compounds from *H. sabdariffa* calyces, such as hibiscus acid and derivatives.	Pimentel-Moral et al. 2019

(Continued)

TABLE 12.4 (CONTINUED)

Sample evaluated	Target compound	Extraction technique, extraction condition, and method	Application	References
Apple pomace	Antioxidant	SFE: 2 h, 45°C, 30 MPa pressure; SC-CO_2: 2 h, 45°C, 30 MPa pressure, 5% ethanol as co-solvent; SE: 6 h; ME: 37 min, 100°C, in boiling water; identification by HPLC-DAD-MS	SFE extracts presented less but more active polyphenols than the extracts processed by Soxhlet and maceration with boiling water.	Ferrentino et al. 2018
Garlic (*Allium sativum* L.)	Polyphenols	SC-CO_2: 9 min, 50°C, 10 Mpa pressure, 30% methanol as co-solvent; quantification by off-line SFC-MS/MS	SFE-SFC-MS/MS was considered as a potential method for the analysis of the phenolic compounds in garlic.	Liu et al. 2018
Asparagus racemosus (shatavari) root	Polyphenols	SC-CO_2: 60 min, 50°C, 200 bar pressure, 10% ethanol as co-solvent; SE: 24 h, 50°C (in water, aqueous ethanol or with pure ethanol); ME: 72 h, 25°C, 150 rpm; identification by HPLC	SC-CO_2-based extract had a larger number of polar compounds and higher antioxidant activities, and the mixture of the different extracts (SC-CO_2, SE, and ME) can be used to enrich the bioactive components of the formulation.	Hasan and Panda 2020

TABLE 12.5
Use of Hydrolysis Methods to Assist the Extraction of Insoluble-Bound Phenolics from Different Plant Matrices, Herbs, and By-Products

Sample evaluated	Sample pretreatment	Hydrolysis technique and conditions	Main phenolic compounds identified	References
Pepper (*Capsicum baccatum*)	Ethanol or butanol solution (both with water 50:50, v/v)	Ethanol: water solution or butanol: water solution, 10 h, 30°C; identification by UPLC ESI-Q-TOF-MS/MS	Quercetin 3-O-rhamnoside, luteolin 7-O-glycoside, and naringenin	Mendes et al. 2019
Wheat (*Triticum aestivum*)	Maceration (PC-free) and alkaline hydrolysis and MAE, followed by acid hydrolysis (PC-bound)	Maceration (celite and 80% ethanol); M: 10 min; AH: 90 min; alkaline: 4 M NaOH; ultrasonic bath: 42 kHz; acid: concentrated HCl; identification by UPLC-QTOF-MS	Ferulic acid, diphyllin, 4-hydroxybenzoic acid, ferulic acid isomer, apigenin 7-O-apiosyl-glucoside isomer, and myricetin isomer	Santos et al. 2019
Apple (*Malus domestica*) (peel and pulp)	Alkaline and acid hydrolysis	Acidified methanol extraction; AH: overnight; AH: 30 min; 85°C; alkaline: 10 M NaOH; acid: HCl; identification by UHPLC ESI-Q-TOF MS/MS	Chlorogenic acid, caffeic acid, p- coumaric acid and protocatechuic acid in the peel, and chlorogenic acid and caffeic acid in the pulp	Lee et al. 2017
Muskmelon (*Cucumis melo* L.)	Ethanol solution	Ethanol: ratio 1:50 w/v; 6 h; 50°C; identification by HPLC-PDA-ESI- MS/MS	Gallic acid, ellagic acid, and kaempferol in the peel; ferulic acid, kaempferol, and gallic acid in the seed	Vella et al. 2019
Green tea (*Camellia sinensis*)	Acid hydrolysis	Sulfuric acid: water; 20 h, 85°C; identification by UPLC – LPG-3400SD	Gallic acid, epigallocatechin-3-gallate, epicatechin-3-gallate, gallocatechin-3-gallate	Yan et al. 2018
Jackfruit (*Artocarpus heterophyllus* Lam.)	Alkaline, acidic, and enzymatic hydrolysis	Alkaline (NaOH), acidic (H_2SO_4), or enzymatic (cellulase and pectinase, the mass ratio was 2:1); concentration and different liquid-solid ratio for a different time; identification by UPLC-ESI-QTOF-MS/MS	10 phenolic acids, 13 flavonoids, 8 organic acid (alkaline); 3 phenolic acids, 7 organic acid (acidic); 7 phenolic acids, 9 organic acid (enzymatic)	Zhang et al. 2020

(Continued)

TABLE 12.5 (CONTINUED)

Sample evaluated	Sample pretreatment	Hydrolysis technique and conditions	Main phenolic compounds identified	References
Brewers' spent grain	Fermentation and acid – alkaline hydrolysis	Fermentation by five strains of *Aspergillus* followed by extraction acid – alkaline; identification by UPLC-ESI-QTOF-MSE	12 PC exclusively in the fermented BSG: irisolidone, schisandrin C, jaceosidin, avenanthramide 2p, rosmarinic acid, salvia-nolic acid D, 3-O-methylgallic acid, 4-O-methylgallic acid, esculin, 6″-O-acetyldaidzin, 3′-O-methylviolanone, and ligstroside	Maia et al. 2020
Black soybean (*Glycine max* (L.) Merr.) (seed coat and cotyledon)	Acid-alkali sequential hydrolysis (A-B-BPE) and alkali- acid sequential hydrolysis (B-A-BPE)	A-B-BPE – 2 M NaOH, 6 M HCl; B-A-BPE – 2 M HCl, 6 M NaOH; identified by UPLC- ESI-QTOF-MS	78 compounds were identified; acid hydrolysis was more effective than alkaline hydrolysis	Peng et al. 2017
Fruit peels: apple (var. Fuji, Golden, and Granny Smith), banana (Del Monte), kiwi (var. Hayward), mandarin (var. Tang Gold), mango (var. Osteen), melon (var. Piel de Sapo or Santa Claus), nectarine (var. Venus), orange (var. Newhall), pear (var. Blanquilla), and watermelon (var. Imperial)	Acid hydrolysis	Hydrolysis with methanol and sulfuric acid for 20 h at 85°C; quantified by HPLC-DAD	Peels made up >40% of total NEPs in four of the samples analyzed (in ascending order: nectarine, orange, watermelon, and mandarin)	Pérez-Jimeénez and Saura-Calixto 2018

12.3 DATA ACQUISITION IN LC-MS/MS

The great analytical challenge for phenolic compounds lies in their vast diversity and structural complexity, with highly polymerized structures, which can also form complexes with various other plant-matrix components (Olalla et al. 2020). Improvements in chromatographic performance in LC column technology and MS instrumentation have been necessary to meet the growing analytical demands for phenolic compounds in terms of resolving power, selectivity, and sensitivity (Kalili and De Villiers 2011; Capriotti et al. 2015). MS has become a fundamental technology for the analysis of polymeric compounds (polyphenols), such as tannins and, especially, proanthocyanidins, as their polydispersity – diversity of polymers, without uniform molecular weights, due to the different sizes of polymer chains – results in poor resolution and detection (Cheynier 2012; Santos et al. 2019).

For the metabolomic approach, LC coupled with MS is one of the most powerful techniques for the elucidation of the structure and the investigation of natural compounds, like phenolic components, for qualitative and quantitative analysis (Piovesana et al. 2020); therefore, this section will focus on this technique. Metabolomics is one of the most applied large-scale approaches to study changes in the metabolome of biological systems (Catalán et al. 2017). Metabolomic platforms allow targeted and untargeted high-throughput analysis to identify various phenolic compounds in different types of samples, enabling the qualitative and quantitative characterization of molecules without the need for standards (Kind et al. 2018; Alvarez-Rivera et al. 2019; Aydoğan 2020).

First, it is necessary to emphasize the importance of using quality control in any metabolomic analysis. Quality control in metabolomics-based applications is related to the stability of the LC-MS system and to the quality of the data during acquisition and post-acquisition handling. For that purpose, it is necessary to analyze quality control samples, preferably a pool of the samples of interest, but also synthetic mixtures or standard compounds, to condition the LC-MS system before starting the batch. Blank samples, both for mobile phases and for extraction solutions and procedures, should also be analyzed and later used to discard not sample-related results. After acquiring the mass spectra data, it is necessary to process them. Spectra processing will be detailed in an ensuing section of this chapter. Below, instruments, techniques, and methods used by the metabolomic approach for the analysis of phenolic compounds will be presented.

12.3.1 LC Types and Columns Used in LC-MS Analysis for Metabolomics

Initially, HPLC was the preferred type of LC technique used in metabolomic approaches for phenolic compounds separation. However, with the emergence of ultra-high-performance liquid chromatography (UHPLC) with sub-2 μm packing materials and ultra-high pressures (up to 5,000 bar or 72,000 psi) it was possible to undertake better analyses of up to 100,000 theoretical plates, and to solve diastereomers which are not resolved by conventional HPLC (Gai et al. 2021). The advantages presented by UHPLC over conventional HPLC (i.e., stationary phases of 3–5 μm particles and pressures up to 400 bar) are manifold: (1) higher separation speed for relatively low plate counts (in HPLC, an analysis lasts between 20 and 80 minutes), (2) enhanced peak efficiency, even in the analysis of complex matrices, (3) improved performance of all kinds of phases, (4) reduced solvent consumption, and (5) lower amounts of sample. Furthermore, the increased instrumental pressure and higher flow rates lead to more uniform flow, with shorter diffusion distances, which increase separation efficiency, in a short time, providing faster analyses (Galuch et al. 2019; Hwang et al. 2019; Jiao et al. 2019; Liu et al. 2019; Lukić et al. 2019; Santos et al. 2019). Undoubtedly, with the emergence of dedicated UHPLC instrumentation and the increased availability of UHPLC stationary phases, a more practical application of this technology became possible. Additionally, UHPLC-MS is less susceptible to matrix effects, contributing to decreased ion suppression, when it is the consequence of the coelution of two different compounds (Motilva et al. 2013). The application of UHPLC instrumentation and its columns, however, has some disadvantages, mostly related to the need for extensive alteration of conventional instrumentation. UHPLC depends on pressures above 400 bar and low-volume detectors providing high (410 Hz) acquisition rates. As such, a rapid separation system needs to be coupled to a mass spectrometer able to provide an equally fast duty cycle, which is only available on the newer-generation MS devices (Kalili and De Villiers 2011; Capriotti et al. 2015).

For phenolic compound separation, identification, and quantification, from a variety of samples, by LC-MS, the most used columns are of reversed-phase mode, mainly reversed-phase fused-core C18 columns, and pentafluorophenyl (PFP), except for BEH (ethylene bridged hybrid) Amide and Luna HILIC (hydrophilic interaction chromatography) columns (Motilva et al. 2013; Kumar 2017; Pertuzatti et al. 2021). The most common stationary phases for phenolic compounds analysis are BEH C18 (the most widely applied) and BEH C8, high strength silica (HSS) T3, BEH shield C18, and BEH amide from Waters; Zorbax SB C18, Zorbax Eclipse Plus C18, and HT C18 from Agilent; Hypersil Gold from ThermoFisher; and Kinetex XB-C18, Kinetex PFP, and Luna HILIC from Phenomenex (Gong and Pegg 2017; Olalla et al. 2020). PFP stationary phase provided higher plate number and superior peak shape for the low-molecular-weight phenolic fractions (Gong and Pegg 2017).

In reverse phase columns, the elution order of phenolic compounds generally follows the pattern of benzoic acids, cinnamic acids, flavonoid glycosides, and flavonoid aglycones, while within individual classes of phenolics, the expected elution is based on the number of hydroxy, and then methoxy substituents, such as caffeic acid (3,4-dihydroxy), ρ-coumaric acid (4-hydroxy), ferulic acid (4-hydroxy-3-methoxy), sinapic acid (4-hydroxy-3,5-dimethoxy), and *trans*-cinnamic acid (no substituents), according to their polarity (Gómez-Romero et al. 2011). For HILIC columns, on the other hand, the non-polar phenolic compounds are eluted before the polar ones, the retention mechanism is mainly governed by hydrophilic partitioning of the compounds between the highly organic mobile phase (mostly acetonitrile) and the surface of the polar stationary phase, where the polar compounds are retained for longer time (Pyrzynska and Sentkowska 2019).

Although LC is the most efficient technique for the separation of polyphenolic compounds from different matrices, unfortunately, to date, there is no single chromatographic method for separating all different kinds of phenolic compounds. Optimizations regarding the stationary and mobile phases, the elution gradient, temperature, and flow rate are relevant. In addition, other factors, such as stereochemistry, molecular weight, polarity, and degree of polymerization of polyphenols, must be considered since they affect the retention of compounds (Olalla et al. 2020). Below are some examples of methodology optimization for the analysis of phenolic compounds.

For anthocyanins, HPLC separation proved to be complex since the various forms of these molecules in solution depend on a pH-dependent equilibrium. To have an efficient chromatographic separation and to represent the different forms of anthocyanins in different peaks, a slow interconversion is necessary between the individual species in relation to the time of the chromatographic run (Olalla et al. 2020). One of the ways to optimize the chromatographic resolution, in this case, is to reduce the size of the column particles and increase the temperature (Villiers et al. 2009). Methods developed for the separation of anthocyanins into red cabbage, grape, and wine extracts using UHPLC-DAD/MS, 1.8 μm or 1.7 μm C18 column, 50°C temperature, using mobile phases of aqueous formic acid-acetonitrile, were successful for detection of various compounds derived from cyanidins with optimization of chromatographic resolution (Pati et al. 2009). For phenolic acids, catechins, stilbenes, tannins, and flavonoids, the methodologies in use included columns with particle sizes around 2.5 μm, 1.8 μm, and 1.7 μm C18 operated at 37, 40, 70°C and acidified water-methanol or acidified water-methanol-acetonitrile mobile phases (Kalili and De Villiers 2011).

For the analysis of many phenolic compounds in complex matrices, as is common in untargeted metabolomic analyses, the multidimensional LC (MDLC) analyses provide high peak and resolution capacity. MDLC consists of a combination of two or more independent and orthogonal separation mechanisms (Motilva et al. 2013; Capriotti et al. 2015). The resolving power (peak capacity) of an LC×LC is the product of peak capacities in each dimension and is even higher than optimized one-dimensional methods (Kalili and De Villiers 2011). LC×LC separations may be performed in three different ways: online (fractions from the first dimension are sequentially transferred to the second dimension for subsequent analysis; a much wider application for phenolic analysis), offline, and stop-flow modes (Sarrut et al. 2014). The drawback of LC×LC is that it produces complex and relatively large datasets (especially when used in combination with MS), which complicates data analysis and quantitative analysis (Sarrut et al. 2014). Therefore, its application should be useful for samples containing compounds of more than one chemical characteristic, which is what occurs with natural phenolic fractions (Kalili and De Villiers 2011). In some of these works with coconut, apple, and tea, the analytical columns employed were HPLC×UHPLC; size exclusion chromatography (SEC) and reversed phase (BEH C18) were used to separate compounds according to their size and polarity, respectively; and HILIC and reversed phase (BEH C18) were used to separate the compounds, based on their hydrophobicity and polarity (Motilva et al. 2013).

12.3.2 LC Tandem High-Resolution Mass Spectrometry (HRMS) or Ultra-High-Resolution Mass Spectrometry (UHRMS)

In the last years, to perform appropriate metabolomics-based techniques (both targeted and untargeted) for studies of plant foods, the use of LC-HRMS and LC-MS/MS approaches has been combined with multivariate statistic analysis. Moreover, for the analysis of phenol metabolome in complex plant food matrices, adequate parameters, such as mass resolution, are crucial. HRMS has high resolving power around 10,000–40,000 FWHM (full width at half maximum) (Lucci et al. 2017; Olalla et al. 2020; Piovesana et al. 2020), while UHRMS afforded by Fourier transform (FT) analyzers has resolving power above 300,000 (FWHM) (Hohenester et al. 2020).

Tandem mass spectrometry (MS/MS or MS^2 first-generation product ion spectra) has become established as a powerful tool that has enabled researchers to elucidate complex phenolic structures, in complex matrices, such as food samples, through the determination of accurate molecular masses and specific fragmentation patterns (Motilva et al. 2013; Capriotti et al. 2015).

Fragmentation studies (MS^2) are essential to corroborate MS data in metabolomic studies, especially when using different bioinformatics software for annotation (Piovesana et al. 2020). Therefore, to improve the reliability of annotations, at least MS^2 spectra (product ion spectra) of corresponding resources from the complete scan need to be acquired to elucidate the structure. These spectra provide information on the structure of the compound, as they involve breaking chemical bonds. MS or MS^1 spectra (precursor ions, which did not undergo fragmentation) with accurate mass or isotopic profile of precursor ions only provide information on atomic composition (De Vijlder et al. 2018).

There are multiple advantages of HRMS over classical unit-mass-resolution tandem MS and low-resolution MS (LRMS), such as (1) differentiation of isobaric compounds, with the same nominal m/z ratio but different elemental composition, which means that LRMS allows for measurements in single-digit mas units, whereas HRMS provides exact mass values with four to six decimals; (2) information collected by a single injection that can be used for quantification and screening purposes, including targeted and undirected analyses; (3) collection of full-scan spectra that can be used in a retrospective posterior stage analysis to check a posteriori hypotheses involving the structural elucidation of unknown or putative compounds; (4) removal of interferences based on accurate mass, which enables the simplification of sample preparation procedures, providing faster analytical methods with less sample manipulation; and (5) possibility of performing both screening and quantitation without an analyte standard.

UHRMS using electrospray ionization Fourier transform ion cyclotron resonance mass spectrometry (ESI-FT-ICRMS) is appropriate to investigate matrices with high chemical complexity (e.g., vegetable oils) (Beneito-Cambra et al. 2020). In addition, for the analysis of complex samples, such as olive oil, the use of ion mobility spectrometry adds another dimension to the m/z separation, representing an interesting alternative. In a recent work for sample authentication, the combined use of electrospray ionization, differential mobility analysis (DMA) – a class of ion mobility spectrometry (IMS) – and mass spectrometry were combined for chemical fingerprinting of olive oils for authentication purposes (ESI- DMA-MS) (Beneito-Cambra et al. 2020).

12.3.3 Mobile Phases for LC-MS/MS

The mobile phases employed in LC-MS (ionization by ESI) are binary systems that include an aqueous phase A and a phase B produced with less polar organic solvents, such as acetonitrile or methanol (an organic solvent modifier). Normally, acetonitrile is preferred because of the lower resulting pressure in comparison to methanol (Arceusz et al. 2013; Motilva et al. 2013). Additionally, an acid is added to both components to maintain a constant acid concentration during gradient runs: formic acid, ammonium acetate, trifluoroacetic acid, or acetic acid (Arceusz et al. 2013; Olalla et al. 2020; Alañón et al. 2021). The decrease of pH of phase A, normally kept below 3 and in low concentration (between 0.005 and 0.2%) (Olalla et al. 2020), helps avoid the dissociation of phenolic compounds, also improving the symmetry of the peak, reducing peak-tailing, and ensuring satisfactory ionization during MS acquisition (Cortina-Puig et al. 2012; Motilva et al. 2013). However, one must be careful, as exceptionally low pH may irreversibly damage silica-based columns (Ruiz et al. 2018).

12.3.4 MS Ionization Sources

The most used ionization source for the analysis of phenolic compounds is electrospray ionization (ESI), both in positive and negative mode, as it is recommended for polar compounds (Motilva et al. 2013). Atmospheric pressure chemical ionization (APCI) is not very applicable for the analysis of phenolics because it has low sensitivity (Motilva et al. 2013). In ESI, in the negative ionization mode, the molecular ion [M + H] – predominates, while in the positive [M + H] +, there is no additional fragmentation (Motilva et al. 2013). For example, ionization in negative mode is recommended for phenolic acids, sometimes after comparison with ionization in positive mode. Both ionization modes can be applied simultaneously (Martini et al. 2021) and, together with chemometric multiblock, they present complementary results, as found in a previous experiment performed to discriminate wines in terms of grape variety (Mazerolles et al. 2010). Briefly, for the analysis of phenolic compounds, the negative mode is used, as these molecules contain numerous hydroxyl groups, which are somewhat acidic. To obtain quasimolecular ions, phenolic compound eluates are often ionized in negative mode ([M – H] –). The exception would be anthocyanins, for which the two ionization modes are used (Santos et al. 2019; Olalla et al. 2020). Anthocyanins and isoflavonoids can be analyzed in the positive mode. Anthocyanins can be detected as flavylium cations under acidic conditions. Isoflavones, which are methoxylated compounds, do not ionize negatively due to the absence of a free hydroxyl group (Motilva et al. 2013). Negative ionization is suitable for the analysis of carboxylic acids and uncharged flavonols (Motilva et al. 2013) In several studies, collision-induced dissociation (CID) has been shown to be very efficient in resolving the structure of flavonoids. ESI made it possible to detect the molecular glycoside mass owing to their prominent [M – H] – ions and fragmentation products of the aglycone arising from Diels-Alder reactions (Motilva et al. 2013).

12.3.5 MS Analyzers

In the ionization sources of the mass spectrometers, ions are produced, and they will be separated according to their masses in the analyzers (Kumar 2017). Several analyzers have been reported to be available for phenol analysis in MS/MS modes (Pereira et al. 2020). MS investigations can be carried out with LRMS, using triple quadrupole (QqQ), or linear ion traps (ITs) used as analyzers, or HRMS, using Orbitrap (Barbera et al. 2017; Lucci et al. 2017; Aydoğan 2020; Nijat et al. 2020). MS methodologies for Orbitrap have been used for the analysis of phenolic compounds in fruit products, artichoke, barberry herb, *Pistacia lentiscus* (var. chia leaves), and alcoholic fermented strawberry products (Lucci et al. 2017). For analysis of phenols in complex samples such as food, when commercial standards cannot be obtained, scan acquisition modes are applied – for example, full scan, product ion scan, and data dependent scan (Nicácio et al. 2021).

The multiple reaction monitoring (MRM) mode of UPLC, coupled with triple quadrupole mass spectrometry (QqQ-MS/MS), has the ability to selectively identify and quantify target compounds in complex mixtures via fast screening of the specific precursor ion-to-product ion transitions, which can significantly shorten analysis time without considering the interference of peak overlapping, and provide excellent sensitivity with an extremely low quantitation limit (Aksay et al. 2021; Gai et al. 2021). Optimizations in various parameters are always necessary to avoid problems with sensitivity and matrix effects – for example, capillary voltage, declustering potential, collision energy, and dwell times (Olalla et al. 2020).

Multistage mass spectrometry (MS^n) information relies on systematically fragmenting product ions from the previous fragmentation step and results in an extensive spectral tree. In the specific case of phenolic compounds, MS^n is extremely useful for the structural characterization of glycoconjugates (it is particularly useful for dereplication of 6-C and 8-C-glycosidic flavonoid isomers in a complex mixture), in which different modifications (hydroxylation, methylation, acylation, prenylation, and O- and C-glycosylation) can possibly produce a complex combination of isomeric and isobaric compounds (Kachlicki et al. 2016; Piovesana et al. 2020). MS^n has been reported to identify phenolic compounds in medicinal plants (Arceusz et al. 2013). In this work, unknown compounds (without standard availability) were characterized based on the information provided by MS^n in the IT analyzer. Good results were found with LC-HRMS, operating in full scan, using a TOF analyzer for identification of polyphenols and flavonoids in grains (Aydoğan 2020). Accurate mass measurements of the product ions generated in the MS^n experiments facilitate the elucidation of the structures of unknown compounds and the differentiation of isomeric compounds, making attractive the use of hybrid mass spectrometers, such as quadrupole-time-of-flight (Q-TOF), ion-trap-time-of-flight (IT-TOF), and linear ion-trap-quadrupole-Orbitrap (LTQ-Orbitrap) (Ofosu et al. 2021). For the analysis of polymeric phenolics and conjugates, preferred choices include hybrid mass analyzers capable of performing acquisition dependent on MS/MS (DDA) data, such as Qlinear ion trap (Q-LIT) (Beldean-Galea et al. 2008), and/or measuring the precise mass of precursor ions or precursor ions and products, such as Q-TOF (Martínez-Busi et al. 2019) or LTQ-Orbitrap (Nijat et al. 2020). Depending on the available instrument scan modes, the survey scan is generally a full MS scan in the m/z range of interest; data are processed on the fly to determine, for each scan cycle, the n candidates of interest based on pre-defined selection criteria. If the selection criteria are satisfied, a second scan, usually a product ion scan, is then performed (Beldean-Galea et al. 2008).

The existing acquisition modes can be dependent or independent. Without acquisition-mode-dependent data (DDA), a precursor ion is selected and fragmented for sequencing. In this sense, independent data acquisition (DIA) is performed using a hybrid system with complete measurement data being recorded on HRMS instruments. In addition, this acquisition mode produces a complex and accurate data structure for intricate data processing. Generally, MS^E for macromolecules and all-ion fragmentation (AIF) for small molecules are used in DIA mode. Regarding processing techniques, they can be categorized into targeted, non-targeted, and suspect screening. Targeted screening is widely used in DDA mode. On the other hand, non-targeted screening strategies, also called untargeted, are based on DIA mode (Aydoğan 2020).

Ultra-high-resolution ($m/\Delta m > 100{,}000$) state-of-the-art mass spectrometers are available commercially, such as Fourier transform mass spectrometers, the Orbitrap Fusion, and the SolariX FT-ICR. However, studies on the metabolomics of phenols using these instruments have not yet been reported (Hohenester et al. 2020). Excellent reviews on the use of LC-MS/MS are available in several articles (Gonzalez-Paramas et al. 2011; Arceusz et al. 2013; Motilva et al. 2013; Santos et al. 2019; Kalogiouri et al. 2020; Olalla et al. 2020).

12.4 BIOINFORMATIC AND CHEMOMETRIC TOOLS FOR THE INTERPRETATION OF METABOLOMIC DATA

The LC-MS/MS-based detection methods make it possible to acquire three-dimensional dataset consisting of mass/charge (m/z), ion intensity, and retention time (RT) distribution (Perez de Souza et al. 2017). However, bioinformatics efforts are needed for data processing, a crucial step to reduce the analysis complexity and extract the most important characteristics. Also, it is possible to prevent human error, to remove artifacts, to decrease working time, and to enable biomarker discoveries from food, medicines, plants, and agro-industrial residues (Rinschen et al. 2019).

Non-targeted metabolomic datasets are usually produced through sample preparation, data acquisition, and data processing. The latter includes pre-processing and identification or annotation of metabolites. The subsequent data are then analyzed by statistical and molecular network approaches, which enable the data interpretation and generation of new testable hypotheses (Figure 12.2) (Castillo et al. 2011). Data

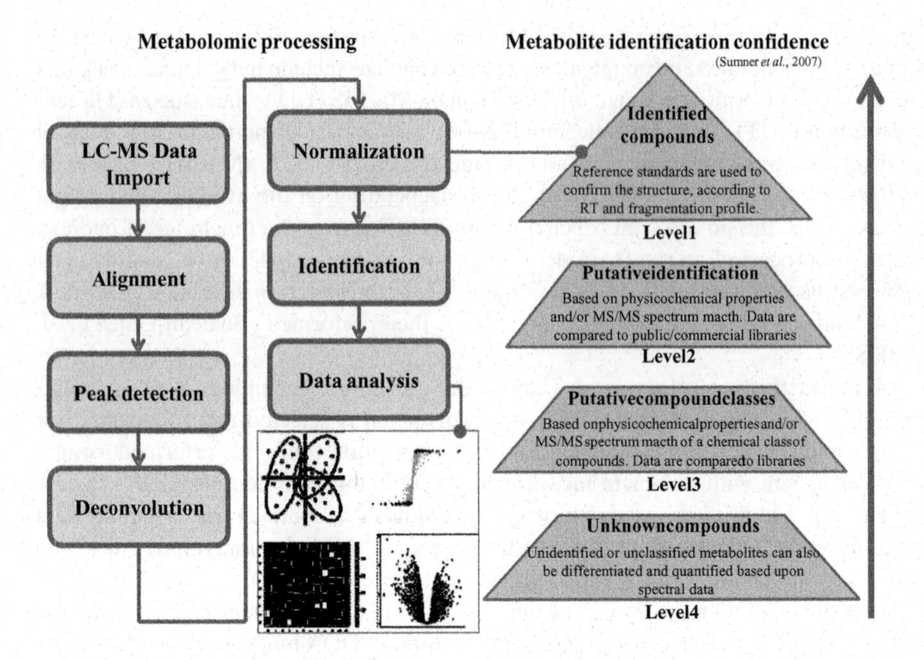

FIGURE 12.2 Schematic overview of the metabolomic in LC-MS data processing. Highlight for the identification stage, in which confidence levels are applied.

pre-processing, normalization, identification, and analysis will be explored in this section of the chapter.

12.4.1 Data Pre-Processing

Data pre-processing includes the initial steps: alignment, peak detection, and deconvolution, and it is a necessary stage to ensure the detection and quantification of high-quality peaks from raw data. The data-pre-processing routine requires algorithms capable of improving signal quality and reducing noise interference, making the data comparable to each other (Antonakoudis et al. 2020). Typically, pre-processing steps are established through pre-processing software packages and databases available to the public commercially or for free. Table 12.6 shows examples of five common software packages reported in literature along with their advantages/disadvantages. Pre-processing exhibits robust functions that comprise, at least, noise filtering, RT alignment, peak deconvolution, peak detection (peak picking), and normalization steps. Before any analysis, acquired raw data are cleaned up by the noise filtration algorithm. This step is based on a mass spectrum without the presence of a bottom line (noise). Thus, compounds with less relative abundance are not discarded during the procedure (Goodacre et al. 2007). In data acquisition, LC-MS chromatograms are also prone to small non-linear variations in the RT and m/z between technical replicates, even with well-calibrated equipment (Burton

TABLE 12.6
Summary of Functions, Advantages, and Disadvantages of LC-MS Data Pre-Processing Tools

Name	Main function	Access	Advantage	Disadvantage	Availability	References
Mzmine	Chromatogram alignment, peak detection, deconvolution, normalization, visualization	Download	It allows the processing of raw data from different mass spectrometry in the same analysis program and free user guide provided (http://mzmine.sourceforge.net/tutorial/).	Two non-related peaks could be matched, or the matching of two related peaks could be omitted.	www.mzmine.github.io/	Pluskal et al. 2010
MetAlign	Chromatogram alignment, peak detection, deconvolution, accurate mass calculations	Download	It can handle peak broadening by a user-defined maximum amplitude threshold.	It does not allow post-processing steps, such as data visualization, normalization, and identification, requiring two software.	www.metalign.nl	Lommen and Kools 2012
XCMS	Chromatogram alignment, peak detection and matching, metabolite identification, structural characterization and statistical analysis	Online	The platform supports high-throughput cloud-based data processing.	It does not have the normalization step.	www.xcmsonline.scripps.edu/	Smith et al. 2006
Progenesis	Chromatogram alignment, peak detection, deconvolution, normalization, structural characterization, and statistical analysis	Commercial	It can perform all processing steps in a single software and supports different raw data formats and easy handling.	License purchase required	www.waters.com/	Nascimento et al. 2019; Santos et al. 2019; Cardoso et al. 2020; Lima et al. 2020; Maia et al. 2020; Brito et al. 2021
Metaboanalyst AuQ1	Chromatogram alignment, peak detection, normalization, statistical analysis, and pathway analysis	Online	It allows easy access and handling, allowing users with little or no experience to perform statistical analysis; it allows the treatment of metabolomic data and transforms them into graphs.	It does not allow the identification of metabolites.	www.metaboanalyst.ca	Xia et al. 2015

et al. 2008; Yi et al. 2016). However, the application of alignment algorithms may compare all compounds in each run and remove shifts among samples to guarantee useful information (Lange et al. 2008; Smith et al. 2015). The greatest challenge of the alignment step is the selection of the reference run since in the most part of software, the selection is manual. Thus, studies highlight the importance of quality control (QC) at this stage, with the aim of obtaining a "ground truth" alignment (Brodsky et al. 2010). QC was briefly addressed in the previous section of this chapter. There are two main approaches for alignment: (1) the feature-based approach that selects a reference run as a basis to align the RT of all other runs and alternatively and (2) the profile-based approach that estimates the variability of signals along the runs. After alignment by any of the approaches, the ion i from run x is superimposed in the same location as the corresponding ion from run y (Want and Masson 2011).

The next step is peak detection, which aims to identify and quantify the signals corresponding to the metabolites present in the sample (Castillo et al. 2011). It is through the peak-picking algorithms that true signals are correctly presented and the record of false positives, caused by noise or column dead volume, is prevented (Yi et al. 2016). For this step, various thresholds must be determined for charge, baseline intensity, peak width, and resolution, for instance. Finally, the deconvolution step recalculates multiple charged mass into the neutral mass (deconvoluted), it means into the accurate molecular weights, improving and resolving also coelution and overlapping of compounds occurring before deconvolution step (Saito and Matsuda 2010).

Usually, the software combines these algorithms into a single function to make easy the separation of structural isomers, to reduce the complexity of the data, and to make feasible the following analysis steps (Castillo et al. 2011; Dias et al. 2016).

12.4.2 Normalization

Multidimensional data do not always show normal distribution. Thus, the use of normalization and scaling approaches are suggested to remove the effect of variability between different runs of the same sample, allowing quantitative comparisons among samples (Yi et al. 2016). In metabolomics, metabolite concentrations can be different in samples due to dilution errors, and the normalization step is important to ensure that variations in analysis are due to changes in metabolic responses and not due to variable dilution (Karaman 2017). Normalization enables the calibration of the data and the quantitative comparison between sample signals (Want and Masson 2011).

A very reliable way of data normalization is through the addition of one or more standards with a known concentration in each sample (Karaman 2017). This approach is widely used in targeted methods of LC-MS. The insertion of the standard may take place in the extractor solvent – to accompany the sampling, extraction, and analysis – or during the injection of the sample in the instrument – to remove variations resulting from the instrumental analysis. As a result, samples may be normalized using the peak intensity/area (Sysi-Aho et al. 2007).

The most common normalization in non-targeted methods of LC-MS is total ion count (or total ion current [TIC]) normalization (Wulff and Mitchell 2018). After the acquisition, the metabolites will be normalized according to the sum of all resources (ion intensity) in the corresponding line (chromatogram) (Veselkov et al. 2011). In other words, the metabolites with higher concentration contribute more to peak intensity/area and, consequently, impact more on normalization when compared to low concentration metabolites. After this process, TIC will be transformed into Base Peak Chromatogram (BPC) (Wulff and Mitchell 2018). This method is more cost-effective, as it does not require the purchase of standards; however, it is important to note that the presence of significant changes in peak intensity/area of highly concentrated metabolites will greatly affect the normalization factor that should be recalculated (Karaman 2017).

In plant samples, normalization is an important step due to the heterogeneity of most matrices (Campmajó et al. 2019). Several plant-based studies applied the normalization step during data processing, which allowed for the relative quantification by total ion abundance, mean, mean fold change (FC), sum, quantile normalization, or log transformation, according to the bioinformatic tool selected (Goodacre et al. 2007; Nascimento et al. 2019; Santos et al. 2019; Cardoso et al. 2020; Lima et al. 2020; Maia et al. 2020; Brito et al. 2021). Figure 12.3 shows the impact of the normalization step on the plant-based food chromatogram after ESI-UPLC-MS^E acquisition.

12.4.3 Strategies for Annotating and/or Identifying Metabolites

The development of robust and effective methods for automating the annotation and identification is still a significant challenge in metabolomic studies, mainly in non-targeted analyses, as the metabolites show high chemo-diversity, such as isomers and co-eluted components. Thus, criteria for the molecular annotation process have been proposed, aiming to refine the annotation according to the types and objectives of each metabolomic study.

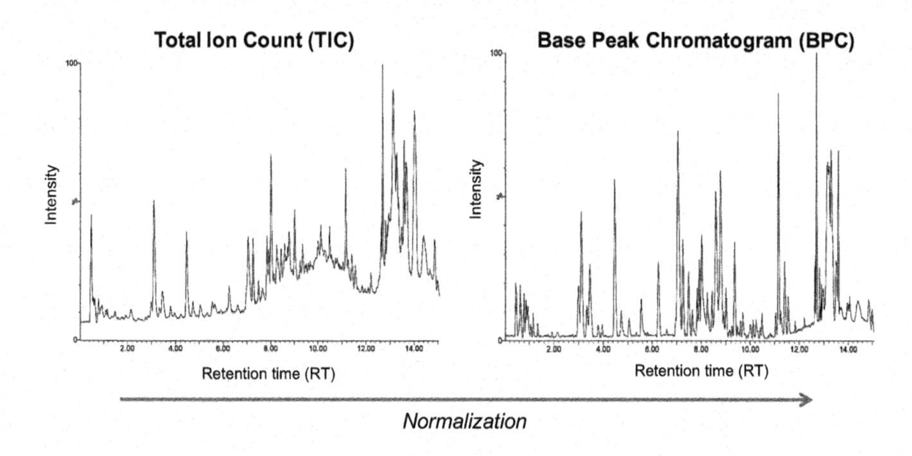

FIGURE 12.3 Representative TIC and BPC plots of ESI-UPLC-MSE data from a plant-based food.

Before the identification/annotation of compounds, it is also important to apply some filters to bring more confidence to the results. There are several studies available that applied different filters, such as maximum mass error value (ppm), minimum isotopic similarity between the analyzed compound and the one reported in the database (%), minimal abundance (to avoid false identification of compounds), and the fragmentation score of the compound (%) (Nascimento et al. 2019; Santos et al. 2019; Cardoso et al. 2020; Lima et al. 2020; Maia et al. 2020; Brito et al. 2021). After applying the filters, processing proceeds to the identification/annotation step. The Chemical Analysis Working Group (CAWG) of the Metabolomics Standards Initiative (MSI) proposed measures that contemplate a four-level confidence scale to the identification/annotation of metabolites from complex extracts (Sansone et al. 2007; Sumner et al. 2007), which are shown in Figure 12.2.

Level 1 indicates that the compound identification was based on comparison with one or more reference standards (commercial or not) under identical analytical conditions and with at least two orthogonal methods (e.g., RT, m/z, MS/MS fragmentation data, and/or collision cross-section). The compound structure is validated, achieving high-reliable criteria (Sumner et al. 2007). Level 2 applies to putatively annotated compounds, in which the standards were not applied for their absolute identification, but predicts the structure from MS/MS spectrum match with a reference fragmentation and orthogonal information (Sumner et al. 2007). In level 2, the annotation is also performed from searches in the MS1 database and orthogonal information, which allow the putative identification of the compounds.

Putative identification of compounds is not always possible, but through the same parameters applied at level 2, the compound may be assigned to a chemical class based on its molecular formula (level 3). Finally, when the characteristics of the metabolite are not sufficient for the putative annotation, it is classified as "unknown compound" according to level 4. Despite the reduced information, annotated compounds may be differentiated based on statistical data. Uni- and multivariate analyses may uncover phenotype features according to the variation of their relative intensity (Sumner et al. 2007; Schrimpe-Rutledge et al. 2016).

Plant products usually show a complex matrix, and several reference standards would be needed to identify all compounds present in the samples. With these levels of identification, the importance of libraries and databases in metabolite identification becomes even clearer. In general, the spectral library and databases contain at least accurate mass, molecular formula, and fragmentation patterns (Schrimpe-Rutledge et al. 2016). The databases frequently used in metabolomics are listed in Table 12.7. During the metabolite structure elucidation process, small molecules databases are indispensable for well-known and well-researched metabolite identification (Blaženović et al. 2018). Among the available databases, PubChem, ChEBI (Degtyarenko et al. 2008), and ChemSpider (Pence and William 2010) stand out for holding a large number of small molecule's chemical structures (Table 7). However, other databases are also important for metabolic identification, such as Kyoto Encyclopedia of Genes and Genomes (KEGG) (Kanehisa et al. 2012), KNApSACK (Afendi et al. 2012), METLIN (Tautenhahn et al. 2012), Phenol Explorer, databases from the Wishart group (HMDB, FooDB) (Wishart 2009; http://foodb.ca/), MassBank (Horai et al. 2010), mzCloud (www.mzcloud.org), LipidBlast (Kind et al.

2013), LipidMaps (Fahy et al. 2009), and GNPS (http://gnps.ucsd.edu/). These data are usually the result of notes from the metabolomics community in previous works, and the size of the spectral database is difficult to measure. MassBank is the greatest example of method success, as it is a website with a wide user base and collaborators from many different countries (Horai et al. 2010). Both validation and putative identification are also useful in integrating metabolites with known biology systems (Schrimpe-Rutledge et al. 2016). For that purpose, MetaboAnalyst (Xia et al. 2015), GNPS (http://gnps.ucsd.edu/), KEGG (Kanehisa et al. 2012), MetaCyc/BioCyc (www.biocyc.org/), and ChemRICH (http://chemrich.fiehnlab.ucdavis.edu/) may assist in the data interpretation through the analysis of metabolic pathways or molecular networks.

12.4.4 Chemometric Analyses

Once the dataset has been refined in the processing step, the data matrix will be produced from raw data, requiring tools that allow statistical analysis and mining of that data in order to select samples or metabolites with significant variations (Sugimoto et al. 2012). Thus, chemometrics is highlighted as a tool capable of analyzing multivariate data in a logical way to design or select ideal measurement procedures and

TABLE 12.7
Available Databases and Their Sizes for Metabolite and Spectral Identification

Name	Databank size	Website
Metabolites Database		
PubChem	>109 million	www.pubchem.ncbi.nlm.nih.gov/
ChemSpider	>98 million	www.chemspider.com/
KEGG	>18.000	www.genome.jp/kegg/ligand.html
ChEBI	>40.000	www.ebi.ac.uk/chebi/
FooDB	>70.000	www.foodb.ca/
KNApSAcK	>53.000	www.knapsackfamily.com/KNApSAcK/
Phenol Explorer	>35.000	www.phenol-explorer.eu/
MS Spectral Library		
MassBank	Undefined	www.massbank.eu/MassBank/Index
ReSpect	Undefined	www.spectra.psc.riken.jp/
METLIN	Undefined	www.metlin.scripps.edu/fragment_search.php
MassBank of North America (MoNA)	Undefined	www.mona.fiehnlab.ucdavis.edu/

experiments and extract or transform the data into relevant chemical information (Pinto 2017). Chemometric analysis encompasses different multivariate methods for data modeling. For this purpose, software-driven data processing, statistical software packages (e.g., R [www.r-project.org/], SAS [SAS Institute Inc.], SPSS [SPSS, Inc.], and MATLAB [www.mathworks.co.uk/]), and web-based bioinformatic tools (such as MetaboAnalyst) (Xia et al. 2015), are employed.

The chemometric methods are divided into two large groups, as presented in Figure 12.4. In unsupervised analyses, no assumptions are made about the samples, in order to explore the general structure and find trends and clusters within the dataset, or supervised analyses, which are based on the construction of classification models to optimize a response using samples with known attributes and then to predict unknown samples classes (Bujak et al. 2016; Yi et al. 2016; Pinto 2017).

12.4.4.1 Unsupervised Method

With the heterogeneity of plant-based matrices, unsupervised analyses are essential when understanding the data since they provide an overview by not using any prior information on sample characteristics during the modeling data (Campmajó et al. 2019). In such matrices, the most commonly used unsupervised data analysis methods

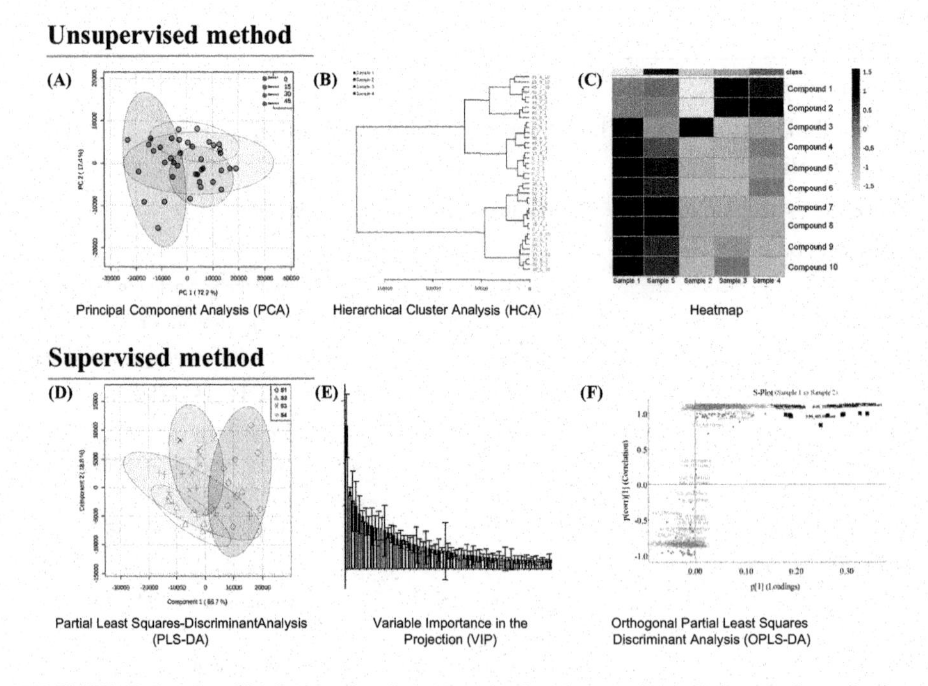

FIGURE 12.4 Graphical example of unsupervised and supervised chemometric methods, in which the first group is represented by (A) principal component analysis, (B) hierarchical cluster analysis, and (C) heatmap, while the second group is represented by (D) partial least squares discriminant analysis, (E) variable importance in the projection, and (F) orthogonal partial least squares discriminant analysis.

are principal component analysis (PCA), hierarchical cluster analysis (HCA), and heatmap (Khakimov et al. 2015).

In PCA, the high-dimensional variables will be transformed into a small number of orthogonal factors called principal components (PCs), providing the projection of samples in the PC space in a two-dimensional or three-dimensional way that explains the maximum variability (Yi et al. 2016). Through PCA's biplot graph (Figure 12.4A), the coordinates of the samples in the projections of the new variables (scores) may be visualized. In addition, PCs show the combination of the original variables and how much of the variability was added to form each PC (loadings) (Gewers et al. 2018). This allows the recognition of behavioral patterns among the samples and the detection of outliers.

Another important unsupervised method is HCA (Figure 12.4B) (Khakimov et al. 2015). This method is based on an agglomerative approach, and it is important to study similarities and differences present among the investigated samples through clusters. From the grouping, HCA allows the separation of samples into groups, and these data are usually presented together with a heatmap (Pinto 2017). Heatmap is the third unsupervised analysis and comprises a graph widely used in bioinformatics (Figure 12.4C). As the name states, it is a colored matrix that visually indicates the distribution of the abundance of metabolites (y-axis) in the analyzed samples (x-axis), and it is normally presented together with HCA, which groups the elements of the x- and y-axis (Ivanisevic et al. 2014).

Several plant-based studies applied these analyses in order to explore the data. Tan et al. (2020) applied the three non-supervised methods mentioned above to observe the differences and similarities between the metabolites of two mango cultivars. Li X et al. (2019) also report the efficiency of these tools for the analysis of five different truffle species. In addition to the differentiation between species/cultivars, these analyses also allow the observation of other factors, such as plant/fruit maturation stages, effects of the processing, and the characterization of plant residues (Nascimento et al. 2019; Santos et al. 2019; Cardoso et al. 2020; Brito et al. 2021).

12.4.4.2 Supervised Method

Supervised techniques are linear methods that are based on the input and output of data, which can be quantitative (e.g., difference between total ion abundance) or qualitative (e.g., discrimination between samples) (Pinto 2017). In plant-based samples, the most commonly used supervised data analysis methods are partial least squares (PLS)–based methods, including partial least squares discriminant analysis (PLS-DA) and orthogonal partial least squares discriminant analysis (OPLS-DA) (Yi et al. 2016). Among them, PLS-DA is the most widely used supervised method for classification in chemometric (Figure 12.4D) (Yi et al. 2016). In foodomics, this PLS regression is used to optimize the discrimination between samples, considering the direct relation between the tentatively identified metabolites (x-data) and the property of interest (y-data or classes) (Khakimov et al. 2015). After regression analysis, it is interesting to discover which variables impact the dissimilarity between the two samples. In other words, in the differentiation, for instance, of a control versus plant-based food, it is interesting to know which metabolites can differentiate these samples. For this purpose, the relevant vectors organization known as the variable importance in the projection (VIP) is applied to measure the contribution of each metabolite on the response (Pinto 2017). Relevant differentiation variables show VIP higher than 1, while less relevant variables present VIP lower than 1 (Figure 12.4E). From the VIP vectors, it is possible to select metabolites capable of influencing the differentiation between samples, allowing the discovery of biomarkers and/or of exclusive metabolites (Favilla et al. 2013; Bujak et al. 2016).

In metabolomic studies, the orthogonal projections to latent structures discriminant analysis (OPLS-DA) are also applied to search biomarkers candidates (Figure 12.4F). The OPLS-DA model is a PLS-DA variant that incorporates an orthogonal signal correction filter (OSC) (Sjoblom et al. 1998). Consequently, the analysis differentiates the groups, highlighting the variability within and between them. In turn, the OPLS-DA model provides maximum class separation and identifies the contribution of each metabolite to the classification (Bujak et al. 2016).

In general, VIP is a parameter also used to summarize the importance of each of the x variables of the OPLS-DA. Maia et al. (2020) and Zhang et al. (2014) used OPLS-DA to compare fermented or non-fermented samples, and VIP was able to select dissimilar metabolites in the samples, indicating synthesis or degradation after fermentation. OPLS-DA and VIP were also essential for the authentication of organic plant-based products through metabolomic analysis (Mie et al. 2014; Cubero-Leon et al. 2018; Xiao et al. 2018). In addition, this technique can also determine age biomarkers in some products, which can impact the final price (Huang et al. 2018).

12.5 CONCLUSION

The awareness of researchers, health professionals, and consumers about the importance of phenolic compounds as bioactive compounds with potential effects on human health has been steadily increasing. However, the available knowledge about the chemistry and variability of these compounds and their natural occurrence is still quite limited. Plant-based food and their residues, as well as medicinal plants, are known important sources of phenolic compounds, but little was unveiled about the influence of growing and harvesting conditions, maturation stage, post-harvest management, industrial and domestic processing, and other many factors of influence on their chemical composition and bioavailability.

Metabolomic tools, such as UPLC-MS/MS followed by chemometric and bioinformatic analysis, preceded by careful and efficient extraction, are a powerful implement through which the variability and the transformations suffered by phenolic compounds may be investigated. Recent advances in instrumentation, software development, and constant updating of databases have made LC-MS high-throughput analysis feasible and the most suitable technique to fully characterize the phenolic composition of food, medicinal plants, and agro-industrial residues, as shown throughout this chapter with an impressive amount of reliable information available to all interested parties. One of the main contributions of metabolomics-based studies has been on the better comprehension, at the molecular level, of the dynamics of secondary metabolism in different organisms. These studies provide a comprehensive dataset of phenolic composition that can improve research on plant breeding and stress adaptation but also on the production of desired high-value biomolecules with industrial, medicinal, and/or ecological applications. Hopefully, the careful explanations and data compilation presented by this chapter will aid future research in this quest.

ACKNOWLEDGMENTS

This work was financed by Coordenação de Aperfeiçoamento de Pessoal de Nível Superior (CAPES) (Code 001) and Conselho Nacional de Desenvolvimento Científico e Tecnológico (CNPq) (310343/2019–4; 401053/2019–9).

REFERENCES

Acosta-Estrada, B. A., Gutiérrez-Uribe, J. A., and Serna-Saldívar, S. O. 2014. Bound phenolics in foods, a review. *Food Chemistry* 152:46–55. https://doi.org/10.1016/j.foodchem.2013.11.093.

Adebo, O. A., and Medina-Meza, I. G. 2020. Impact of fermentation on the phenolic compounds and antioxidant activity of whole cereal grains: A mini review. *Molecules* 25(4):927. https://doi.org/10.3390/molecules25040927.

Afendi, F. M., Okada, T., Yamazaki, M., et al. 2012. KNApSAcK family databases: Integrated metabolite-plant species databases for multifaceted plant research. *Plant and Cell Physiology* 53(2):12. https://doi.org/10.1093/pcp/pcr165.

Ahmad, R., Ahmad, N., and Shehzad, A. 2019. Solvent and temperature effects of accelerated solvent extraction (ASE) with Ultra-high pressure liquid chromatography (UHPLC-PDA) technique for determination of Piperine and its ICP-MS analysis. *Industrial Crops and Products* 136:37–49. https://doi.org/10.1016/j.indcrop.2019.04.016.

Aires, A. 2017. Phenolics in Foods: Extraction, analysis and measurements. In: *Phenolic Compounds – Natural Sources, Importance and Applications*, eds. M. Soto-Hernández, M. Palma-Tenango, and M. del R. Garcia-Mateos, 61–88. InTechOpen, Rijeka.

Aires, A., and Carvalho, R. 2020. Kiwi fruit residues from industry processing: Study for a maximum phenolic recovery yield. *Journal of Food Science and Technology* 57:4265–76. https://doi.org/10.1007/s13197-020-04466-7.

Aksay, O., Selli, S., and Kelebek, H. 2021. LC-DAD-ESI-MS/MS-based assessment of the bioactive compounds in fresh and fermented caper (*Capparis spinosa*) buds and berries. *Food Chemistry* 337:127959. https://doi.org/10.1016/j.foodchem.2020.127959.

Alañón, M. E., Pimentel-Moral, S., Arráez-Román, D., and Segura-Carretero, A. 2021. HPLC-DAD-Q-ToF-MS profiling of phenolic compounds from mango (*Mangifera indica* L.) seed kernel of different cultivars and maturation stages as a preliminary approach to determine functional and nutraceutical value. *Food Chemistry* 337:127764. https://doi.org/10.1016/j.foodchem.2020.127764.

Alcântara, M. A., Polari, I. L. B., Meireles, B. R. L. A., et al. 2018. Effect of the solvent composition on the profile of phenolic compounds extracted from chia seeds. *Food Chemistry* 275:489–96. https://doi.org/10.1016/j.foodchem.2018.09.133.

Alvarez-Rivera, G., Ballesteros-Vivas, D., Parada-Alfonso, F., Ibañez, E., and Cifuentes, A. 2019. Recent applications of high-resolution mass spectrometry for the characterization of plant natural products. *Trends in Analytical Chemistry* 112:87–101. https://doi.org/10.1016/j.trac.2019.01.002.

Ameer, K., Shahbaz, H. M., and Kwon, J. H. 2017. Green extraction methods for polyphenols from plant matrices and their byproducts: A review: Polyphenols extraction by green methods. *Comprehensive Reviews in Food Science and Food Safety* 16(2):295–315. https://doi.org/10.1111/1541-4337.12253.

Antonakoudis, A., Barbosa, R., Kotidis, P., and Kontoravdi, C. 2020. The era of big data: Genome-scale modelling meets machine learning. *Computational and Structural Biotechnology Journal* 18:3287–300. https://doi.org/10.1016/j.csbj.2020.10.011.

Arceusz, A., Wesolowski, M., and Konieczynski, P. 2013. Methods for extraction and determination of phenolic acids in medicinal plants: A review. *Natural Product Communications* 8(12). https://doi.org/10.1177/1934578X1300801238

Aune, D., Giovannucci, E., Boffetta, P., et al. 2017. Fruit and vegetable intake and the risk of cardiovascular disease, total cancer and all-cause mortality-A systematic review and dose-response meta-analysis of prospective studies. *International Journal of Epidemiology* 46(3):1029–56. https://doi.org/10.1093/ije/dyw319.

Aydoğan, C. 2020. Recent advances and applications in LC-HRMS for food and plant natural products: A critical review. *Analytical and Bioanalytical Chemistry* 412(9):1973–91. https://doi.org/10.1007/s00216-019-02328-6.

Barbera, G. L., Capriotti, A. L., Cavaliere, C., et al. 2017. Liquid chromatography-high resolution mass spectrometry for the analysis of phytochemicals in vegetal-derived food and beverages. *Food Research International* 100(1):28–52. https://doi.org/10.1016/j.foodres.2017.07.080.

Barros, L., Dueñas, M., Carvalho, A. M., Ferreira, I. C. F. R., and Santos-Buelga, C. 2012. Characterization of phenolic compounds in flowers of wild medicinal plants from North-eastern Portugal. *Food and Chemical Toxicology* 50(5):1576–82. https://doi.org/10.1016/j.fct.2012.02.004.

Belayneh, H. D., Wehling, R. L., Reddy, A. K., Cahoon, E. B., and Ciftci, O. N. 2017. Ethanol-modifed supercritical carbon dioxide extraction of the bioactive lipid components of *camelina sativa* seed. *Journal of the American Oil Chemists Society* 94(6):855–65. https://doi.org/10.1007/s11746-017-2993-z.

Beldean-Galea, M. S., Jandera, P., and Hodisan, S. 2008. Retention and separation selectivity of natural phenolic antioxidants on zirconia based stationary phases. *Journal of Liquid Chromatography and Related Technologies* 31(6):807–18. https://doi.org/10.1080/10826070801890454

Belwal, T., Pandey, A., Bhatt, I. D., and Rawal, R. S. 2020. Optimized microwave assisted extraction (MAE) of alkaloids and polyphenols from Berberis roots using multiple-component analysis. *Scientific Reports* 10:917. https://doi.org/10.1038/s41598-020-57585-8.

Benabderrahim, M. A., Yahia, Y., Bettaieb, I., Elfalleh, W., and Nagaz, K. 2019. Antioxidant activity and phenolic profile of a collection of medicinal plants from Tunisian arid and Saharan regions. *Industrial Crops and Products* 138:111427. https://doi.org/10.1016/j.indcrop.2019.05.076

Beneito-Cambra, M., Moreno-González, D., García-Reyes, J. F., Bouza, M., Gilbert-López, B., and Molina-Díaz, A. 2020. Direct analysis of olive oil and other vegetable oils by mass spectrometry: A review. *Trends in Analytical Chemistry* 135:116046. https://doi.org/10.1016/j.trac.2020.116046

Bezerra, F. De. S., Da Costa, D. F., and Koblitz, M. G. B. 2020. Aproveitamento integral de matérias-primas oleaginosas com “solventes verdes”: Revisão e oportunidades. *Research, Society and Development* 9(8):e372985388. https://doi.org/10.33448/rsd-v9i8.5388.

Bhuyan, D. J., and Basu, A. 2017. Phenolic compounds: Potential health benefits and toxicity. In: *Utilisation of Bioactive Compounds from Agricultural and Food Production Waste*, eds. S. Azeez, C. K. Narayana, and H. S. Oberoi, 27–59. CRC Press, Boca Raton.

Bijttebier, S., Van der Auwera, A., Foubert, K., Voorspoels, S., Pieters, L., and Apers, S. 2016. Bridging the gap between comprehensive extraction protocols in plant metabolomics studies and method validation. *Analytica Chimica Acta* 935:136–150. https://doi.org/10.1016/j.aca.2016.06.047.

Bingol, K. 2018. Recent advances in targeted and untargeted metabolomics by NMR and MS/NMR methods. *High-Throughput* 7(2):9. https://doi.org/10.3390/ht7020009.

Blaženović, I., Kind, T., Ji, J., and Fiehn, O. 2018. Software tools and approaches for compound identification of LC-MS/MS data in metabolomics. *Metabolites* 8(2):31. https://doi.org/10.3390/metabo8020031.

Bordoloi, A., and Goosen, N. 2020. Green and integrated processing approaches for the recovery of high-value compounds from brown seaweeds. *Advances in Botanical Research* 95:369–413. https://doi.org/10.1016/bs.abr.2019.11.011.

Brito, T. B. N., Lima, L. R. S., Santos, M. C. B., et al. 2021. Antimicrobial, antioxidant, volatile and phenolic profiles of cabbage-stalk and pineapple-crown flour revealed by GC-MS and UPLC-MSE. *Food Chemistry* 339:127882. https://doi.org/10.1016/j.foodchem.2020.127882.

Brodsky, L., Moussaieff, A., Shahaf, N., Aharoni, A., and Rogachev, A. 2010. Evaluation of peak picking quality in LC–MS metabolomics data. *Analytical Chemistry* 82:9177–87. https://doi.org/10.1021/ac101216e.

Bujak, R., Daghir-Wojtkowiak, E., Kaliszan, R., and Markuszewski, M. J. 2016. PLS-based and regularization-based methods for the selection of relevant variables in non-targeted metabolomics data. *Frontiers in Molecular Biosciences* 3:10. https://doi.org/10.3389/fmolb.2016.00035.

Burton, L., Ivosev, G., Tate, S., Impey, G., Wingate, J., and Bonner, R. 2008. Instrumental and experimental effects in LC-MS-based metabolomics. *Journal of Chromatography B – Analytical Technologies in the Biomedical and Life Sciences* 871(2):227–35. https://doi.org/10.1016/j.jchromb.2008.04.044.

Cai, Y. Z., Mei, S., Xing, J., Luo, Q., and Corke, H. 2006. Structure – radical scavenging activity relationships of phenolic compounds from traditional Chinese medicinal plants. *Life Sciences* 78(25):2872–88. https://doi.org/10.1016/j.lfs.2005.11.004.

Campmajó, G., Núñez, N., and Núñez, O. 2019. The role of liquid chromatography-mass spectrometry in food integrity and authenticity. In: *Mass Spectrometry: Future Perceptions and Applications*, ed. G. Kamble, 3–24. InTechOpen, London.

Capriotti, A. L., Cavaliere, C., Foglia, P., Piovesana, S., and Ventura, S. 2015. Chromatographic methods coupled to mass spectrometry detection for the determination of phenolic acids in plants and fruits. *Journal of Liquid Chromatography and Related Technologies* 38(3):353–70. https://doi.org/10.1080/10826076.2014.941263.

Cardoso, R. R., Neto, R. O., D'Almeida, C. T. D. S., Nascimento, T. P., Pressete, C. G., Azevedo, L., et al. 2020. Kombuchas from green and black teas have different phenolic profile, which impacts their antioxidant capacities, antibacterial and antiproliferative activities. *Food Research International* 128:108782. https://doi.org/10.1016/j.foodres.2019.108782.

Casas, M. P., and González, H. D. 2017. Enzyme-assisted aqueous extraction processes. *Water Extraction of Bioactive Compounds* 333–68. https://doi.org/10.1016/B978-0-12-809380-1.00013-9.

Castillo, S., Gopalacharyulu, P., Yetukuri, L., and Orešič, M. 2011. Algorithms and tools for the preprocessing of LC-MS metabolomics data. *Chemometrics and Intelligent Laboratory Systems* 108(1):23–32. https://doi.org/10.1016/j.chemolab.2011.03.010.

Catalán, Ú., Barrubés, L., Valls, R. M., Solà, R., and Rubió, L. 2017. *In vitro* metabolomic approaches to investigating the potential biological effects of phenolic compounds: An update. *Genomics, Proteomics and Bioinformatics* 15(4):236–45. https://doi.org/10.1016/j.gpb.2016.12.007.

Chanioti, S., and Tzia, C. 2018. Extraction of phenolic compounds from olive pomace by using natural deep eutectic solvents and innovative extraction techniques. *Innovative Food Science and Emerging Technologies* 48:228–39. https://doi.org/10.1016/j.ifset.2018.07.001.

Chew, K. K., Khoo, M. Z., Ng, S. Y., Thoo, Y. Y., Wan Aida, W. M., and Ho, C. W. 2011. Effect of ethanol concentration, extraction time and extraction temperature on the recovery of phenolic compounds and antioxidant capacity of *Orthosiphon stamineus* extracts. *International Food Research Journal* 18(4):1427–35.

Cheynier, V. 2012. Phenolic compounds: From plants to foods. *Phytochemistry Reviews* 11(2):153–77. https://doi.org/10.1007/s11101-012-9242-8.

Chohra, D., Ferchichi, L., Cakmak, Y. S., Zengin, G., and Alsheikh, S. M. 2020. Phenolic profiles, antioxidant activities and enzyme inhibitory effects of an Algerian medicinal plant (*Clematis cirrhosa* L.). *South African Journal of Botany* 132:164–70. https://doi.org/10.1016/j.sajb.2020.04.026.

Cortina-Puig, M., Gallart-Ayala, H., and Lacorte, S. 2012. Liquid chromatography coupled to electrochemical detection and mass spectrometry for the determination of phenolic compounds in food and beverages. *Current Analytical Chemistry* 8(4):436–55. https://doi.org/10.2174/157341112803216681.

Cubero-Leon, E., De Rudder, O., and Maquet, A. 2018. Metabolomics for organic food authentication: Results from a long-term field study in carrots. *Food Chemistry* 239:760–70. https://doi.org/10.1016/j.foodchem.2017.06.161.

Cvetanović, A., Zengin, G., Zeković, Z., et al. 2018. Comparative *in vitro* studies of the biological potential and chemical composition of stems, leaves and berries *Aronia melanocarpa's* extracts obtained by subcritical water extraction. *Food and Chemical Toxicology* 121:458–66. https://doi.org/10.1016/j.fct.2018.09.045.

de Falco, B., Fiore, A., Rossi, R., Amato, M., and Lanzotti, V. 2018. Metabolomics driven analysis by UAEGC-MS and antioxidant activity of chia (*Salvia hispanica* L.) commercial and mutant seeds. *Food Chemistry* 254:137–43. https://doi.org/10.1016/j.foodchem.2018.01.189.

De Vijlder, T., Valkenborg, D., Lemière, F., Romijn, E. P., Laukens, K., and Cuyckens, F. 2018. A tutorial in small molecule identification via electrospray ionization-mass spectrometry: The practical art of structural elucidation. *Mass Spectrometry Reviews* 37(5):607–29. https://doi.org/10.1002/mas.21551.

Degtyarenko, K., De Matos, P., Ennis, M., et al. 2008. ChEBI: A database and ontology for chemical entities of biological interest. *Nucleic Acids Research* 36:344–50. https://doi.org/10.1093/nar/gkm791.

Del Coco, L., Girelli, C. R., Angilè, F., et al. 2021. NMR-based metabolomic study of *Apulian coratina* extra virgin olive oil extracted with a combined ultrasound and thermal conditioning process in an industrial setting. *Food Chemistry* 345:128778. https://doi.org/10.1016/j.foodchem.2020.128778.

Dias, D. A., Jones, O. A. H., Beale, D. J., et al. 2016. Current and future perspectives on the structural identification of small molecules in biological systems. *Metabolites* 6(4):46. https://doi.org/10.3390/metabo6040046.

Djemaa-Landri, K., Hamri-Zeghichi, S., Valls, J., et al. 2020. Phenolic content and antioxidant activities of *Vitis vinifera* L. leaf extracts obtained by conventional solvent and microwave-assisted extractions. *Food Measure* 14:3551–64. https://doi.org/10.1007/s11694-020-00596-w.

Domínguez-Rodríguez, G., Marina, M. L., and Plaza, M. 2017. Strategies for the extraction and analysis of non-extractable polyphenols from plants. *Journal of Chromatography* 1514:1–15. https://doi.org/10.1016/j.chroma.2017.07.066.

Dorta, E., Lobo, M. G., and Gonzalez, M. 2012. Reutilization of mango byproducts: Study of the effect of extraction solvent and temperature on their antioxidant properties. *Journal of Food Science* 71(1):80–8. https://doi.org/10.1111/j.1750-3841.2011.02477.x.

Duba, K. S., and Fiori, L. 2015. Extraction of bioactives from food processing residues using techniques performed at high pressures. *Current Opinion in Food Science* 5:14–22. https://doi.org/10.1016/j.cofs.2015.06.009.

Dudzik, D., Barbas-Bernardos, C., Garcia, A., and Barbas, C. 2018. Quality assurance procedures for mass spectrometry untargeted metabolomics. A review. *Journal of Pharmaceutical and Biomedical Analysis* 147:149–73. https://doi.org/10.1016/j.jpba.2017.07.044.

Dzah, C. S., Duan, Y., Zhang, H., Serwah Boateng, N. A., and Ma, H. 2020. Latest developments in polyphenol recovery and purification from plant by-products: A review. *Trends in Food Science and Technology* 99:375–88. https://doi.org/10.1016/j.tifs.2020.03.003.

Fahy, E., Subramaniam, S., Murphy, R. C., et al. 2009. Update of the LIPID MAPS comprehensive classification system for lipids. *Journal of Lipid Research* 50:9–14. https://doi.org/10.1194/jlr.R800095-JLR200.

Favilla, S., Durante, C., Vigni, M. L., and Cocchi, M. 2013. Assessing feature relevance in NPLS models by VIP. *Chemometrics and Intelligent Laboratory Systems* 129:76–86. https://doi.org/10.1016/j.chemolab.2013.05.013.

Fernández, M. de los Á., Espino, M., Gomez, F. J. V., and Silva, M. F. 2018. Novel approaches mediated by tailor-made green solvents for the extraction of phenolic compounds from agro-food industrial by-products. *Food Chemistry* 239:671–8. https://doi.org/10.1016/j.foodchem.2017.06.150.

Ferrentino, G., Morozova, K., Mosibo, O. K., Ramezani, M., and Scampicchio, M. 2018. Biorecovery of antioxidants from apple pomace by supercritical fluid extraction. *Journal of Cleaner Production* 186:253–61. https://doi.org/10.1016/j.jclepro.2018.03.165.

Filho, P. J. S., Silveira, L. A., Betemps, G. R., Oliveira, P. K., Sampaio, D. M., and Santos, D. G. 2019. Use of lyophilization as analytical strategy for chromatographic characterization of aqueous phase of bio-oil produced by rice husk pyrolysis. *Microchemical Journal* 152:104457. https://doi.org/10.1016/j.microc.2019.104457.

Gai, Q. Y., Jiao, J., Wang, X., et al. 2021. Simultaneous quantification of eleven bioactive phenolic compounds in pigeon pea natural resources and *in vitro* cultures by ultra-high performance liquid chromatography coupled with triple quadrupole mass spectrometry (UPLC-QqQ-MS/MS). *Food Chemistry* 335:127602. https://doi.org/10.1016/j.foodchem.2020.127602.

Gallego, R., Bueno, M., and Herrero, M. 2019. Sub- and supercritical fluid extraction of bioactive compounds from plants, food-by-products, seaweeds and microalgae – An update. *Trends in Analytical Chemistry* 116:198–213. https://doi.org/10.1016/j.trac.2019.04.030.

Galuch, M. B., Magon, T. F. S., Silveira, R., Nicácio, A. E., Pizzo, J. S., Bonafe, E. G., and Visentainer, J. V. 2019. Determination of acrylamide in brewed coffee by dispersive liquid – liquid microextraction (DLLME) and ultra-performance liquid chromatography tandem mass spectrometry (UPLC-MS/MS). *Food Chemistry* 282:120–6. https://doi.org/10.1016/j.foodchem.2018.12.114.

Gálvez-Ranilla, L. 2020. The application of metabolomics for the study of cereal corn (*Zea mays* L.). *Metabolites* 10(8):300. https://doi.org/10.3390/metabo10080300.

García-Salas, P., Gómez-Caravaca, A. M., Morales-Soto, A., Segura-Carretero, A., and Fernández-Gutiérrez, A. 2014. Identification and quantification of phenolic compounds in diverse cultivars of eggplant grown in different seasons by high-performance liquid chromatography coupled to diode array detector and electrospray-quadrupole-time of flight-mass spectrometry. *Food Research International* 57:114–22. https://doi.org/10.1016/j.foodres.2014.01.032.

Gewers, F. L., Ferreira, G. R., Arruda, H. F., et al. 2018. Principal component analysis: A natural approach to data exploration. *ACM Computing Surveys* 54(4):1–34. https://doi.org/10.1145/3447755.

Gil-Chávez, J. G., Villa, J. A., Fernando Ayala-Zavala, J., et al. 2013. Technologies for extraction and production of bioactive compounds to be used as nutraceuticals and food ingredients: An overview: Production of nutraceutical compounds. *Comprehensive Reviews in Food Science and Food Safety* 12(1):5–23. https://doi.org/10.1111/1541-4337.12005.

Gómez-Romero, M., Zurek, G., Schneider, B., Baessmann, C., Segura-Carretero, A., and Fernández-Gutiérrez, A. 2011. Automated identification of phenolics in plant-derived foods by using library search approach. *Food Chemistry* 124(1):379–86. https://doi.org/10.1016/j.foodchem.2010.06.032.

Gonçalves, E. C. B. A., Lozano-Sanchez, J., Gomes, S., Ferreira, M. S. L., Cameron, L. C., and Segura-Carretero, A. 2018. Byproduct generated during the elaboration process of isotonic beverage as a natural source of bioactive compounds: Byproduct generated during the elaboration. *Journal of Food Science* 83(10):2478–88. https://doi.org/10.1111/1750-3841.14336.

Gong, Y., and Pegg, R. B. 2017. Separation of ellagitannin-rich phenolics from U.S. pecans and Chinese hickory nuts using fused-core HPLC columns and their characterization. *Journal of Agricultural and Food Chemistry* 65(28):5810–20. https://doi.org/10.1021/acs.jafc.7b01597.

Gong, Z. G., Hu, J., Wu, X., and Xu, Y. J. 2017. The recent developments in sample preparation for mass spectrometry-based metabolomics. *Critical Reviews in Analytical Chemistry* 47(4):325–31. https://doi.org/10.1080/10408347.2017.1289836.

Gonzalez-Paramas, A., Santos-Buelga, C., Duenas, M., and Gonzalez-Manzano, S. 2011. Analysis of flavonoids in foods and biological samples. *Mini Reviews in Medicinal Chemistry* 11(14):1239–55. https://doi.org/10.2174/138955711804586720.

Goodacre, R., Broadhurst, D., Smilde, A. K., et al. 2007. Proposed minimum reporting standards for data analysis in metabolomics. *Metabolomics* 3:231–41. https://doi.org/10.1007/s11306-007-0081-3.

Görgüç, A., Özer, P., and Yılmaz, F. M. 2019. Microwave-assisted enzymatic extraction of plant protein with antioxidant compounds from the food waste sesame bran: Comparative optimization study and identification of metabolomics using LC/Q-TOF/MS. *Journal Food Processing and Preservation* 44(1):e14304. https://doi.org/10.1111/jfpp.14304.

Harrigan, G. G., Venkatesh, T. V., Leibman, M., et al. 2016. Evaluation of metabolomics profiles of grain from maize hybrids derived from near-isogenic GM positive and negative segregant in breds demonstrates that observed differences cannot be attributed unequivocally to the GM trait. *Metabolomics* 12(5):82. doi:10.1007/s11306-016-1017-6

Hasan, M., and Panda, B. P. 2020. Chemometric analysis of selective polyphenolic groups in *Asparagus racemosus* (Shatavar) root extracts by traditional and supercritical fluid (CO_2) based extractions. *Separation Science and Technology* 55(7):1339–55. https://doi.org/10.1080/01496395.2019.1594896.

Hazarika, U., and Gosztola, B. 2020. Lyophilization and its effects on the essential oil content and composition of herbs and spices – A review. *Acta Scientiarum Polonorum Technologia Alimentaria* 19(4):467–73. https://doi.org/10.17306/J.AFS.2020.0853.

Heavisides, E., Rouger, C., Reichel, A., et al. 2018. Seasonal variations in the metabolome and bioactivity profile of *Fucus vesiculosus* extracted by an optimised, pressurised liquid extraction protocol. *Marine Drugs* 16(12):503. https://doi.org/10.3390/md16120503.

Hohenester, U. M., Barbier Saint-Hilaire, P., Fenaille, F., and Cole, R. B. 2020. Investigation of space charge effects and ion trapping capacity on direct introduction ultra-high-resolution mass spectrometry workflows for metabolomics. *Journal of Mass Spectrometry* 55(10):e4613. https://doi.org/10.1002/jms.4613.

Horai, H., Arita, M., Kanaya, S., et al. 2010. MassBank: A public repository for sharing mass spectral data for life sciences. *Journal of Mass Spectrometry* 45:703–14.

Huang, B. M., Zha, Q. L., Chen, T. B., et al. 2018. Discovery of markers for discriminating the age of cultivated ginseng by using UHPLC-QTOF/MS coupled with OPLS-DA. *Phytomedicine* 45(7):8–17. https://doi.org/10.1002/jms.1777.

Hwang, I. M., Park, B., Dang, Y. M., Kim, S. Y., and Seo, H. Y. 2019. Simultaneous direct determination of 15 glucosinolates in eight *Brassica* species by UHPLC-Q-Orbitrap-MS. *Food Chemistry* 282:127–33. https://doi.org/10.1016/j.foodchem.2018.12.036.

Ibrahim, N. A., and Zaini, M. A. A. 2018. Dielectric properties in microwave-assisted solvent extraction – Present trends and future outlook. *Asia-Pacific Journal of Chemical Engineering* 13(4):e2230. https://doi.org/10.1002/apj.2230.

Ivanisevic, J., Benton, P., Rinehart, D., et al. 2014. An interactive cluster heat map to visualize and explore multidimensional metabolomic data. *Metabolomics* 11:1029–34. https://doi.org/10.1007/s11306-014-0759-2.

Jiao, Y., Chen, D., Fan, M., and Quek, S. Y. 2019. UPLC-QqQ-MS/MS-based phenolic quantification and antioxidant activity assessment for thinned young kiwifruits. *Food Chemistry* 281:97–105. https://doi.org/10.1016/j.foodchem.2018.12.062.

Kachlicki, P., Piasecka, A., Stobiecki, M., and Marczak, L. 2016. Structural characterization of flavonoid glycoconjugates and their derivatives with mass spectrometric techniques. *Molecules* 21(11):1494. https://doi.org/10.3390/molecules21111494.

Kalili, K. M., and De Villiers, A. 2011. Recent developments in the HPLC separation of phenolic compounds. *Journal of Separation Science* 34(8):854–76. https://doi.org/10.1002/jssc.201000811.

Kalogiouri, N. P., Aalizadeh, R., Dasenaki, M. E., and Thomaidis, N. S. 2020. Application of high-resolution mass spectrometric methods coupled with chemometric techniques in olive oil authenticity studies – A review. *Analytica Chimica Acta* 1134:150–73. https://doi.org/10.1016/j.aca.2020.07.029.

Kanehisa, M., Goto, S., Sato, Y., Furumichi, M., and Tanabe, M. 2012. KEGG for integration and interpretation of large-scale molecular data sets. *Nucleic Acids Research* 40:109–14. https://doi.org/10.1093/nar/gkr988.

Kang, J., Price, W. E., Ashton, J., Tapsell, L. C., and Johnson, S. 2016. Identification and characterization of phenolic compounds in hydromethanolic extracts of sorghum wholegrains by LC-ESI-MSn. *Food Chemistry* 211:215–26. https://doi.org/10.1016/j.foodchem.2016.05.052.

Karaman, I. 2017. Preprocessing and pretreatment of metabolomics data for statistical analysis. In: *Metabolomics: From Fundamentals to Clinical Applications*, ed. A. Sussulini, Vol. 965, 145–61. Springer. https://doi.org/10.1007/978-3-319-47656-86

Khakimov, B., Gürdeniz, G., and Engelsen, S. 2015. Trends in the application of chemometrics to foodomics studies. *Acta Alimentaria* 44:4–31. https://doi.org/10.1556/aalim.44.2015.1.1.

Kim, H. K., and Verpoorte, R. 2009. Sample preparation for plant metabolomics. *Phytochemical Analysis* 21(1):4–13. https://doi.org/10.1002/pca.1188.

Kind, T., Liu, K. H., Lee, D. Y., DeFelice, B., Meissen, J. K., and Fiehn, O. 2013. LipidBlast *in silico* tandem mass spectrometry database for lipid identification. *Nature Methods* 10:755–58. https://doi.org/10.1038/nmeth.2551.

Kind, T., Tsugawa, H., Cajka, T., et al. 2018. Identification of small molecules using accurate mass MS/MS search. *Mass Spectrometry Reviews* 37(4):513–32. https://doi.org/10.1002/mas.21535.

Kumar, B. R. 2017. Application of HPLC and ESI-MS techniques in the analysis of phenolic acids and flavonoids from green leafy vegetables (GLVs). *Journal of Pharmaceutical Analysis* 7(6):349–64. https://doi.org/10.1016/j.jpha.2017.06.005.

Lange, E., Tautenhahn, R., Neumann, S., and Gröpl, C. 2008. Critical assessment of alignment procedures for LC-MS proteomics and metabolomics measurements. *BMC Bioinformatics* 9:375. https://doi.org/10.1186/1471-2105-9-375.

Lee, J., Chan, B. L. S., and Mitchell, A. E. 2017. Identification/quantification of free and bound phenolic acids in peel and pulp of apples (*Malus domestica*) using high resolution mass spectrometry (HRMS). *Food Chemistry* 215:301–10. https://doi.org/10.1016/j.foodchem.2016.07.166.

Li, H. Z., Zhang, Z. J., Xue, J., et al. 2016. Optimization of ultrasound-assisted extraction of phenolic compounds, antioxidants and rosmarinic acid from perilla leaves using response surface methodology. *Food Science Technology* 36(4):686–93. https://doi.org/10.1590/1678-457X.13516.

Li, J., Zhang, S., Zhang, M., and Sun, B. 2019. Novel approach for extraction of grape skin antioxidants by accelerated solvent extraction: Box – Behnken design optimization. *Journal of Food Science Technology* 56:4879–90. https://doi.org/10.1007/s13197-019-03958-5.

Li, X., Zhang, X., Ye, L., et al. 2019. LC-MS-based metabolomic approach revealed the significantly different metabolic profiles of five commercial truffle species. *Frontiers in Microbiology* 10:2227. https://doi.org/10.3389/fmicb.2019.02227.

Lima, L. G. B., Montenegro, J. A. O., Abreu, J. A. O., et al. 2020. Metabolite profiling by UPLC-MS(E), NMR, and antioxidant properties of amazonian fruits: Mamey Apple (*Mammea americana*), Camapu (*Physalis angulata*), and Uxi (*Endopleura uchi*). *Molecules* 25(2):342. https://doi.org/10.3390/molecules25020342.

Liu, J., Ji, F., Chen, F., et al. 2018. Determination of garlic phenolic compounds using supercritical fluid extraction coupled to supercritical fluid chromatography/tandem mass spectrometry. *Journal of Pharmaceutical and Biomedical Analysis* 159:513–23. https://doi.org/10.1016/j.jpba.2018.07.020.

Liu, J., Yong, H., Yao, X., Hu, H., Yun, D., and Xiao, L. 2019. Recent advances in phenolic – protein conjugates: Synthesis, characterization, biological activities and potential applications. *RSC Advances* 9(61):35825–40. doi:10.1039/C9RA07808H

Lommen, A., and Kools, H. J. 2012. MetAlign 3.0: Performance enhancement by efficient use of advances in computer hardware. *Metabolomics* 8:719–26. https://doi.org/10.1007/s11306-011-0369-1.

Lou, X., Xu, H., Hanna, M., and Yuan, L. 2020. Identification and quantification of free, esterified, glycosylated and insoluble-bound phenolic compounds in hawthorn berry fruit (*Crataegus pinnatifida*) and antioxidant activity evaluation. *LWT Food Science and Technology* 130:109643. https://doi.org/10.1016/j.lwt.2020.109643.

Lucci, P., Saurina, J., and Núñez, O. 2017. Trends in LC-MS and LC-HRMS analysis and characterization of polyphenols in food. *Trends in Analytical Chemistry* 88:1–24. https://doi.org/10.1016/j.trac.2016.12.006.

Lukić, I., Radeka, S., Budić-Leto, I., Bubola, M., and Vrhovsek, U. 2019. Targeted UPLC-QqQ-MS/MS profiling of phenolic compounds for differentiation of monovarietal wines and corroboration of particular varietal typicity concepts. *Food Chemistry* 300:125251. https://doi.org/10.1016/j.foodchem.2019.125251.

Luna-Guevara, M. L., Luna-Guevara, J. J., Hernández-Carranza, P., Ruíz-Espinosa, H., and Ochoa-Velasco, C. E. 2018. Phenolic compounds: A good choice against chronic degenerative diseases. *Studies in Natural Products Chemistry* 59:79–108. https://doi.org/10.1016/B978-0-444-64179-3.00003-7.

Maia, I. C., D'Almeida, C. T. S., Freire, D. M. G., et al. 2020. Effect of solid-state fermentation over the release of phenolic compounds from brewer's spent grain revealed by UPLC-MSE. *LWT Food Science and Technology* 133:110136. https://doi.org/10.1016/j.lwt.2020.110136.

Mallmann, L. P., Tischer, B., Vizzotto, M., Rodrigues, E., and Manfroi, V. 2020. Comprehensive identification and quantification of unexploited phenolic compounds from red and yellow araçá (*Psidium cattleianum* Sabine) by LC-DAD-ESI-MS/MS. *Food Research International* 131:108978. https://doi.org/10.1016/j.foodres.2020.108978.

Martínez-Busi, M., Arredondo, F., González, D., et al. 2019. Purification, structural elucidation, antioxidant capacity and neuroprotective potential of the main polyphenolic compounds contained in *Achyrocline satureioides* (Lam.) DC. (Compositae). *Bioorganic and Medicinal Chemistry* 27(12):2579–91. https://doi.org/10.1016/j.bmc.2019.03.047.

Martini, S., Conte, A., Cattivelli, A., and Tagliazucchi, D. 2021. Domestic cooking methods affect the stability and bioaccessibility of dark purple eggplant (*Solanum melongena*) phenolic compounds. *Food Chemistry* 341:128298. https://doi.org/10.1016/j.foodchem.2020.128298.

Mazerolles, G., Preys, S., Bouchut, C., et al. 2010. Combination of several mass spectrometry ionization modes: A multiblock analysis for a rapid characterization of the red wine polyphenolic composition. *Analytica Chimica Acta* 678(2):195–202. https://doi.org/10.1016/j.aca.2010.07.034.

Meini, M. R., Cabezudo, I., Boschetti, C. E., and Romanini, D. 2019. Recovery of phenolic antioxidants from Syrah grape pomace through the optimization of an enzymatic extraction process. *Food Chemistry* 283:257–64. https://doi.org/10.1016/j.foodchem.2019.01.037.

Mendes, N. S., Santos, M. C. P., Santos, M. C. B., Cameron, L. C., Ferreira, M. S. L., and Gonçalves, É. C. B. A. 2019. Characterization of pepper (*Capsicum baccatum*)–A potential functional ingredient. *LWT – Food Science and Technology* 112:108209. https://doi.org/10.1016/j.lwt.2019.05.107.

Mie, A., Laursen, K. H., Åberg, K. M., et al. 2014. Discrimination of conventional and organic white cabbage from a long-term field trial study using untargeted LC-MS-based metabolomics. *Analytical and Bioanalytical Chemistry* 406:2885–97. https://doi.org/10.1007/s00216-014-7704-0.

Motilva, M. J., Serra, A., and Macià, A. 2013. Analysis of food polyphenols by ultra high-performance liquid chromatography coupled to mass spectrometry: An overview. *Journal of Chromatography* 1292:66–82. https://doi.org/10.1016/j.chroma.2013.01.012.

Mushtaq, M. Y., Choi, Y. H., Verpoorte, R., and Wilson, E. G. 2014. Extraction for metabolomics: Access to the metabolome: Extraction for metabolomics: Access to the metabolome. *Phytochemical Analysis* 25(4):291–306. https://doi.org/10.1002/pca.2505.

Nascimento, T. P., Santos, M. C. B., Abreu, J., et al. 2019. Effects of cooking on the phytochemical profile of breadfruit as revealed by high-resolution UPLC-MSE. *Journal of the Science of Food and Agriculture* 100(5):1962–70. https://doi.org/10.1002/jsfa.10209.

Nazir, S., and Azad, Z. R. A. A. 2019. Ultrasound: A food processing and preservation aid. In: *Health and Safety Aspects of Food Processing Technologies*, eds. A. Malik, Z. Erginkaya, and H. Erten, 613–32. Springer, Cham. https://doi.org/10.1007/978-3-030-24903-8_22.

Nicácio, A. E., Rodrigues, C. A., Visentainer, J. V., and Maldaner, L. 2021. Evaluation of the QuEChERS method for the determination of phenolic compounds in yellow (*Brassica alba*), brown (*Brassica juncea*), and black (*Brassica nigra*) mustard seeds. *Food Chemistry* 340:128162. https://doi.org/10.1016/j.foodchem.2020.128162.

Nijat, D., Abdulla, R., Liu, G. Y., Luo, Y. Q., and Aisa, H. A. 2020. Identification and quantification of Meiguihua oral solution using liquid chromatography combined with hybrid quadrupole-orbitrap and triple quadrupole mass spectrometers. *Journal of Chromatography* 1139:121992. https://doi.org/10.1016/j.jchromb.2020.121992.

Ofosu, F. K., Elahi, F., Daliri, E. B. M., et al. 2021. UHPLC-ESI-QTOF-MS/MS characterization, antioxidant and antidiabetic properties of sorghum grains. *Food Chemistry* 337:127788. https://doi.org/10.1016/j.foodchem.2020.127788.

Olalla, L., Dominguez, R., Pateiro, M., Munekata, P. E. S., Rocchetti, G., and Lorenzo, J. M. 2020. Determination of polyphenols using liquid chromatography–tandem mass spectrometry technique (LC-MS/MS): A review. *Antioxidants* 9(6):479. https://doi.org/10.3390/antiox9060479.

Oliveira, J. P. S., Hakimi, O., Murgu, M., et al. 2018. Tissue culture and metabolome investigation of a wild endangered medicinal plant using high-definition mass spectrometry. *Plant Cell, Tissue and Organ Culture* 134(1):153–62. https://doi.org/10.1007/s11240-018-1408-7.

Oliveira, J. P. S., Koblitz, M. G. B., Ferreira, M. S. L., Cameron, L. C., and Macedo, A. F. 2018. Comparative metabolomic responses to gibberellic acid and 6-benzylaminopurine in *Cunila menthoides* Benth. (Lamiaceae): A contribution to understand the metabolic pathways. *Plant Cell Reports* 37:1173–85. https://doi.org/10.1007/s00299-018-2303-8.

Palafox-Carlos, H., Yahia, E. M., and González-Aguilar, G. A. 2012. Identification and quantification of major phenolic compounds from mango (*Mangifera indica* cv. Ataulfo) fruit by HPLC – DAD – MS/MS-ESI and their individual contribution to the antioxidant activity during ripening. *Food Chemistry* 135(1):105–11. https://doi.org/10.1016/j.foodchem.2012.04.103.

Pati, S., Liberatore, M. T., Gambacorta, G., Antonacci, D., and La Notte, E. 2009. Rapid screening for anthocyanins and anthocyanin dimers in crude grape extracts by high performance liquid chromatography coupled with diode array detection and tandem mass spectrometry. *Journal of Chromatography* 1216(18):3864–68. https://doi.org/10.1016/j.chroma.2009.02.068.

Pence, H. E., and Williams, A. 2010. ChemSpider: An online chemical information resource. *Journal of Chemical Education* 87(11):1123–24. https://doi.org/10.1021/ed100697w.

Peng, H., Li, W., Li, H., Deng, Z., and Zhang, B. 2017. Extractable and non-extractable bound phenolic compositions and their antioxidant properties in seed coat and cotyledon of black soybean (*Glycine max* (L.) merr). *Journal of Functional Foods* 32:296–312. https://doi.org/10.1016/j.jff.2017.03.003.

Pereira, G. A., Arruda, H. S., de Morais, D. R., Araujo, N. M. P., and Pastore, G. M. 2020. Mutamba (*Guazuma ulmifolia* Lam.) fruit as a novel source of dietary fibre and phenolic compounds. *Food Chemistry* 310:125857. https://doi.org/10.1016/j.foodchem.2019.125857.

Perez de Souza, L., Naake, T., Tohge, T., and Fernie, A. R. 2017. From chromatogram to analyte to metabolite. How to pick horses for courses from the massive web resources for mass spectral plant metabolomics. *GigaScience* 6:1–20. doi:10.1093/gigascience/gix037

Pérez-Jiménez, J., and Saura-Calixto, F. 2018. Fruit peels as sources of non-extractable polyphenols or macromolecular antioxidants: Analysis and nutritional implications. *Food Research International* 111:148–52. https://doi.org/10.1016/j.foodres.2018.05.023.

Pertuzatti, P. B., Barcia, M. T., Gómez-Alonso, S., Godoy, H. T., and Hermosin-Gutierrez, I. 2021. Phenolics profiling by HPLC-DAD-ESI-MSn aided by principal component analysis to classify Rabbiteye and Highbush blueberries. *Food Chemistry* 340:127958. https://doi.org/10.1016/j.foodchem.2020.127958.

Pimentel-Moral, S., Borrás-Linares, I., Lozano-Sánchez, J., Arráez-Román, D., Martínez-Férez, A., and Segura-Carretero, A. 2019. Supercritical CO_2 extraction of bioactive compounds from Hibiscus sabdariffa. *The Journal of Supercritical Fluids* 147:213–21. https://doi.org/10.1016/j.supflu.2018.11.005.

Pinto, D., Cádiz-Gurrea, M. de la L., Sut, S., et al. 2020. Valorisation of underexploited *Castanea sativa* shells bioactive compounds recovered by supercritical fluid extraction with CO_2: A response surface methodology approach. *Journal of CO_2 Utilization* 40:101194. https://doi.org/10.1016/j.jcou.2020.101194.

Pinto, R. 2017. Chemometrics methods and strategies in metabolomics. In: *Metabolomics: From Fundamentals to Clinical Applications. Advances in Experimental Medicine and Biology*, ed. A. Sussulini, Vol. 965, 163–90. Springer. https://doi.org/10.1007/978-3-319-47656-8_7.

Piovesana, S., Cavaliere, C., Cerrato, A., Montone, C. M., Laganà, A., and Capriotti, A. L. 2020. Developments and pitfalls in the characterization of phenolic compounds in food: From targeted analysis to metabolomics-based approaches. *Trends in Analytical Chemistry* 133:116083. https://doi.org/10.1016/j.trac.2020.116083.

Pluskal, T., Castillo, S., Villar-Briones, A., and Oresic, M. 2010. MZmine 2: Modular framework for processing, visualizing, and analysing mass spectrometry-based molecular profile data. *BMC Bioinformatics* 11:395. https://doi.org/10.1186/1471-2105-11-395.

Pyrzynska, K., and Sentkowska, A. 2019. Chromatographic analysis of polyphenols. In: *Polyphenols in Plants – Isolation, Purification and Extract Preparation*, ed. R. R. Watson, 353–64. Academic Press, London.

Radenkovs, V., Püssa, T., Juhnevica-Radenkova, K., et al. 2020. Wild apple (*Malus* spp.) by-products as a source of phenolic compounds and vitamin C for food applications. *Food Bioscience* 38:100744. https://doi.org/10.1016/j.fbio.2020.100744.

Rajput, M., and Kumar, N. 2020. Medicinal plants: A potential source of novel bioactive compounds showing antimicrobial efficacy against pathogens infecting hair and scalp. *Gene Reports* 21:100879. https://doi.org/10.1016/j.genrep.2020.100879.

Ramon, B. M. R., Figueroa-Espinoza, M. C., and Durand, E. 2017. Application of deep eutectic solvents (DES) for phenolic compounds extraction: Overview, challenges, and opportunities. *Journal of Agricultural and Food Chemistry* 65(18):3591–601. https://doi.org/10.1021/acs.jafc.7b01054.

Rinschen, M. M., Ivanisevic, J., Giera, M., and Siuzdak, G. 2019. Identification of bioactive metabolites using activity metabolomics. *Nature Reviews Molecular Cell Biology* 20:353–67. https://doi.org/10.1038/s41580-019-0108-4.

Rocchetti, G., Blasi, F., Montesano, D., et al. 2019. Impact of conventional/non-conventional extraction methods on the untargeted phenolic profile of *Moringa oleifera* leaves. *Food Research International* 115:319–27. https://doi.org/10.1016/j.foodres.2018.11.046.

Ruiz, A., Sanhueza, M., Gómez, F., et al. 2018. Changes in the content of anthocyanins, flavonols, and antioxidant activity in *Fragaria ananassa* var. Camarosa fruits under traditional and organic fertilization. *Journal of the Science of Food and Agriculture* 99(5):2404–10. https://doi.org/10.1002/jsfa.9447.

Saito, K., and Matsuda, F. 2010. Metabolomics for functional genomics, systems biology, and biotechnology. *Annual Review of Plant Biology* 61(S):463–89. https://doi.org/10.1146/annurev.arplant.043008.092035.

Sansone, S. A., Schober, D., Atherton, H. J., et al. 2007. Metabolomics standards initiative: Ontology working group work in progress. *Metabolomics* 3:249–56. https://doi.org/10.1007/s11306-007-0069-z.

Santos, M. C. B., Barouh, N., Durand, E., et al. 2021. Metabolomics of pigmented rice coproducts applying conventional or deep eutectic extraction solvents reveal a potential antioxidant source for human nutrition. *Metabolites* 11(2):110. https://doi.org/10.3390/metabo11020110.

Santos, M. C. B., Lima, L. R. S., Nascimento, F. R., Nascimento, T. P., Cameron, L. C., and Ferreira, M. S. L. 2019. Metabolomic approach for characterization of phenolic compounds in different wheat genotypes during grain development. *Food Research International* 124:118–28. https://doi.org/10.1016/j.foodres.2018.08.034.

Sarrut, M., Crétier, G., and Heinisch, S. 2014. Theoretical and practical interest in UHPLC technology for 2D-LC. *Trends in Analytical Chemistry* 63:104–12. https://doi.org/10.1016/j.trac.2014.08.005.

Schrimpe-Rutledge, A. C., Codreanu, S. G., Sherrod, S. D., and McLean, J. A. 2016. Untargeted metabolomics strategies-challenges and emerging directions. *Journal of the American Society for Mass Spectrometry* 27:1897–905. https://doi.org/10.1007/s13361-016-1469-y.

Shahidi, F., and Yeo, J. 2016. Insoluble-bound phenolics in food. *Molecules* 21(9):1216. https://doi.org/10.3390/molecules21091216.

Sjoblom, J., Svensson, O., Josefson, M., Kullberg, H., and Wold, S. 1998. An evaluation of orthogonal signal correction applied to calibration transfer of near infrared spectra. *Chemometrics and Intelligent Laboratory Systems* 44:229–44. https://doi.org/10.1016/S0169-7439(98)00112-9.

Smith, C. A., Want, E. J., O'Maille, G., Abagyan, R., and Siuzdak, G. 2006. XCMS: Processing mass spectrometry data for metabolite profiling using nonlinear peak alignment, matching, and identification. *Analytical Chemistry* 78(3):779–87. https://doi.org/10.1021/ac051437y.

Smith, R., Ventura, D., and Prince, J. T. 2015. LC-MS alignment in theory and practice: A comprehensive algorithmic review. *Brief Bioinformatics* 16(1):104–17. https://doi.org/10.1093/bib/bbt080.

Sonar, M. P., and Rathod, V. K. 2020. Microwave assisted extraction (MAE) used as a tool for rapid extraction of Marmelosin from *Aegle marmelos* and evaluations of total phenolic and flavonoids content, antioxidant and anti-inflammatory activity. *Chemical Data Collections* 30:100545. https://doi.org/10.1016/j.cdc.2020.100545.

Sugimoto, M., Kawakami, M., Robert, M., Soga, T., and Tomita, M. 2012. Bioinformatics tools for mass spectroscopy-based metabolomic data processing and analysis. *Current Bioinformatics* 7(1):96–108. https://doi.org/10.2174/157489312799304431.

Sumner, L. W., Amberg, A., Barrett, D., et al. 2007. Proposed minimum reporting standards for chemical analysis: Chemical analysis working group (CAWG) metabolomics standards initiative (MSI). *Metabolomics* 3(3):211–21. https://doi.org/10.1007/s11306-007-0082-2.

Sut, S., Dall'Acqua, S., Zengin, G., et al. 2019. Influence of different extraction techniques on the chemical profile and biological properties of *Anthemis cotula* L.: Multifunctional aspects for potential pharmaceutical applications. *Journal of Pharmaceutical and Biomedical Analysis* 173:75–85. https://doi.org/10.1016/j.jpba.2019.05.028.

Sysi-Aho, M., Katajamaa, M., Yetukuri, L., and Orešič, M. 2007. Normalization method for metabolomics data using optimal selection of multiple internal standards. *BMC Bioinformatics* 8:93. https://doi.org/10.1186/1471-2105-8-93.

Sytar, O., Hemmerich, I., Zivcak, M., Rauh, C., and Brestic, M. 2018. Comparative analysis of bioactive phenolic compounds composition from 26 medicinal plants. *Journal of Biological Sciences* 25(4):631–41. https://doi.org/10.1016/j.sjbs.2016.01.036.

Tan, L., Jin, Z., Ge, Y., et al. 2020. Comprehensive ESI-Q TRAP-MS/MS based characterization of metabolome of two mango (*Mangifera indica* L.) cultivars from China. *Scientific Reports* 10:20017. https://doi.org/10.1038/s41598-020-75636-y.

Tang, Y., Zhang, B., Li, X., et al. 2016. Bound phenolics of quinoa seeds released by acid, alkaline, and enzymatic treatments and their antioxidant and α-glucosidase and pancreatic lipase inhibitory effects. *Journal of Agricultural Food Chemistry* 64(8):1712–19. https://doi.org/10.1021/acs.jafc.5b05761.

Tautenhahn, R., Cho, K., Uritboonthai, W., Zhu, Z. J., Patti, G. J., and Siuzdak, G. 2012. An accelerated workflow for untargeted metabolomics using the METLIN database. *Nature Biotechnology* 30:826–28. https://doi.org/10.1038/nbt.2348.

Valdés, A., Cifuentes, A., and León, C. 2017. Foodomics evaluation of bioactive compounds in foods. *Trends in Analytical Chemistry* 96:2–13. https://doi.org/10.1016/j.trac.2017.06.004.

Vázquez-Rodríguez, B., Gutiérrez-Uribe, J. A., Antunes-Ricardo, M., Santos-Zea, L., and Cruz-Suárez, L. E. 2020. Ultrasound-assisted extraction of phlorotannins and polysaccharides from *Silvetia compressa* (Phaeophyceae). *Journal of Applied Phycology* 32:1441–53. https://doi.org/10.1007/s10811-019-02013-2.

Vella, F. M., Cautela, D., and Laratta, B. 2019. Characterization of polyphenolic compounds in cantaloupe melon by-products. *Foods* 8(6):196. https://doi.org/10.3390/foods8060196.

Veselkov, K. A., Vingara, L. K., Masson, P., et al. 2011. Optimized preprocessing of ultra-performance liquid chromatography/mass spectrometry urinary metabolic profiles for improved information recovery. *Analytical Chemistry* 83(15):5864–72. https://doi.org/10.1021/ac201065j.

Vieira, V., Prieto, M. A., Barros, L., Coutinho, J. A. P., Ferreira, O., and Ferreira, I. C. F. R. 2017. Optimization and comparison of maceration and microwave extraction systems for the production of phenolic compounds from *Juglans regia* L. for the valorization of walnut leaves. *Industrial Crops and Products* 107:341–52. https://doi.org/10.1016/j.indcrop.2017.06.012.

Villiers, A. de, Cabooter, D., Lynen, F., Desmet, G., and Sandra, P. 2009. High performance liquid chromatography analysis of wine anthocyanins revisited: Effect of particle size and temperature. *Journal of Chromatography* 1216(15):3270–9. https://doi.org/10.1016/j.chroma.2009.02.038.

Vinatoru, M., Mason, T. J., and Calinescu, I. 2017. Ultrasonically assisted extraction (UAE) and microwave assisted extraction (MAE) of functional compounds from plant materials. *Trends in Analytical Chemistry* 97:159–78. https://doi.org/10.1016/j.trac.2017.09.002.

Vuong, Q. V. 2017. Utilisation of bioactive compounds from agricultural and food production waste. In: *Utilisation of Bioactive Compounds from Agricultural and Food Production Waste*, eds. S. Azeez, C. K. Narayana, and H. S. Oberoi, 27–46. CRC Press, Boca Raton.

Wang, D., Zhang, L., Xu, Y., et al. 2019. Optimization of an ultrasound-assisted extraction for simultaneous determination of antioxidants in sesame with response surface methodology. *Antioxidants* 8:321. https://doi.org/10.3390/antiox8080321.

Wang, Z., Li, S., Ge, S., and Lin, S. 2020. Review of distribution, extraction methods, and health benefits of bound phenolics in food plants. *Journal of Agricultural Food Chemistry* 68(11):3330–43. https://doi.org/10.1021/acs.jafc.9b06574.

Want, E., and Masson, P. 2011. Processing and analysis of GC/LC-MS-based metabolomics data. In: *Metabolic Profiling Methods and Protocols*, ed. T. O. Metz, 277–98. Humana Press, New York.

WHO. 2020. *Promoting Fruit and Vegetable Consumption Around the World*. World Health Organization, Geneva. Available from: www.who.int/dietphysicalactivity/fruit/en/.

Wishart, D. S. 2009. Computational strategies for metabolite identification in metabolomics. *Bioanalysis* 1(9):1579–96. https://doi.org/10.4155/bio.09.138.

Wulff, J., and Mitchell, M. 2018. A comparison of various normalization methods for LC/MS metabolomics data. *Advances in Bioscience and Biotechnology* 9:339–51. https://10.4236/abb.2018.98022.

Xia, J. G., Sinelnikov, I. V., Han, B., and Wishart, D. S. 2015. MetaboAnalyst 3.0-making metabolomics more meaningful. *Nucleic Acids Research* 43:251–57. https://doi.org/10.1093/nar/gkv380.

Xiao, R., Ma, Y., Zhang, D., and Qian, L. 2018. Discrimination of conventional and organic rice using untargeted LC-MS-based metabolomics. *Journal of Cereal Science* 82: 73–81. https://doi.org/10.1016/j.jcs.2018.05.012.

Xu, D. P., Li, Y., Meng, X., et al. 2017. Natural antioxidants in foods and medicinal plants: Extraction, assessment and resources. *International Journal of Molecular Sciences* 18:2–32. https://doi.org/10.3390/ijms18010096.

Yan, S., Shao, H., Zhou, Z., Wang, Q., Zhao, L., and Yang, X. 2018. Non-extractable polyphenols of green tea and their antioxidant, anti-α-glucosidase capacity, and release during in vitro digestion. *Journal of Functional Foods* 42:129–36. https://doi.org/10.1016/j.jff.2018.01.006.

Yi, L., Dong, N., Yun, Y., et al. 2016. Chemometric methods in data processing of mass spectrometry-based metabolomics: A review. *Analytica Chimica Acta* 914:17–34. https://doi.org/10.1016/j.aca.2016.02.001.

Yuan, Y., Zheng, S., Zeng, L., Deng, Z., Zhang, B., and Li, H. 2019. The phenolic compounds, metabolites, and antioxidant activity of propolis extracted by ultrasound-assisted method. *Journal of Food Science* 84:3850–65. https://doi.org/10.1111/1750-3841.14934.

Zengin, G., Mahomoodally, F., Picot-Allain, C., et al. 2019. Metabolomic profile of *Salvia viridis* L. root extracts using HPLC-MS/MS technique and their pharmacological properties: A comparative study. *Industrial Crops and Products* 131:266–80. https://doi.org/10.1016/j.indcrop.2019.01.060.

Zhang, B., Zhang, Y., Li, H., Deng, Z., and Tsao, R. 2020. A review on insoluble-bound phenolics in plant-based food matrix and their contribution to human health with future perspectives. *Trends in Food Science and Technology* 105:347–62. https://doi.org/10.1016/j.tifs.2020.09.029.

Zhang, L., Deng, W. W., and Wan, X. C. 2014. Advantage of LC-MS metabolomics to identify marker compounds in two types of Chinese dark tea after different post-fermentation processes. *Food Science and Biotechnology* 23:355–60. https://doi.org/10.1007/s10068-014-0049-9.

Zhang, Y., Zhang, Y., Taha, A. A., et al. 2018. Subcritical water extraction of bioactive components from ginseng roots (*Panax ginseng* C.A. Mey). *Industrial Crops and Products* 117:118–27. https://doi.org/10.1016/j.indcrop.2018.02.079.

Index

Note: Page numbers in *italic* indicate a figure and page numbers in **bold** indicate a table on the corresponding page.

N

O

P

Q

R

S

W

Y

Z